Recollections

—The NHS story- a GPs view—

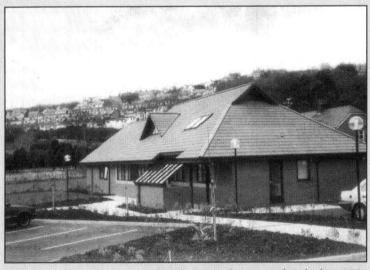

Penrhyn Bay Surgery, Llandudno 1991

Dr Idris Humphreys

First published June 2007

ISBN 978-0-9556262-0-3

Designed, Printed & Published by Fineline Printing & Stationery Ltd.
on behalf of the
North Wales Local Medical Committee
nwlmc@btinternet.com

Dedication

Dedicated to my wife Marian and our family for their support and patience during my frequent absences.

And to the many colleagues, medical and others, with whom I have had the pleasure and privilege to work with, and sometimes cross swords with, over many years and without them this book would not have been written.

Personal Details

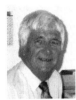

Dr Idris Humphreys was born in Penygroes, Caernarfonshire, in 1932 but moved immediately to live in Cornwall, the family moving to Llangefni on Anglesey in 1944 and to Mold, Flintshire in 1947. He trained at the Welsh National School of Medicine in Cardiff and has been in general practice in Ruabon and in Penrhyn Bay, Llandudno.

Welsh-speaking, married with two children and five grandchildren, he now lives in retirement at Gellifor, near Ruthin in the Vale of Clwyd but remains a member of the North Wales Local Medical Committee and retains an active interest in all matters medical and political.

Acknowledgments

The support and encouragement of the North Wales Local Medical Committee and its members past and present has been invaluable in bringing this book to fruition. In particular its medical secretary Dr Gruff Jones and its Executive secretary Mrs Elaine Jones have provided invaluable guidance and assistance.

I am grateful to all who have racked their brains to recall details of events and of individuals.

Introduction

Much has been written about the Health Service, its perceived strengths and weaknesses, its successes and failures, its politics and the various re-organisations over the years but much of this is specifically topic related and little has been written about its history as a whole. Very little if anything has been written about the personalities, individual doctors and others, who have tried to make it work, often in spite of political decisions driven by dogma, and who deserve to have their contribution acknowledged and preserved. It is hoped that the following chapters will provide an interesting, informative and an enjoyable read resulting in a better understanding of where we are now and how we have reached there.

My medical career had started when I entered medical school in 1950, very soon after the introduction of the NHS in 1948 so my personal path and that of the NHS have run alongside each other. Certainly much has changed during these five decades, both in the clinical management of patients and diseases, in the development and organisation of the Health Service, and in the way that general practice provides for its patients.

It is now nearly a hundred years since the first attempt at a state-organised health service took place in 1911. Many of the younger generation of doctors know little of the detailed history of the NHS or of the struggles which have been necessary to achieve the relative benefits which they now enjoy. Administrators and politicians also are unaware of past history and events, of ideas which were tried and failed in the past but which are sometimes resurrected, and of other ideas which were perhaps ahead of their time and which now need to be dusted off and reconsidered. Nor is it generally appreciated by how much medical treatment has advanced both in treatment and in the delivery systems within practices and hospitals and how much of the changes have necessarily arisen from this.

It seemed appropriate to try to record these and at the same time to set down one's personal recollections and views, making use also of the memories of others who have been through the same period. Since it is a personal account it is of necessity an incomplete and possibly inaccurate record highlighting and changes which I have personally been involved in or have knowledge of.

I have not kept detailed diaries as most politicians seem to do and this account is necessarily sketchy and dependent on my memory and that of colleagues, assisted by access to some documents and records. Readers may notice where my prejudices show in the narrative and I apologise for these. It needed to be written now while many of these active doctors remain fresh in the memories of colleagues who can add their own contributions to preserve their memory. What has become clear is that records of events within the history of the NHS are already very scattered, are not easily located and many have been lost or destroyed during the many organisational changes which have taken place, perhaps a further reason for trying to record one's recollections of them. Other researchers have found it easier to access records from the first half of the century than from the later years.

I was conscious that a number of doctors I had known and worked with over my career had devoted a tremendous amount of effort and time into helping their colleagues both individually and collectively through the BMA, the RCGP and other organisations. This had often been at considerable personal sacrifice of time and of their family life, and their efforts have never been adequately recognised and documented. GPs are often very well known and respected within their individual practices and communities but the extent of their work in other spheres is often unknown to their community or even to the colleagues for whom they are trying to seek improvements. The medical profession, like the other older professions, the dentists, lawyers and teachers, were until very recently strictly forbidden by the General Medical Council to advertise their expertise in any way, a small plate setting out their name and qualifications at their home and practice premises being all that was allowed. At a higher level the Honours System frequently fails to recognise their contributions and even if honoured it is more often for service to official bodies or for non-medical contributions to their community rather than for services directly to patients or colleagues. In these writings I have attempted to rectify this to some extent by recalling those who I have had the pleasure to know and to work with personally. In doing so I have concentrated to some extent on those who have retired from the work and in some instances who have died, while recognising that there are others currently doing equally good work and whose efforts should perhaps be chronicled by someone else at a later date. This narrative is written from personal experiences working in practices across North Wales since the late fifties and from active involvement over that period in the medico-political and administrative structures in North Wales, in Wales as a whole and on a United Kingdom-wide basis.

It is autobiographical only to the extent necessary to illustrate the topics. The layout of the narrative does of necessity lead to a degree repetition at times.

The 1940`s during the latter stages of the World War and at a time when great plans for the future were being conceived, amongst them the concept of a comprehensive National Health Service available to all and free at the point of delivery, saw major proposals for medical training. Two reports by Sir Henry Cohen, later Lord Cohen of Birkenhead, identified the need for GP education and proposed specific training for general practitioners, although it took a couple of decades before this was available.

One of the things which I have come to appreciate during my various contacts with doctors and with practices across the UK is that there is no "standard GP or standard practice". The variation is enormous and arises partly from the need to adapt to the environment in which they are located. To quote from one of the first books to be published about general practice "There is nothing stereotypical about general practice, the variety is enormous, the scope infinite and the men and women who conduct it are as individual as the patients they serve ".

CHAPTER ORDER

Medical school days

To begin at the beginning, or at least at the relevant beginning since what came previously while interesting is not pertinent. My medical career started at the Cardiff medical school in October 1950. Why Cardiff? Probably at that time most medical students from North Wales went to Liverpool, some to London schools and others to Manchester or Edinburgh.

Liverpool as a venue did not appeal for some reason, perhaps it was too close to home, and I applied to Cardiff, Manchester and some of the London colleges. Entry to medical school at that time was not easy, there were still a number of ex-services candidates as well as those of us applying directly from school. Cardiff accepted me and I was very happy to accept and study at the Welsh National School of Medicine as it was then called.

There were only about fifty students in each year at Cardiff, about half direct from school and the rest ex-service, either with war experience or having done two years National Service. The year ahead of us had quite a few "elderly" students who had war experience and some had even spent time in prisoner-of-war camps. The number of women was very low, quite different from the current intake which has at least 60% women, a proportion which is causing some disquiet about how exactly medical services will be run in future but more of that later.

There were four of us from North Wales new in our year, Tudor Jones from Cricieth, Gwen Price from Bethesda, Jos Jones from Llangefni, and myself from Mold. Gwyn Thomas from Denbigh, Tom Lloyd from Deeside and Tudor Williams from Wrexham were already there.

The medical course was quite different from the one presently organised. The first three years was a preclinical course studying anatomy, physiology, and pharmacology but with no contact with patients and leading to a B.Sc degree. It was possible to be exempted from the first year on the results of the Higher Certificate, the equivalent to today's A levels, and most of us arrived in this way. The downside was that one was then formally in the University of Wales for only two years (the clinical years were considered to be postgraduate ones) and therefore ineligible to be awarded the degree.

Disappointing because it meant less letters after one's name, but it also had a possible practical consequence - if one at any time should fall foul of the General Medical Council and be struck off the medical register one would at least have a BSc degree which would allow one to teach or enter industry. Luckily none of us has found ourselves in this unfortunate position.

Since we started in the second year we were in at the deep end from the start. The first day was practical anatomy and we all entered the dissecting room laid out with a number of cadavers. For youngsters just out of school and who had never seen a dead body or had any real contact with death this was a sobering experience. Four of us, complete strangers, were assigned to our cadaver, two to each arm. Two girls Judy Evans and Anna Morgan on one arm, and Bryan Wilcox and myself on the other. Bryan, who later became a GP in Abersychan, remained a close friend for the whole of our medical course and afterwards. Its strange how one makes one's friends.

I forget which of the four of us actually made the first tentative skin incision but it was only after spending much time contemplating and plucking up courage. After that it was much easier, but there were many complex Latin names of muscles and nerves which we had to learn and place with Gray's Anatomy being the ever-present bible. Curriculum changes in recent years following Tomorrows Doctors published by the GMC in 1993 have resulted in an integrated cross-disciplinary course with much less practical anatomy and dissection.

Physiology was somewhat more familiar after biology at school and more open to logical thought in places. Pharmacology completely divorced from patients and from diseases was very boring with much time being spent learning about making pills and tablets and making up medicines, none of which one ever had occasion to do after qualifying. At least I now know that when using tea-bags (unknown at that time) to make a pot of tea I am making an infusion.

Since the purpose of this work is to record and comment on events after qualification the medical school years will be dealt with very briefly. Suffice it to say we duly completed the two years, considered to be the most difficult part of the course, and moved on to clinical work, hospitals, patients … and nurses.

Clinical ward work was interesting and one felt one was getting towards one's goal but in the context of this narrative there was little to note. Highlights worth recording were perhaps the first taste of general practice, a day in a Cardiff practice with of all people Dr Jack Mathews, the great Cardiff and Wales rugby centre of the post-war years, Later a week was spent in the practice of Dr Ianto Clifford Jones at Llanbadarn Fawr, Aberystwyth, who also doubled as an anaesthetist at Aberystwyth General Hospital. It was an eye-opener to see how different a non-teaching hospital was from the attitudes of a teaching hospital. These were very early days in the recognition that students needed to learn anything about general practice and the world outside hospitals and that practices had much to offer as teaching venues. Perhaps by definition the early GP teachers were enthusiasts. The wheel has turned so much since then with the greatly increased numbers of students and the change in hospital practice with very short length of stays and the focus on more complex cases more and more of the course will be of necessity be arranged away from the centre and in the periphery and the major implications of this will be considered later.

The other memorable occasion was when I arrived in my final year to spend a few days studying paediatrics at Wrexham. The department consisted of a Consultant, a registrar and a house officer. When I arrived both the juniors were off sick with flu so I as a final year student had three days running a busy department with Dr Gerry Roberts, the Paediatrician, dashing in and out at great pace as was his wont, often between domiciliary visits, to check all was well. Great experience which held me in great stead later and which would never be possible now.

Qualification duly came on time in August 1955. At that time the sole mandatory requirement was to undertake two pre-registration house-doctor posts. I returned north to do six months paediatrics at the Wrexham Maelor, and then back to Cardiff to do surgery with Mr Hugh "Spot" Jenkins at Llandough Hospital along with some cardiac surgery with Mr Dillwyn Thomas and Mr Hugh Harley. How cardiac surgery has advanced, then they used to separate mitral and aortic valves with a finger inside the heart, and post-operative analgesia was a maximum of 25 mg of pethidine.

How communication technology has advanced as well. When working at Wrexham where my sole off-duty time was a half day a week after finishing whatever had to be done and until I arrived back in the hospital that evening, and with alternate weekends from finishing on Saturday mornings. There being no bleeps or mobile phones I had to continually inform the switchboard as to my whereabouts within the hospital. Nor was there a phone in my bedroom so that I had to be personally fetched by a member of staff whenever required, which did not provide much privacy. We were however well looked after in the doctor' mess.

In 1956 National Service was still a requirement, although it was gradually being phased out. I went for my medical along with another great pal from my year Dr Keith Fowler. As a result of an x-ray diagnosed duodenal ulcer, found only as a result of an insurance medical a few months before and blamed on long hours and very irregular hospital meals, I was graded three but told I would be required to serve as I would go in as a doctor with a commission. One week later the government announced that no more recruits in Grade three would be accepted and I was spared. Had I had my medical a couple of weeks later I would possibly have been given a different grade and required to enlist.

What to do now? I had decided against a career in hospital medicine and under the regulations at that time I could go straight into general practice if I wished. However because I was not to spend two years in the Armed Forces I decided to spend more time in hospital posts and had six months in general medicine at St David's Hospital Cardiff with the incomparable Dr Byron Evans who I had clerked for as a student and then on to Neath in the Obstetrics and Gynaecology department with Mr Garfield Evans. Towards the end of the latter job I was persuaded by a fellow resident Dr. Roy Halsall who had just returned from a period at sea that I should spend some time on the ocean wave and join the P&O shipping company as a ship's doctor which I duly did in August 1957.

It was around this time that the doctor turned writer, Richard Gordon was publishing his hilarious books Doctor in the House and Doctor at Sea and which were later turned into films. Many of the incidents described were very familiar to all medical students.

A year at sea

Having joined P&O for an unspecified period I was posted to Tilbury docks in London to provide medical cover for the Company crews and workers in the docks while awaiting a vacancy on a ship. P&O because of its origins and history had traditionally recruited crews from the Indian sub-continent, cabin crews and stewards from Goa, an area at that time virtually unknown but now becoming popular for holidays from the UK. Deck and engine room crew came largely from northern India, many of the latter particularly looking considerably older and frailer than their official documents showed. Soon after I arrived in the docks so did the influenza outbreak of 1957. Conditions on board during turnaround and any necessary repairs are not the best at any time, certainly not ideal for looking after and treating many sick crew members on a number of different ships.

Soon however I received a posting to the S.S.Sunda, one of the company's fast cargo liners carrying 100 crew and up to 12 passengers. Marine regulations required any ship carrying more than 99 persons to have a ship's doctor. The advantage of these ships for passengers was that they spend several days in port loading and unloading, allowing time for touring the local sights. Since the number both of passengers and of Senior Officers was small contact was close and fairly intimate. One could either be lucky or unlucky with the company one was stuck with for some months.

The first trip was across to northern Europe to pick up cargoes for the Far East. On my first day we left London for Hamburg with the holds virtually empty, the ship riding high in the water, and promptly ran into a Force eight gale. Not a good start. Hamburg with all its infamous night spots and its red-light area was a revelation but luckily did not result in any additional work for the doctor in the following days.

Visits to Bremen, Rotterdam, and Antwerp followed with reasonable time to look round, and then back to London to prepare for the three month trip to Japan and China via Suez, Colombo, Penang, Singapore and Hong Kong, and returning by the same route. Work for the doctor was light, mainly minor injuries and mild infections and sorting out the work dodgers. Since at that time I had no experience of medicine outside hospitals there was need for a sharp learning curve. Passengers with serious illnesses did not tend to go on such vessels but they were on the whole middle aged or older and at potential risk. The doctor is the only person with any medical knowledge and has no one available for a second opinion. Ships without a doctor had to rely on "The Ship Captains' Medical Guide" and in specified circumstances the Captain was allowed to administer morphine.

Luckily serious problems were infrequent but caused anxieties when they arose. The Suez canal had only recently been reopened. It had been closed by President Nasser during the Suez crisis, a number of ships had been scuttled in the canal and these had just been cleared away. When ships traversed the Suez canal during the night the Ship's Electrician was required to be in the bows of the ship for some hours with searchlights highlighting the canal sides and looking for possible obstructions. As a perk for this work and to keep him warm the electrician received a fairly generous issue of rum. This was not consumed at the time but shared around later, following which he fell down a companionway and sustained a nasty fracture of his lower leg. Trying to get this into a reasonable shape and apply plaster without skilled assistance and without the assistance of anaesthetic, other than the alcohol, was not easy. We were due to put in at Aden which was then a British base and a refuelling stop the next day and he was then transferred to more capable care.

After leaving Aden there was a five day uninterrupted sail across the Indian Ocean to Colombo in Ceylon (now Sri Lanka). On the second day one of the engineers developed a very high temperature which was very resistant to treatment and which persisted for more than 48 hours. In the absence of other causes I presumed it was heatstroke although I had never seen a case. It was a very worrying time as at that time communication with land from the middle of the Indian Ocean was far more difficult and less sophisticated than it is today with modern satellite communication systems.

The ship was not scheduled to visit Calcutta on this particular trip or I would have had to certify most of the crew, myself included, as alcoholics. Prohibition was in force there at that time and the only way one could get a drink ashore was if one was a certified alcoholic.

Apart from these episodes the trip passed fairly uneventfully from a medical point of view. From a "tourist doctor" viewpoint the Far East was fascinating and unforgettable. We spent the Christmas period in Tokyo and other Japanese ports and the New Year in Shanghai. We were still to some extent in the post-war period and Communist China was still closed to foreigners. We were one of the first ships to enter Shanghai to trade and had armed guards on board day and night. Everyone was in the standard Chinese Mao-type blue serge trouser suits and we only saw two skirts during the five days we were there, at the French Embassy which was our only contact base and where New Years Eve celebrations were to be held. Before the latter I, together with the Captain and other senior officers, had to attend an official dinner at the Peace Hotel with Chinese officials. Later I left the hotel with the intention of meeting up with our junior officers at the French Embassy, jumped into a rickshaw and said where I wanted to go and off we went. After some time the "driver" stopped, asked again where I wanted to go and set off again, repeating this again a few minutes later. I was completely isolated and lost in a foreign city after curfew hour. Normally in a city abroad even if the street names and signs are in the local language one can understand some and have some sense of direction, not so in Shanghai where all signs were in Chinese writing and literally no-one spoke a word of English. In a considerable panic I managed to convey to him partly by sign language the word "ship" and eventually found myself back safely on board. Lesson learnt.

Arriving back in London three months later saw another short spell in the docks and then a transfer to the S.S.Arcadia which was the flagship of the company at that time and due to sail to Australia. The ship carried about 2800 passengers, first and second class, and crew and the medical set-up was quite different. There was a senior surgeon, myself as the junior and two experienced nursing sisters. Practice on board was private so he saw most of the passengers while I saw mainly the crew, except in emergencies and out-of-hours. But I was happy with this, never being very keen on treating private patients.

Smartness at all times was the word on P&O ships. Caps always had to be worn or carried while on board. It was often said within the company that there were three navies, the Royal Navy, the P&O, and the rest of the merchant navy, and one did see a difference when visiting ships of other lines when in port on our travels. The name POSH has been used to describe the P&O and in fact the term originated from its passengers travelling on board to India in the early days of the Raj and well before air-conditioning. To avoid the worst of the heat the more expensive cabins were on the side away from the sun as far as possible, **P**ortside **O**ut and **S**tarboard **H**ome

Arcadia travelled via the Mediterranean, stopping at Athens to pick up a number of migrants going to Australia and paying the subsidised £10 fare current at the time to encourage new settlers, and then on via Suez and the Indian Ocean to Freemantle, Adelaide, Melbourne and finally Sydney where we spent a week before turning round and returning home by the same route. While there I was able to meet up with my uncle Hugh Evans who was a pillar of the Welsh chapel in Sydney.

An interesting sight when in port, especially in the European ports, was that of the Indian and Pakistani crew members coming back to the ship carrying old Singer treadle sewing machines to take back home where they were much in demand. One of the perks of sailing to these parts was the ability to have clothing, suits and shirts especially, made to measure within hours and at a very cheap price at a time when post-war effects were still being felt at home.

During my spell on Arcadia we occasionally had to pull out all the stops and we had the need to perform three appendicectomies, a problem which seemed more prevalent then than now, sometimes but not always enlisting the help of an anaesthetist from amongst the passengers. Anaesthesia was of course much less sophisticated then. It was policy to try to treat and keep patients on board rather than put them ashore for treatment for two reasons, our facilities were often likely to be better than the local facilities in some ports visited, and secondly if patients were put ashore there was a problem for those travelling with them and of repatriating them later at considerable expense and inconvenience. One appendicectomy was performed on board with the ship tied up in Palma Harbour in Majorca

Deaths do occur at sea from time to time and traditionally a committal over the side was the routine procedure. On our way back from Australia a day out from Freemantle a distinguished passenger, a paramount chief from one of the South Pacific Island groups had a stroke and died. The traditional burial procedure was not appropriate as it was wished to give him a ceremonial send-off back in his home-land. Riots were taking place in Colombo at the time so no stop was scheduled there and the next port, Bombay, was three days sailing away. Refrigeration was not as developed then, particularly to transport a corpse part way round the world and the only practical alternative was to attempt some amateurish embalming with formalin which was duly done. He was delivered to his fellow countrymen in good condition, dressed in his finery. Some months later while reading a magazine in my local dentist's waiting room I came across several pages of pictures of his funeral celebrations and felt some pride that I had contributed to the occasion.

Arrival back in the London was followed by the short sail to Southampton to start the summer cruise season. We on Arcadia did two two-week cruises to the Mediterranean and one to the Scandinavian Capitals with quick turnarounds between each, hectic for the crew but great for sightseeing for me.

Quite apart from the medical and social aspects of life on board it was fascinating to observe at first hand and at close quarters the running of the ship and the intricacies of getting safely into and out of ports in various parts of the world.

Towards the end of my time at sea I received an offer, very informally and halfway around the world, to become a trainee assistant at Prestatyn with a view to partnership after twelve months. This sounded a very good offer in those days and I accepted. Otherwise I would probably have spent at least another twelve months at sea, and perhaps everything later would have turned out quite differently. As I had taken up the offer at Prestatyn in September 1958 it was time to bring my seafaring period to an end and to start my career in general practice. I had been extremely fortunate in the variety of experiences I had had in the twelve months and the wonderful places visited while at the same time being well rewarded and living a life of comparative luxury. Other doctors who did a similar period often had three or four trips on the same ship to Australia and back. I managed to leave without having put on much weight, in spite of the high-living, both the rich food and cheap alcohol.

The late 50's was at a time when there was a still lot of uncertainty and unhappiness within general practice in the UK and when a number of my contemporaries were emigrating to Australia or Canada. I did think about it for a while but family ties proved too strong. I have not regretted the decision.

Ruabon and before

In the late 1950's and 60's general practice was seen very much as inferior to consultant and hospital career posts and morale was very low. Lord Moran, the Queen's physician and a pillar of the London establishment famously remarked that GP's were "doctors who had fallen off the consultant ladder". Many practices were still single-handed and competing with each other for patients. There were frequent reports of apparent abuse of the newly available benefits such as spectacles, dentures and corsets, all of which many patients had never previously been able to afford. Stories of NHS cotton wool being used to stuff cushions and of patients asking for tubes of liniment or ointment and then taking them back to the chemist to exchange for toothpaste circulated.

Many doctors were very disillusioned by the way the NHS had turned out in regard to their conditions of work and their pay, both in the amount and in the way the global sum was divided up. There had already been several major crises between GPs and government since the start in 1948 leading to threats of resignation from the NHS.

The infamous "pool" system of payment was in operation. Briefly there was a global sum or pool of remuneration calculated from the total number of GPs working in the NHS, together with the total sum of their allowable expenses. This Pool was subsequently divided into capitation fees for each patient and fees for certain other services such as immunisation. Since the total number of doctors, items of service and expenses from Inland Revenue returns could not be known for some time a sum on account was paid with a balancing amount two years later. When the total figure was eventually known and since the Pool was a fixed amount there was usually an under or an overpayment. Monies earned by GPs from other official sources such as for services to government departments, hospitals or local health authorities had to be deducted from the pool before it was distributed. As a result of the massive immunisation programme and other work carried out by GPs with the newly available vaccine, there was in 1963 a large paper overpayment and the agreed fees were reduced to bring the total into the Pool calculated figure. This obviously created massive disquiet and unrest with very stormy meetings across the country and certainly in the Flintshire and Denbighshire LMC area with demands for changes to the system. Undated resignations were collected through the BMA Guild but the threat led to negotiations which produced the 1966 Charter and in the end made it unnecessary to use them.

The abject state of many general practices in the early fifties soon after the setting up of the National Health Service in 1948 was highlighted in the Collings report written by an Australian and published in the BMJ in 1951 and which created shock waves and lead amongst other things to the setting up of the College of General Practitioners. Working arrangements in some of the better practices were later well set out in the report of a survey by Stephen Taylor for the Nuffield Trust in 1954 which makes fascinating reading and was one of the first books about general practice to be published. It looked in a non-statistical way at a number of practices and at GPs recognised as good doctors by their colleagues highlighting good ideas as well as showing where improvements could be made and it gives a very clear account of the medical and social situation and problems at that time.

It was into this situation that I came into general practice in 1960, having finished my training at Prestatyn. In 1958, as previously described while working with the P&O as a ships surgeon, I received indirectly through family contacts an offer to become a trainee doctor with Dr Gwyn Davies at Prestatyn for twelve months with a view to a partnership at the end. I must admit I knew nothing about traineeships at that time but since I was sailing back to the UK from Australia on the SS Arcadia at the time it was difficult to find out more details. It seemed a very good opportunity in a nice part of North Wales and I accepted the invitation to start in September.

Gwyn's senior partner, Dr Elizabeth Armstrong, was much respected by her patients and in particular by the mineworkers at Point of Air Colliery in Ffynnongroew where she first started the practice. It was quite something at that time for a lady doctor to have become so involved in the very male-oriented mining industry. She was unmarried but well supported by her elderly non-medical father who ran the practice very rigidly but well. The practice still ran the Ffynongroew practice, as it does to this day, but the centre had moved to Prestatyn giving a completely different practice population. The two areas were some eight miles apart and on many evenings when on call the doctors went backwards and forwards between the two villages and as far as Greenfield because of the absence of mobile communication and the limited number of homes with telephones at that time.

The traineeship was in fact an assistantship with a view but financed partly by the NHS, with training being no more than what a senior doctor would normally pass on to a junior assistant. It certainly was entirely different to the vocational training organisation developed from 1971 onwards and discussed later in another chapter Approval of a doctor as a trainer was given by the Local Medical Committee. Oddly enough I have never met another doctor who participated in the scheme.

Apart from Ffynnongroew there was another branch surgery at Gronant two miles away, held twice a week in the front parlour of a small cottage, with no facilities except a jug and basin to wash one's hands, and no equipment other than that carried in the car.

Branch surgeries were common in many practices at this time and reflected to some extent a move by patients from the practice into new development areas but also the absence of transport by many patients at that time. Many were held in the front room of a village house lived in at non-surgery times, while in many other villages and hamlets there were "calling-houses" where requests for visits were collected and medicines were dropped off. Many branch surgeries have gradually been reduced in frequency and then closed over the years but often after strenuous local resistance. Of course if the doctor is at a branch surgery he or she cannot also be available at the main surgery at the same time, and if a partner is away another partner may have to cover and therefore not be available for consultation at his usual times so the convenience of some was the inconvenience of others. Things have now moved on so much that branch surgery consultations are no longer medically safe and many more practices are now being given permission to close them.

Further surgeries were held in the summer months at the Bastion Road caravan park. The whole of the coastal strip from Talacre to Abergele contained a mass of caravan parks served, and in many cases also owned, by local G.Ps. These provided a host of temporary patients often with very trivial complaints such as wasp stings but attending the doctor because they were away from home and their domestic remedies, or because they wanted a quick cure so that their holidays were not spoiled. Such was the concentration of such temporary patients in some parts of the country including the N.Wales coastal strip that at one time only half the NHS fee was paid for seeing patients at a surgery on a camp site. GPs being ever resourceful, a number of new surgeries were opened not on the campsite itself but immediately across the road thus attracting full fees. At one time the income claimed by one practice in particular was so large that an official investigation was undertaken by the Executive Council but no evidence of any culpable malpractice was found.

A similar massive concentration of camps occurred elsewhere, in particular on the west coast in the Barmouth area where the winter population of some 4000 residents would rise to a peak of 80,000 in August. Obviously summer holidays for the doctors were out of the question. Since then many of these holiday makers have shifted their allegiance and go to Benidorm and other Spanish resorts instead. Responding to visit requests on caravan sites was always difficult, callers often not knowing even the name of the site correctly or the location of their van. Usually the description was of a car parked alongside the van but if one did not manage to get there very soon one sometimes found the car had been moved to the camp bar area.

The year at Prestatyn passed quickly and pleasantly but as the promised partnership did not materialise. At the time I was unmarried and shared digs (as lodgings were then called) with a young veterinary assistant Gordon McArthur. Being unmarried contributed to the decision not to stay on in the Prestatyn practice. A new branch surgery was being opened in the developing Ffrith Beach area of Prestatyn and a house had been bought as a surgery with a doctor's flat upstairs. At that time no one would think about living in a flat and looking after themselves, and there was always the need to have someone to answer the phone. These days it would probably be relatively easy to acquire a live-in girlfriend and solve the problem, but not in the social climate of the fifties. I moved on and began to look for locum appointments or an assistantship.

Within weeks a single handed practice was advertised in Benllech on Anglesey, a Welsh-speaking area. Having spent three years in school six miles away in Llangefni it was of considerable interest. I applied to the Anglesey Executive Council and was short listed although obviously not a strong candidate as I was young, unmarried and with no experience of general practice other than as a trainee. In due course the practice was given to an English speaking doctor from Darwen in Lancashire. To say this did not go down at all well with the local population because of the language was an understatement and appeals against the decision were submitted. We all trooped down to the Medical Practices Committee in London for a re-hearing. The strength of local feeling expressed was reflected in the decision to have an oral hearing which was very unusual. Normally some two hundred single-handed practice vacancies would be dealt with by the MPC in a year and only in one or two would an oral hearing be held. The MPC reversed the decision and appointed Dr W. Parry-Jones of Llangefni who had applied to amalgamate the Benllech and Llangefni practices bringing in his son, Chas, who was currently doing National Service and employing an assistant until he was free to start. In the circumstances this seemed an eminently sensible solution and most were happy. Chas was actually in the same class as me in school in Llangefni, a class which also boasted John Henry Jones who became Professor of Medicine at Cardiff, Gwilym Owen the broadcaster and writer, J.O.Roberts the actor, Gwyn Morris Jones who served on the Gwynedd FHSA and WJ Williams, leader of Ynys Mon County Council amongst others.

Pre-NHS and in the fifties and sixties it was not unusual for practices to take a series of assistants who would do a major part of the practice work, and much of the night and weekend work, uncomplainingly in the hope that they would in time be offered a partnership but often this did not materialise and they moved on. Some practices even employed several assistants at the same time. If in time a partnership was offered it was usually on a small share moving up to parity in three to five years, sometimes much longer, and of course at that time it was often necessary to buy into the share of the practice premises and fixtures and fittings.

Doctors did not however have to buy a share of the goodwill in the practice as in pre-NHS days. The Government had at the inception of the NHS in 1948 assessed the nominal goodwill of each practice and agreed to pay this amount to the doctor on retiring or leaving the practice, adding 2 ½% interest p.a. Since some doctors did not retire until twenty or thirty years later when inflation and interest rates had risen considerably higher this was a great coup on the government's part.

After several short locum appointments in the Wrexham area including one with Dr Wesley Hill, one of the most respected GPs in the area and a BMA activist, I was taken on in January 1960 as an assistant by the Ruabon practice of Drs. John Lawton Roberts and Glyn Roberts. They had had a couple of assistants before me but to be fair had not exploited them in the way some others had.

It was an interesting set-up, based on the mining area west of Wrexham together with some very pleasant countryside going down to the River Dee at Overton Bridge, all within a radius of three or four miles of the centre. A complete contrast to the affluent retirement area of Prestatyn.

The practice had originally been developed pre-1911 and the Insurance Act by Dr John's great-grandfather based on a Friendly Society arrangement with the local colliery mineworkers and their families. At some time afterwards a young Dr Turner was brought in by another group from the mines undercutting the going rate of two-pence a week per family by charging one penny-halfpenny a week. Dr Turner set up premises across the road and for many years, and indeed it was still on-going at the time I arrived, an intense animosity and rivalry for patients went on. Personal relationships between the practices were non-existent.

The National Insurance Act introduced in 1911 by Lloyd George was a considerable step forward but was limited in its scope. Becoming known as the Lloyd George 9d for 4d it covered one sixth of all male employees, those earning less than £160 per annum. The employee contributed four pence, the employer three pence and government two pence. It did not include women, children, retired workers, the self-employed and the unemployed and did not cover hospital treatment.

The scheme operated through a series of Clubs and Friendly Societies who employed the doctors. Many of them extended the scope of benefits to other members of the family and other income groups. One of the bigger ones, the Tredegar Medical Aid Society covered all services including treatment at the Cardiff Royal Infirmary. Aneurin Bevan was associated with this scheme in his constituency and probably used it as a template when planning his new National Health Service.

Miners are a close knit community and generally had big extended families locally, brothers and sisters and of several generations, all intensely close. Payment at this time was based almost entirely on a capitation system based on the number of patients registered on the list. If the practice upset and lost one member of the family then there was a significant chance of losing many others. Many patients would use this as a lever to pressurise the doctor to obtain services which they would otherwise not have received, including pressure for sick notes, prescriptions and for home visits.

In complete contrast the other part of the practice was largely the area of the Wynnstay estate and its farms stretching down to the Dee, although the Hall had for some years been a private residential school, Lindisfarne College, which the practice also serviced

I had only been there as an assistant for three months when Dr Turner, who by this time was elderly, had to retire. Since the practice was single-handed it had to be advertised by and an appointment made by the Executive Council, with no input by the retiring GP. I applied stating I would wish to amalgamate the two practices to form a group working from the same premises. At the end of the process I was duly appointed to take over on April 1st 1960 and Dr Turner was incandescent. When the take-over day arrived the Clerk to the Executive Council, Mr Hugh Tunnah, had to personally collect the medical records from the surgery on a Saturday afternoon and deliver them across the road to me. He was kept waiting for a considerable time while Dr Turner "finished writing up his notes".

The whole area was one of high morbidity arising from working in the mines, many of the men markedly disabled and breathless from lung disease and requiring much support with little in the way of effective treatment to offer. They were often housebound in front of a coal fire, they still received an allocation of cheap coal, and were often dead by the age of sixty. On the whole they had few outside interests and of course in the early 60's there was no television in most homes. My immediate impression when moving to Penrhyn Bay years later was the tremendous difference in the health status between patients of the same age in the two areas.

The practice itself had recently moved from a surgery in the house of Dr Jack Roberts, Dr John's late father and which had at one time been the local hospital, into a purpose-built surgery in the centre of the village with two consulting rooms, a waiting room and a reception office area with a receptionist and a patient call system. Really state of the art in the early sixties. It also ran branch surgeries in two adjoining villages, Penycae and Johnstown, both about two miles away. These were of a completely different standard but were justified at that time because of the lack of private cars and the general morbidity of the population. Wales has always been at the top of morbidity statistics lists and levels of prescribing costs in the UK, and our practice with its history of mining and its associated morbidity contributed its share.

The arrival of a young eligible bachelor doctor in the practice led to some interest amongst a section of the female population and this was not without its problems, particularly in a single-practice village. Luckily I was able to resolve the problem fairly soon, meeting my future wife Marian from sufficiently far away in Denbigh and we were married the following Easter, significantly on the anniversary of becoming a principal on April 1st, a date which has figured considerably in my life and career.

I arrived to my first surgery at Penycae which was in a traditional Welsh stone cottage, a "Ty a Siambr", with a waiting room with wooden benches and a door leading directly into a consulting room, both with smoking coal fires. If the wind was in the wrong direction, and it was that day, one came out quite black. The only contents were a table, two chairs, and a jug and basin to wash ones hands. Confidentiality was impossible because only a door divided them, there was no couch and if anything other than a cursory examination was required then the patient was sent home to await a visit or asked to attend the Ruabon Surgery. Surgeries lasted from 8.30 a.m to 9.30 three mornings a week. Interestingly enough the practice recently applied to close the Penycae surgery but were refused permission.

The other branch surgery at Johnstown, again on three mornings a week, was of similar standard and held in part of a large wooden building with a waiting area and a consulting area which had a sloping writing desk at which both doctor and patient stood. I did not go to this surgery except to provide cover when Dr Glyn was away.

Branch surgeries usually had multiple quick consultations, a repeat prescription or a repeat medical sickness certificate. There was no access to notes or hospital correspondence, although these were much less bulky than at present as referrals were less frequent and tests carried out directly by GPs were non-existent as there was no direct access to laboratories. Detailed examination requiring undressing was impossible and patients were sent home to undress for examination. Even then it was not always easy as old ladies wore the so-called "combinations" with access from the back and rarely took these off. Children were at times reputedly sewn into their vests for the winter. Patients were often reluctant to undress and Scruffy's triangle, an area accessed by opening one or sometimes two buttons of a shirt or blouse and inserting the stethoscope, allowed a token examination to take place satisfying both parties. The development of the diaphragm end to the stethoscope in addition to the traditional bell-end was a major advance in examinations in practice.

Both allowed different sounds and signs to be heard better. The old bell-end required it to be held at right angles to the chest wall whereas the diaphragm was applied flat, allowing it to be slipped down the back of a patient's blouse or shirt without undressing. This saved time when the doctor was really only undertaking a token examination and also allowed for some modesty in an era when patients were less inclined to flaunt large areas of their bodies than at present. It must be remembered that at this time intimacy was always referred to as "making love" whatever the circumstances, not as having sex, and often took place in the dark. Many husbands had never seen their wives completely naked. Contraception was confined to condoms which were available from barbers who offered "something for the week-end Sir", and from some but not all chemists where they were kept strictly under the counter.

Branch surgeries were usually fairly short and one could start visiting early. This in marked contrast to the present situation where surgeries can last all morning and when visits even when requested early may not be done until quite late in the day. Of course there were many more visits to do, I once did a total of thirty-seven in one day during a flu epidemic. The poor state of health of many of the patients meant that it was necessary to visit and assess simple flu symptoms and often to revisit more than once. The drugs available at the time were very limited and often ineffective. Although there were district nurses the doctor visited to give injections of the diuretic Mersalyl and often to inspect wounds and change dressings. There were no disposable syringes, each patient had his or her own glass syringe and needle which they carefully boiled up after each use.

Home visits often required the dog to be tied up as there was nothing worse than to have a dog sniffing round when one bent over to examine a patient. In later years there was often a battle to have the TV switched off as well. Near-patient pathology tests were in their infancy but the need to boil up urine to test for sugar and protein had gone and Clinitest tablets for glucose testing were a great improvement. Only later did the variety of Stix tests become available, starting with sugar and protein and now in recent years covering a whole batch of tests. Virtually all referrals were to the Wrexham Maelor Hospital and having worked at the hospital I knew all the consultants, not that there were that many.

An important feature of the NHS was the system of domiciliary visits by consultants accompanied by the GP to a patient's home. It was seen as having three important aspects, to give an opportunity for a specialist opinion to be given in the home at no cost to the patient, to possibly avoid unnecessary admissions, and thirdly to form a useful part of the GPs postgraduate training. This form of consultation preceded the NHS at a time when both GP and consultant were dependent on private fees for their income. It was not without its dangers as suggested in a cynical letter in the BMJ in 1886 which read "In order to be fairly successful in their efforts they (consultants) must, like other men, be fairly dishonest. If he be called in by friends to consult with the usual medical adviser he must necessarily try to find out what points of difference exist between the friends and their medical man. Then, if he is a fairly dishonest man and wishes to be a successful consultant, he will strongly back up the relatives"

To get round any dangers of possible competition the general practitioner introduced the consultants and remained while the examination took place, they then retired to consult in private as hands were washed on what was to be said and done, and then stayed together while the consultant advised the patient and family. This format continued into the NHS and it was one which we found very useful at times. Some GPs, either from lack of confidence or because they wished to impress patients used the system to excess. There was one GP in the Wrexham area who obviously felt very uncertain about children's illnesses and sometimes requested more than one domiciliary visit in a day. Consultants were paid a fee, the GP was not. Gradually over the years the difficulty in arranging for the consultant and the GP to attend at the same time led to a telephone conversation and then the consultant visiting alone. Later still it became much more difficult to persuade consultants to do D.V.s and many would suggest that the patient be admitted. Psychiatry was perhaps the area in which domiciliary visits were the most useful as it allowed the consultant to get a taste of the home situation and the attitudes of the relatives while it was much more socially acceptable and relaxing than a psychiatric out-patient appointment.

Terminal care at home meant that one did develop close relationships with the district nurse and similarly home confinements which were common led to many hours spent with the district midwife, the patient and her family. There was no need for the now fashionable weekend team-building and bonding sessions at that time. With no bleeps or mobile phones one was often unreachable except on foot on these occasions, but then patients were not so unreasonably demanding for an immediate response in those days.

Postgraduate education was very rudimentary at the time, there were the occasional lectures at the Maelor Hospital but no extended courses locally. I asked permission of the partners to go on a week's course to Manchester and after discussion this was agreed but only if I personally employed a locum. I found a GP from Canada who was visiting his family in Colwyn Bay and went off to my course. On the first morning he started at 8.30 a.m, called for coffee and at 10 a.m. decided he had had enough and left, not to be seen again. The partners were not too pleased when I arrived back the following week.

Some three years later the practice joined with that of Dr Arnold Barlow, a single-handed practitioner working in Rhosllanerchrugog, reputed to be the largest village in Wales, of similar population characteristics but with its own unique community and patois. It had one street with three no.1s and uniquely a number naught as addresses. Arnold and I had worked together as house officers in the Maelor Hospital in the mid fifties. The amalgamation changed little in the organisation of the practice except that it meant a one-in-four rota instead of a one-in-three, a significant improvement socially and for the family. Before mobile phones when on call the doctor was confined to the house and garden or had to arrange for messages to be taken and relayed. Being on call meant someone else had to be in the home at all times to look after the phone and also the children if called out on a visit. The development of technology allowing telephone calls to be transferred was a major advance but still did not solve the problem of the children.

Obviously all the doctors had to live within the practice area and with the limited number of private phones and with public kiosks often out-of -order it was not unusual to find patients turning up at the door, which could be quite frightening for the family at night if the doctor was out. One of a previous generation of doctors, a Dr Davies in Rhosllanerchrugog, was reputed to open the window and throw a bucket of water on anyone knocking on his door when he was in bed.

An early development was the answer-phone at the surgery with the recorded message telling patients what alternative number to ring. My wife took a call one evening from a very irate man who said he "couldn't get any sense from that bloody woman at the surgery."

Time went by happily with no problems or friction in the practice but after six years I felt that I did not wish to spend the rest of my professional life there. The new 1966 contract was just being implemented and we started to look around. At about the same time Arnold Barlow, born and bred in Rhosllanerchrugog, also felt the need for a change and moved to a country practice at Llansantffraid in Powys.

A single-handed practice was advertised at Betws-y-coed and we went over to see it twice. The weather on both days were very fine and the place appeared idyllic. I did not mind the practice being single-handed but off duty cover was a problem. The practice covered a large area up into the Penmachno area although there was another elderly doctor with a small list there. I talked to the Llanrwst practice but they were not interested in a rota at that time as the total area to be covered was too large, although they did start one with Dr Mike Jeffries at Betws-y-coed some years later.

Soon afterwards the vacancy at Penrhyn Bay came up and as described later I moved on.

The British Medical Association

Since throughout this account there will be frequent mention of the BMA and its various structures, the LMC, the Royal College of General Practitioners and the GMC perhaps there is a need now to look at these and explain how they function.

The BMA as an organisation is well known and respected by the population at large. It was founded by Sir Charles Hastings in a meeting at Worcester Infirmary attended by fifty doctors on 19th July 1832 as "an Association both friendly and scientific" and called the Provincial Medical and Surgical association (PMSA). It later expanded and covered the whole country. In 1840 it was known as the Provincial Medical Association. Now some 75% of all doctors are members.

The BMA still holds a very definite status and recognition in the eyes of the public because it is seen as the professions' face and voice, whether discussing national or local issues and whether they be relating to health care and the public health or discussing difficulties within the service. It has since 1925 had its headquarters in a prestigious building designed by Sir Edwin Lutyens and located in Tavistock Square on the site of the home of Charles Dickens, just a few hundred yards from Euston station, which was a great advantage to those of us from North Wales rushing to meetings or to catch the infrequent trains home.

It has over the years provided educational, social and medico-political guidance and support for all branches of the profession, its role and constitution changing to suit new situations and needs. Since its start it has published a weekly Journal, originally known as the Transactions of the Provincial Medical and Surgical Association, by 1840 it was the Provincial Medical Association Journal and by 1857 it had become the British Medical Journal. Together with The Lancet, it has always been rated amongst the most prestigious Journals in the world. In 1981 it was considered that its existing format with many research papers was too specialised for general practitioners and three versions were produced each week, research, overseas, and Practice Observed and this led to a more widely read Journal. Over recent years the extent of other BMA publications, journals and books for both professionals and for the public has expanded enormously.

The BMA has at the centre of its constitution and activities the Representative Body (the R.B) which meets annually, sometimes more frequently, as the Annual Representative Meeting (the A.R.M) which usually creates considerable media interest and an elected Council. Within the BMA centrally are the powerful craft committees, the Central Consultants and Specialists Committee (the CCSC) representing the consultants and specialists, and the General Medical Services Committee (the GMSC and more recently known as the GPC) representing general practitioners and discussed in detail later. The BMA has over the years had differences and sometimes difficult relationships with the Royal Colleges, particularly so in the early years of the NHS. A Joint Consultants Committee (the JCC) with one member representing each of the six Royal Colleges and an equal number from the CCSC had to be developed to allow them to speak to government with one voice, at times at least.

The BMA was not initially a trade union and in fact its Articles of Association specifically forbid this. When political activity was required such as in the various potential resignation crises over the years its ability to act to protect members interests was restricted. A shadow organisation called the British Medical Guild had to be established to undertake any trade union activities should they be necessary.

In 1930 the BMA had produced plans for a scheme for general medical services and this was reissued in 1938. The government Medical Planning Commission was charged in 1940 with considering the future of British Medical Services and its findings were incorporated into the Beveridge Report (A National Health Service) and into the publication of a White Paper in 1944 which led to the creation of the NHS Act in 1946 and its introduction in 1948.

The BMA is organised into local Divisions, the number of doctors in each division varies across the UK from a few hundred up to several thousand. One of the Division's important functions is to appoint representatives to the Annual Representative Meeting (the A.R.M,) where policy is discussed and where the Executive (the BMA Council) is often criticised for its actions or lack of action. Divisions used to have an important social function providing opportunities for doctors and their spouses to become involved and to meet up with the names that their partners kept talking about. Dinners and dinner dances were well attended and were often the social highlight of the year but as these became less popular and fashionable they gradually disappeared. In part this also reflected the tendency as social barriers were dropped for younger doctors and their partners to mix with a much broader cross-section of society than previously.

During this same period the medico-political functions previously carried out through the Divisions and the Council centrally have largely been taken over by the two separate Craft Committees, the CCSC and the GMSC and more recently central committees for other groups also. The craft committees themselves hold Annual Conferences where their own issues are debated and when necessary these are then debated again at the ARM to become Association policy.

North Wales is no different from other areas in its lack of enthusiasm for divisional activities and the local secretaries have for years had a thankless job. Many doctors wonder what the purpose of the Divisions are. In my professional lifetime the British Medical Association has never been an active local organisation in North Wales except in times of crisis within the profession In the early sixties when resignation from the Health Service was very much under consideration many stormy meetings were held under the banner of the British Medical Guild. The scattered nature of the area has not helped. The pattern is mirrored in most parts of the country although some BMA Divisions do continue an active social function. It is estimated that only half of the two hundred divisions in the UK are "active" and this has caused considerable anxiety and debate within the higher echelons of the BMA.

A working group was set up to review the position as part of a root-and-branch reform of the BMA decision-making structures and at the 2004 ARM, which incidentally was held at Llandudno, four options were debated. None of the new proposals were considered acceptable and the option of retaining the status quo was accepted, allowing for further discussions and in particular the opportunity to find out more about what members wanted at a local level. A conference of divisional secretaries met to discuss the problems, agreed that the way forward was not clear, but suggested improved electronic communication from the centre and more devolution to regions, a situation we already enjoy in Wales but which may not prove to be as effective in English regions Whether or not the divisional structure is still functioning adequately the core central structures are still very active and well-organised.

Wales has its own BMA Council, which is the senior committee in the Principality. In earlier years I was a representative on the Council. At that time it met in mid-Wales on a Sunday, appeared to function poorly with no great vision or success and my attendances were sporadic. I was very junior in medico-politics then and probably did not appreciate what went on behind the scenes. Now since devolution the BMA Wales has a much wider remit with devolved functions and has a new headquarters in Cardiff Bay. The Council and its chairman plays a very important part in relationships with the Welsh Assembly Government (WAG) as the civil service in Wales is now called as well as with other professional organisations.

Members are frequently asked by the media to comment on topical issues on behalf of the BMA, often on reports that have been published only that day or on comments that others just have made on air. Media reporters get to know who to approach and I have done my share of this in the past. Not infrequently one is required to make a response in the middle of a surgery on something which one has not seen or a discussion not heard and in reply to the slant put on them by the interviewer. As always with the media only selected parts of what one says is broadcast or published. Dr Phil White, the Gwynedd Division secretary is the current spokesman and does it very well, in both Welsh and

English. He seems to be able to quote facts generally unknown to the rest of us to support his case.

The BMA centrally has had a very efficient and powerful media and parliamentary lobby department and if time allowed one could ring them to get the official line. They also provided training in television interviews but unfortunately too late in my career for me to benefit fully.

The BMA has had a Welsh office in Cardiff for many years and during my time had a number of excellent and popular Welsh Secretaries, the first of my acquaintance being Dr Maldwyn Catell, who unfortunately died tragically early and suddenly in 1981. The Association has funded a Prize for students in the Medical School in his memory. Miss Rosemary Roberts acted up for nearly two years, followed briefly from 1982 to 1983 by Mr Roger Doherty, a consultant gynaecologist who then moved on to the Medical Defence Union (the MDU), and then in 1984 by Dr Bryan Davies, a GP from Maerdy in the Rhondda, a great character and fixer with an infectious laugh and perpetual, if rather edentulous, smile. Bryan at the time was chairman of WGMSC and had to relinquish this on appointment, propelling me into the chair earlier than anticipated.

Bryan was followed in 1993 by Dr Bob Broughton, one-time consultant radiologist and later active in the development of audit in Wales and in management in the secondary services. Bob had a GP wife so he had a broad base of contacts to call on and he did so very effectively. Personality and the ability to get on with others, on both sides of the table, is vital in these positions. Bob retired in 2003 to be replaced by the current secretary Dr Richard Lewis but this was after my time of activity in the BMA.

Very capably assisting the Welsh Secretaries as well as acting as administrative secretary to all the Welsh BMA committees from 1981 to her retirement to west Wales in 2000 was Miss Rosemary Roberts. For the whole of my time on the central committees she provided invaluable support and advice to successive chairmen and committees under the BMA Wales umbrella. As the administrative support for all the committees and in particular the GP, the Public Health, and the Consultants ones she was a font of knowledge on current thinking and potential problems including inter-craft issues.

Contractual problems, more common in hospital than in general practice, for doctors individually or in groups were for many years in the very capable hands of Tony Chadwick, the Industrial Relations Officer, who latterly was seconded to the London Office and who retired in 2006.

Many of the personalities of the BMA in North Wales have also active in other spheres and will feature when these are discussed later. One who does merit special mention and who does not appear elsewhere was Dr Bill Hughes from Amlwch who did sterling work as secretary for the old Anglesey division in the sixties and seventies and who was a regular attender at BMA functions and ARMs over many years, accompanied by his wife Jo.

The Medical Practitioners Union - the MPU.

The only active alternative to the BMA in the Fifties and Sixties was a much smaller organisation known as the Medical Practitioners Union. It was a radical left-wing orientated organisation which always was very cagey about admitting its membership base but it was good at producing new and radical ideas and blueprints. It produced the Medical World Newsletter which set out views which the more conservative BMJ and The Lancet would not cover. The latter in February 1965 under the heading "No Withdrawal" took general practitioners to task for threatening to terminate their contracts with the Executive Councils expressing the view that "practitioners should not use their independence collectively as a weapon of mass pressure to secure their demands". The MPU saw considerable advantages in a salaried service as a means of ensuring an equality of access to GP services in all areas and published them in its Blue Book. In 1991 it produced a further document again putting forward the concept of a salaried service. The MPU is now part of the Manufacturing Science and Finance Union (the MSF) which includes the Health Visitors Association and the Guild of Healthcare Pharmacists and it is particularly active in recruiting amongst the non-principal GPs.

In order for the GMSC to maintain its sole negotiating rights with government the MPU were allocated two seats on the committee and these are still there today. The MPU members have always been very effective in their contributions to GMSC debates. Dr Arnold Elliott from London and Dr Helen Groom were the members I recall from the start of my time on GMSC. Arnold at that time was nearing retirement but was a very effective debater and persuader. Later Brian Gibbons from Blaengwynfi in South Wales took his place. Brian who I knew well from sitting on Welsh GMSC worked with great dedication in a blind-end mining community in the Afan valley, an area of great deprivation over many years. He is now a Labour member of the Welsh Assembly and at the time of writing is struggling to correct the problems of health in Wales as Minister for Health. His dedication to his community was such that, while discussing his candidacy for the Assembly elections, he told me that if elected and then the quite likely possibility of being unable to find a replacement for his practice occurred he would not take up his seat.

Another very influential member and thinker was the socialist GP Julian Tudor Hart who worked in Glyncorrwg, a neighbouring and equally deprived valley. He was responsible for formulating in 1971 his Inverse Care Law which suggested that those most in need received the poorest care. The Black Report of 1980 and the Acheson Report on Inner London in 1981 had both drawn attention to the link between poverty and deprivation and poor health and morbidity but insufficient attention had been paid to these and insufficient resources allocated to the problem. Welsh GMSC drew attention to the problems in South Wales in their report on Underprivileged areas formulated in 1980. In 1997 Julian produced his blueprint Going for Gold and published by the Socialist Medical Association setting out his concepts for improved care in the South Wales valleys.

Local Medical Committees

Local Medical Committees, the LMCs, are the lynchpin of all medico-political activity associated with general practice. They were set up following pressure from the British Medical Association in Lloyd George's National Insurance Act of 1911 as representatives of the "panel" doctors, although in the original Bill no provision had been made for general practitioners participation in the administration of the scheme.

The government were however happy to agree these arrangements as the success of the health insurance scheme depended on the cooperation of the large number of independent practitioners. The concept of a State medical scheme was supported by the profession but it was strongly opposed to a salaried service as doctors believed that the loss of the independent contractor status would undermine the ability to practice without state interference and so put patient care at risk This independence has persisted over the years but in my opinion is very near to being lost in the recent reorganisations and contracts.

LMCs were given statutory recognition and the Local Insurance Committee (the forerunner of the NHS Executive Council and its successors) was required to consult with the LMC on a wide range of issues. Since then they have been the source of advice to a succession of health service organisational structures, the only constant factor in a sea of changes over nearly a hundred years. The first Annual Conference of Local Medical Committees was held in the Royal Pavilion in Brighton in 1913.

After they were set up a national committee, the Insurance Acts Committee which later became the General Medical Services Committee, (more recently renamed the General Practitioners Committee) was established within the BMA structure to represent the panel doctors in negotiations with government and this committee has always been recognised by government as the sole authoritative voice of general practitioners.

The LMC links into the BMA and into the central GPC (the General Practitioners Committee), and also with the Welsh Medical infrastructure, committees and organisations means that they have vast collective and individual experience which is not otherwise available (the so-called "herd memory") and which is vital when ideas which have been floated and rejected previously reappear years later in a slightly different guise.

LMCs are usually based on County, County Borough or sometimes other NHS administrative areas. They vary very considerably in the number of GPs they cover. I recall that on one occasion when sitting in London on a committee reviewing the constitution of the BMA and its representative structure I was trying to make a point about representation of GPs in Wales. Dr John Marks, a very powerful member of GMSC, and later BMA Council chairman, informed me in no uncertain terms that he had more GPs in his Hertfordshire LMC than we had in the whole of Wales.

LMCs have always been democratically elected by vote of all GPs within the area and members obviously need to ensure that they retain the confidence of their colleagues for the next election. Every effort has been made to ensure that the LMC can claim to be representative of all GPs and they have always been recognised by statute in successive NHS Acts as the local professional organisations representing General Medical Practitioners.

LMCs provide input and guidance to the central organisation of the BMA through elected representatives to the GPC and also through the Annual Conference of LMCs, of which more later. The detailed history of LMCs has been very well set out in a pamphlet by Dr John Marks in 1972 on which I have drawn extensively and in another by Dr John Chisholm

The Scharr Report prepared by the University of Sheffield in 2003 stated that "it is widely acknowledged that general practice is the cornerstone of the NHS. However because of its history of contractor status and tradition of independence, general practice is perhaps the most precariously supported element of the Health Service." It also recognised the LMC as being "the memory of the NHS" and that all should recognise that effective LMCs are in everyone`s interests and should continue to support them as they address new changes". One response to their consultation stated "LMCs are unique because they are paid for and owned by GPs".

All active GPs finance the LMCs through a statutory levy which pays the running costs of the LMC and a voluntary levy which amongst other things pays into the central GMS Defence Fund originally set up in 1913 Both levies are based on the number of patients on their list of patients. The Defence Fund covers all central committees functions and expenses, including honoraria to members attending and the very considerable legal fees arising from studying the proposed changes and legislation, and from checking various pronouncements. The existence of a very substantial reserve in the GMS Defence Fund has always given GPs more of a fall-back position during negotiations and disputes than the consultant body has had.

Consultations based on the LMC structure has considerable advantages for all parties. Sometimes however bodies try to circumvent the system and seek opinions from others, perhaps hoping to get different answers. Practising doctors without LMC involvement and experience may have considerable valuable and specialised experience in certain fields and can be a valuable source of advice, but if consulted direct by Health Authorities they may not always be aware of the implications of their advice and decisions, nor of other ongoing discussions which may be taking place on a UK, Wales or North Wales level. Doctors themselves if nominated to various organisations or committees often feel happier in knowing that they have an organisation behind them to whom they may turn, particularly so if the advice which they give is being rejected inappropriately or out-of-hand.

The Annual Conference of LMCs

The LMCs of the UK meet in London over two days for an Annual Conference at which the report on the activities of the GMSC/GPC over the year is discussed and further issues for them to consider over the coming year are debated. While the GMSC is not strictly bound by conference resolutions the oft-repeated words are "that GMSC ignores the wishes of Conference at its peril". At one LMC conference which I attended in the seventies the chairman of GMSC, Dr A.B.Davies, was forced to resign after persistent criticism of GMSC actions. Election to the Chair of Conference is a high honour within the BMA executive structure and requires a considerable in-depth knowledge of the constitution and procedures as well as a quick wit. I particularly recall the chairmanship of George Rae in this respect.

For many years the Conference was held in the impressive high-ceilinged Great Hall in BMA House. This was an impressive structure but its high ceiling led to poor acoustics and difficulty in heating. As BMA House was a grade-two listed building modifications were difficult but in 1986 the Hall had a new ceiling built at balcony level two thirds of the way up allowing for two floors, one which retained many of the original features and which housed the new Nuffield Library and an upper one which provided much needed office space. Subsequent conferences have been held in the nearby Logan Hall. At one of the last Conferences held in the Great Hall a photograph published in the BMJ showed the Gwynedd representatives Drs John Griffiths and Arthur Kenrick actively voting on a motion while the lay secretary Brian Jones looked on.

Some four hundred motions are on the agenda and while similar ones are now grouped into composite motions by the agenda committee (membership of this is an important stepping stone to the Chair) this is not to the extent of the composite motions of the Trades Union Conferences. One point was frequently emphasised, that in contrast to Union delegates doctors were attending as representatives who had been briefed by their peers but who could decide on the debate which way to vote. If someone referred in discussion to delegates they were rapidly corrected.

In my early years of attendance at Conference there was no grouping of motions and many agenda items had a series of amendments, sometimes six or seven on one motion, attached to them. Motions had to be formally proposed then each amendment had to be debated separately. This in itself gave rise to numerous "points of order" and rulings about "if amendment A is passed then B falls" and motions that the Conference "move to next business" before returning to the original motion as amended. Many of the amendments appeared trivial such as whether the working day should be defined as until 6pm, to 6.30pm or to 7pm but feelings often ran high about these and reflected the tension about terms of service at the time. Nowadays amendments are not allowed for debate although sometimes a motion can be changed beforehand with the agreement of the proposers and of Conference. The standard of debate is usually very high with some representatives becoming favourites of Conference. David Williams was one of these and he always had the ear of Conference which would listen carefully to his arguments, which were sometimes far seeing and often related to the medico-legal minutiae of the Regulations on which he was an expert. One agenda item recurring for years was whether London Weighting payments should be introduced into the pay structure to compensate for additional costs in the Capital, something which existed for the civil service and other public servants such as teachers. Obviously most of the non-London representatives were against this as any payment would reduce their own pay since it would all come from a fixed total sum. David made a memorable and telling tongue-in-cheek speech advocating additional payments for doctors living in rural Wales to compensate for the additional cost of petrol and food and because of the deprivation of the absence of theatres and concert-halls. The motion was always lost.

Andrew Dearden, now chairman of Welsh G.P.C., was another darling of the conference from his early days when he was a mere young representative. His witty and rabble-rousing speeches would receive thunderous applause. The oratorical skills of Lloyd George are still alive and well in Wales, although personally and sadly they passed me by.

Some sections of the agenda were taken by the sub-committee chairmen. When in the GMSC Education Chair I found this a very daunting experience as one had to respond off the cuff to issues raised without warning by representatives, taking care not to make any unwise commitments. The GMSC chairman and the Conference chairman were always at hand to save the day if necessary. The WGMSC chairman slot was usually much less of an effort as the controversial issues were on the main agenda and the slot was always immediately after lunch before many representatives had returned to the chamber.

The tenor of Annual Conferences was very much dependent on the political situation and relationships with government at the time but were always interesting to attend. On occasions when problems were great Special Conferences were necessary, sometimes more than one in a year.

LMCs in North Wales

North Wales has during my clinical lifetime had a number of different configurations of the LMC structure, based on the changing local government and administrative health structures in force at the time.

In my early days at Ruabon there were four LMCs in North Wales co-terminous with the four administrative Executive Councils (later the Family Practitioner Committees). The eastern end was served by a single Denbigh and Flintshire Executive Council covering the two counties, whereas in the northwest Caernarfonshire, Anglesey as it was then known, and Merioneth all had there own Councils. The smaller Executive Council areas were largely rural and had few GPs. In Anglesey and Merioneth all the GPs were members of the LMC whereas Caernafonshire being larger did have an elected membership. The three were amalgamated to form the Gwynedd LMC in 1974. Usually relationships with the Executive Council chairmen and their Clerks (later to be renamed Administrators) have always been close and co-operative.

Initially administration was relatively simple and LMCs usually had a medical secretary and some professional outside support. Caernarfonshire were supported for many years by W. Mathews and Son, a firm of accountants, initially by Trefor Mathews and later from 1970 to 1994 his partner Brian Jones provided the herd memory and valuable advice, as well as a fair degree of humour. On his retirement in 1994 Mrs Litton from Llanberis was appointed as lay secretary and continued until the merger into the North Wales LMC in 1996.

April 1989 saw the medical secretary of Gwynedd Dr Arthur Kenrick appointed to the chair of the new FHSA and Dr John Roberts of Dolgellau took over as medical secretary. In 1992, following the resignation from the FHSA of Dr Ian Roberts of Bala due to pressure of work, John was appointed by the Secretary of State as a member of the FHSA and had to resign as medical secretary. Dr Jonathan Jones of Penygroes was appointed and continued until the merger into a North Wales LMC in 1996.

The eastern area of North Wales was much more varied with industrial urban areas including Wrexham and Deeside and large rural areas and was much the most politically active of the LMC`s. Dr D.B.Evans from Coedpoeth was a powerful figure who I just remember and in fact one of my locums before joining the Ruabon practice was with his partner, Dr Elgan Evans, following on his death in 1959. D.B.Evans had been elected a member of the Panel Committee for Denbighshire in 1923 and was its secretary from 1928 to 1948, continuing as secretary of the new Local Medical Committee at the outset of the NHS. He was one of the two Welsh representatives on the Central Insurance Acts Committee (later the GMSC) until 1955. Dr Ivor Davies from Cerrig-y-drudion took over in 1954 and had an encyclopaedic knowledge of the NHS Regulations. This was particularly important because this committee, unlike the other LMCs, appointed a new chairman every year on a "buggin's turn" basis. Sometimes they were good, occasionally disastrous and in any case they did not stay long enough to make their mark. Ifor continued until 1972 when Dr Eddie Lewis of Mold took over as secretary. He continued as secretary until his retirement in 1990 when he was succeeded by Dr Gruff. Jones of Holywell who was in post when the LMCs amalgamated in 1996 and who has continued as a very active secretary ever since in addition to his wide GPC and WGPC commitments and involvement. Relationships with the administrative bodies in Clwyd varied considerably over the years and was sometimes strained by unnecessary inflexibility and attention to detail by individual officers

The first dedicated administrative secretary, Mrs Janet Capper, was appointed to Clwyd LMC in 1979 and provided valuable support and assistance to members until her retirement. Mrs Elaine Jones is proving to be a worthy successor and her developing administrative support to other medical committees in North Wales will prove mutually beneficial.

I was first elected to the Denbighshire and Flintshire LMC in 1963 when working in Ruabon and there first met a number of colleagues, doctors such as David Williams from Holywell, John Lynch from Denbigh, and Eddie Lewis from Mold who became my mentors in medical politics over the next thirty years. There were a number of other senior members who left lasting impressions, in particular Dr B.D.Chowdhury, an Indian doctor who had come to this country and set up a practice in Penyffordd near Holywell. He established himself as a very powerful figure in the area, becoming chairman of Flintshire County Council and also chairman of the Clwyd Family Practitioner Committee.

In the early sixties the Flintshire doctors had their own little caucus, the Flintshire Practitioners Union, led by Drs Chowdhury, Gavin, Godlove, and Hamilton of the Deeside coastal strip, and which would meet to discuss policy and tactics before LMC meetings. Dr Chowdhury would then ring round members canvassing, or coercing, support. At meetings Dr Chowdhury would sit in the front row and turn round and glare at members and dare them to speak out of turn. For reasons discussed later there was much more controversy in LMC meetings at that time, in later years decisions were usually easily reached by consensus and voting was rarely required. Perhaps it was because in the earlier years the changes and the issues tended to be big and dramatic, involving possible resignations, and affected all the doctors whereas later on changes were more frequent and often less major, affecting only some doctors and practices. Major crises did arise from time to time and are discussed later in the narrative.

A major geographical reorganisation took place in Wales in 1974 with the merger of the three western counties into Gwynedd (not the present and smaller Gwynedd which was formed in the later reorganisation in 1996) and with the amalgamation of Flintshire and Denbighshire to form Clwyd. It saw the formation of two Area Health Authorities, Gwynedd and Clwyd, and for the first time saw the hospital services and the practitioner services coming under one Authority. Family Practitioner Committees were created in the 1980 reorganisation to replace the Executive Councils, technically as sub-committees of the Health Authority although in practice they had a wide degree of autonomy.

Further reorganisation in 1990 saw the abolition of FPCs and the introduction of FHSA's with a reduction in the GP representation but with Dr Arthur Kenrick of Llanrwst being appointed chairman in Gwynedd by the Secretary of State.

1996 saw a yet another re-organisation (someone has called these repeated changes re-disorganisations) in Wales with five new Authorities being formed from the previous eight and with Gwynedd and Clwyd Health Authorities being merged into a North Wales Health Authority with Dr Kenrick again appointed chairman. He was the only medically qualified chairman appointed in Wales. In order to be co-terminous the LMCs also merged.

The North Wales LMC following the reorganisation of Health Authorities was elected by postal ballot and held its first meeting in February 1996. Following the amalgamation and prior to the meeting I had been elected to the chair by postal ballot. Dr Huw Lloyd of Old Colwyn and Dr Wally Murfin of Tywyn, Merioneth, were elected deputy chairmen. Dr Gruff. Jones of Holywell who had previously been the Secretary of Clwyd LMC was appointed its secretary, with Mrs Janet Capper continuing as his administrative assistant. Janet retired in 2004 just before completing 25 years service to the LMC. Tragically Wally, who had also been elected founder chairman of the North Wales District Medical Committee but who had to resign soon afterwards when he was appointed as a medical adviser by the Health Authority and who was starting to develop a significant presence in the Welsh Office, died tragically early in 2001, which was a great loss to the committee and to the NHS in Wales as a whole.

Although I had been a member on LMC's since the early 1960's I had not previously held office in an LMC, partly I suppose because of commitments on the all-Wales scene. I have however over the years served on a total of five LMC's which could be some sort of record, mainly because of the various administrative changes and boundary reorganisations. I originally was elected to the Denbighshire and Flintshire LMC in 1963 when in the Ruabon practice. After I moved to the Penrhyn Bay practice in 1967 I was elected to the then Caernarfonshire LMC and following on the 1974 reorganisation to the Gwynedd LMC until 1996. As our practice in Penrhyn Bay actually straddled the border between Caernarfonshire and Denbighshire with many patients in both counties I retained an interest in both LMCs over the years and remained an elected or co-opted member on Clwyd LMC for most of the time, ensuring I had a knowledge of the problems of the whole of North Wales which was useful on the all-Wales level. Perhaps for this reason it was appropriate that I became the first chairman of the North Wales LMC in 1996 and I considered this a great honour.

The term of office was for four years and even though I am now retired from practice I have remained on the LMC as immediate past-chairman, although I realise increasingly that with all the changes arising from the new 2004 GP contract I am no longer as familiar with details as I once was. There is not the same incentive to spend hours checking all the small print in the many documents. Dr Eddie Lewis of Mold, for years the secretary of Clwyd LMC, is also a co-opted member and we do have contributions to make from time to time, sometimes making use of our combined herd memory. We also represent the interests of retired GPs.

An interesting minute indicating tensions at the time records that there were three observers at the count of the Denbighshire and Flintshire LMC ballot papers in 1964. At the most recent election, at which I was ineligible to vote, I acted as Returning Officer and did the count unsupervised.

Having written at length about the history of the LMC perhaps it is appropriate to describe in some detail exactly what LMC's do.

The Sixties was certainly a period of change and development within the relatively young Health Service whose development in the early years was held back by the aftermath of the war and its financial implications. In addition to local issues the Sixties particularly saw a series of major Reports to do with the organisation of the Health Service both for general practice and on the development of the hospital service and these provided lively discussion and sometimes polarised opinions.

An early and significant one was that by Porritt in 1967 proposing one administrative unit, the Area Health Board, which should be the focal point of all medical services in an appropriate area and that doctors and other personnel should be under contract with it (the blueprint for Area Health Authorities)

The Hospital Plan for England and Wales introduced the concept of the District General Hospital serving an extended locality and supported by community hospitals based on the old cottage hospitals and by major centres of excellence in the larger conurbations. The Bonham Carter Report on the Functions of the District General Hospital followed in 1969. Three DGHs were proposed for North Wales and in due course these were established at Bodelwyddan, Wrexham, and at Bangor. The changes would have significant effects on local hospitals and services in which the LMC had a considerable interest and view.

Other major Reports were those by Dame Annis Gillie in 1963 on The Field of Work of the Family Doctor, the Bruce Fraser Joint Working Party, the Willink Report which disastrously resulted in a ten per cent reduction in the intake of medical students, the Todd Report on Medical Education, the Sheldon Report on Child Health Services, and the Peel Report on domiciliary midwifery. All needed very careful study and debate locally and centrally as they had major implications for general practice.

Reviewing old minutes emphasises the recurrence of the same problems and local issues year after year in spite of attempts to solve them. Many of these could have been solved relatively easily given the will, the requirement for individuals to stick to agreed protocols plus a moderate amount of finance which could have been easily recouped elsewhere.

Significant changes were achieved from time to time, either locally or nationally, and North Wales can feel justifiably proud of the major contributions of its national representatives, in particular Drs David Williams of Holywell and John Lynch of Denbigh.

A recurring LMC agenda item was a determination under Schedule 16 of the NHS Regulations as to whether an item which had been prescribed for a patient was a food or a drug. If it was thought to be the former the cost was deducted from the doctor's remuneration. Items included corn oil for cooking (new at the time) which was advised for high cholesterol and heart disease, whisky which was sometimes prescribed to improve circulation in peripheral vascular disease, and later gluten-free products. This was of course at a time when specific remedies and drugs were often not available. Another interesting recurring item was an ethyl chloride spray used to freeze the skin before incision of boils and abscesses, the administration seemed to believe (probably correctly) that any left over was being used for other patients which was considered a crime. Doctors obviously objected to themselves paying for items used directly for patients and usually appealed so the LMC had to adjudicate. It has always been a rule that a prescription is for one patient and one patient only, very time consuming and expensive when a large family of children all needed the same medication for head lice or similar conditions. The wrath of authority was incurred if the family was included in a single prescription form.

Later a Ministerial committee was set up to make central determinations on the medical conditions and the circumstances when so-called borderline substances could be prescribed. If the GP endorsed the prescription with ACBS (**A**ccording to the **C**ommittee on **B**orderline **S**ubstances) signifying that it fell within the guidance then the prescription was not queried, a great advance as the number of available borderline substances has grown markedly in recent years.

Dispensing formed another important topic for discussion, either central proposals affecting dispensing in practices, or local issues either within an individual practice or local disputes with pharmacies, and these are discussed elsewhere.

Agendas included giving approval for an extension of pensionable age for doctors reaching age sixty-five. At that time there was no bar to continuing in practice to a ripe old age and I recall that in the seventies there was one elderly single-handed doctor in Clwyd still practicing, in his nineties, reputedly seeing patients from his bed towards the end. The 1990 contract brought in a compulsory retirement age as a principal of seventy, although doctors could continue as an assistant or locum indefinitely. The present generation of GPs now seem to be considering and planning for retirement in their fifties rather than in their seventies.

Another role was the approval of the adequacy of practice premises, in three categories, main surgery, branch surgery, and calling places.

Payment for temporary residents formed a fairly regular discussion item, especially for those in holiday camps and in nursing and residential homes. Those in Homes were paid for at half-rate, presumably on the basis that one was likely to see several on one visit, although by definition and the fact they were in a Home it is probable that they required more rather than less care. The problems with holiday camps has already been discussed.

Problems associated with admission to hospitals, especially Denbigh with chronic alcoholics particularly difficult, and poor or absent communication on patient discharge figured frequently and recurringly (and still does). Waiting times were an issue then as now with orthopaedics at Wrexham particularly bad and patients were opting to go privately. Doctors were warned not to accept statements of waiting times second or third hand but to contact the hospital administrator rather than the consultant to cover themselves legally when advising patients on waiting times and private referrals. There was often the feeling that some departments were keeping a long waiting list to encourage private referrals.

The Abortion Act of 1967 frequently gave rise to discussion as local consultants were not enthusiastic about performing the operation and one usually had to have a one-to-one discussion with the consultant before patients were seen. The setting up of a private BPAS (British Pregnancy Advisory Service) clinic at Chester made things easier but there was a financial cost which was a difficulty for some patients, often those who perhaps needed a termination the most.

More recently and with newer and more complex contracts with administrative issues and targets featuring large and with Health Boards increasingly strapped for money much time has been spent on ensuring that arrangements follow the guidance correctly.

Regrettably LMCs like many other medical committees have over the years been male-dominated areas and it has been very difficult to persuade women doctors to put their names forward, if nominated they would certainly have been elected. One or two names do merit inclusion and praise for their contributions. In the early years Dr Meira Pritchard from Penygroes was a regular member. In the east there was Dr Anne McLeod from Prestatyn and in Gwynedd Dr Gwen Richards from Beaumaris, both of whom contributed greatly to the LMCs over a number of years and by nomination on a variety of other committees and working groups. In addition to standing up forcefully for the interests of women doctors they also oversaw the feminine areas of maternity, child health, cervical screening and family planning. Others have come and gone, perhaps not finding the work to their taste but have contributed in other ways.

The other major group of doctors who were not officially represented on the LMC were the Non-principals. This disparate group has increased significantly in size and in importance in recent years and covers locums, sessional doctors and assistants, and doctors on the Retainers Scheme. Their contractual issues and their continuing education needs have assumed greater significance and an attempt has been made to establish an electorate so that they can be represented on the LMC

It has been the constantly changing scene and the need to react to it that has made the work of the LMC so fascinating and absorbing over the years.

The Royal College of General Practitioners

The College of General Practitioners was set up by a steering group of enthusiasts from across the UK in November 1952, soon after the inception of the NHS in 1948. It followed the publication as a supplement to the BMJ of two separate memoranda by Dr Fraser Rose and by Dr John Hunt which had been discussed in the General Practice Review Committee of the BMA, and was started at a time when general practice was in a state of decay and disorganisation with morale at rock bottom. An even greater crisis was facing general practice in the United States and an Academy of General Practice had been set up there in 1947, although it failed to halt the decline.

Other specialties such as the surgeons and the physicians had had a Royal College structure overseeing its members and controlling entry into the specialties for very many years while other newer specialties were starting to clamour for their own colleges. The trend to hospitalisation and specialisation was accelerating after the start of the NHS and the voice of the three specialist Royal Colleges was progressively diminishing general practice.

The new College became the first academic body for general practitioners in Europe and was set up against considerable opposition from the three existing Royal Colleges culminating in a final attempted put-down letter from Sir Russell Brain, the President of the Physicians, the tone of which is so stern as to be worth quoting in full. On 11 Jan 1952 Sir Russell, writing with the effective support of Sir Cecil Wakely for the Royal College of Surgeons and Dame Hilda Lloyd for the Royal College of Obstetricians and Gynaecologists wrote -

"I think I ought to make it quite plain that this College, and I am sure I can here speak for the other two Colleges as well, would not be able to support in any way an organisation which aimed at establishing another college or which it seemed to us might seek to do so at some future date. I can say this with confidence because this very point has just been settled by the three Royal Colleges jointly in connection with another matter. I want to make this plain now because, while as you know, the three Royal Colleges would view sympathetically the establishment of a Joint Faculty for General Practice, I do not want those now considering the formation of an institution of general practice to go forward feeling that the three Royal Colleges would be likely to support an independent body without very stringent safeguards against it ever becoming a College.

Yours sincerely

W Russell Brain.

Another consultant reputedly said "a proposed College of GPs, nonsense, we will be having a College of Toenails next", while yet another is reported as saying that GPs should not handle hypertension which was becoming treatable but refer them because "consultants needed grateful patients".

The founders were not so easily put down. Wales was represented at the Foundation of the College by Dr Trevor Hughes of Ruthin, incidentally one of the few GPs who have written about their times in practice, while South Wales was represented by Drs David Hughes from St Clears and Wilfred Howells from Swansea.

The stated objectives of the steering committee included the words "To improve the quality, the art, the skill of general practitioners by setting a high standard and by encouraging and helping general practitioners to reach and maintain it".

The new College did not attempt to usurp the functions of the BMA and concentrated its efforts on improving quality and setting and raising standards within practice. The tone of this emphasis towards Quality and further statements from the new College were seen by many GPs as being elitist and "holier than thou" and this feeling persisted amongst many doctors for years. Indeed some still see it this way although this attitude has diminished markedly in recent years, particularly since most GP registrars now sit the entrance examination at the end of their training. Many within the BMA and in the profession generally saw the laying down of standards to be reached without at the same time achieving any negotiated benefits or concessions from Government in return as dangerous and unwise.

Initially membership of the new College was open to all GPs who had been in practice for at least twenty years, or for five years if they gave a commitment to continuing professional development, but in 1965 the College set a requirement of admission by examination only, gaining the letters MRCGP (member of the RCGP), although this was not initially accepted as registrable with the GMC. While this provided a feeling of status the introduction of an entrance examination did have the effect of excluding many very good but older and established GPs who had not already joined and who would not on principle sit another examination. It was felt that it tested factual knowledge more readily available to the recently qualified rather than that resulting from practical experience, and this did add to the antagonism against the College. I had completed the necessary five years in practice and joined the College in 1965 shortly before the compulsory examination came in, and since it was already ten years since I had qualified luckily avoiding the hassle of taking an exam.

The College had a variety of headquarters in the early years but in 1961 established its headquarters at 14 Princes Gate, London, overlooking Hyde Park in a house which had at one time been the residence of Joseph Kennedy, the American Ambassador to Britain and where JFK spent part of his childhood. In 1980 it had its excitement by being next door to and involved in the siege and the storming of the Iranian Embassy by the SAS. For years afterwards the building suffered damp and other structural problems arising from the extensive structural damage to the Embassy while disputes over insurance and compensation went on. It has remained at Princes Gate although it is now recognised as no longer being adequate for its purpose and a move to purpose built premises is under discussion. Princes Gate provided overnight accommodation for doctors visiting London and I have made use of this on numerous occasions, in so doing meeting informally many of the College Officers, and especially during my time at the JCPTGP which had its office within the building and held its meetings at the College.

The College received Royal Status and a Charter in 1967 and became the Royal College of General Practitioners. Both Prince Phillip in 1972 and Prince Charles twenty years later have held the position of President.

Since 1967 the College has recognised merit and service by the award of Fellowship, FRCGP, which was awarded centrally on the secret recommendation of existing Fellows and the Provost within the local Faculty. Membership as in other Colleges allowed the wearing of an academic gown, of black silk with silver facings but uniquely recognisable by the large College Badge on the right lapel which could be added on election to Fellowship. This was to be worn on all ceremonial and academic functions and during College council meetings.

In 1968 a ceremonial mace was presented by Dame Annis Gillie on behalf of Scottish members and for years was carried into Council and general meetings ahead of the President. The development of regalia and status symbols in the early years was part of a process within the College of developing parity with older academic institutions and colleges but by the nineties the increasing informality of dress within the profession and within society as a whole made the place of formal gowns and regalia less appropriate and the mace and wearing of gowns in Council meetings was stopped in 1991.

The College has over the years set out to define the differences between general practice and care in hospital, later well enunciated by Dr. Marshall Marinker as "the role of the GP is to tolerate uncertainty, explore probability and marginalize danger. In contrast the role of the secondary care specialist is to reduce uncertainty, explore possibility and marginalize error. It deals with undifferentiated presentations of illness. General practice's strength is that it does manage uncertainty and get it right most of the time when symptoms are inconclusive". It set out to make clear how the different role can best be carried out and to provide guidance and training for this. In particular members of the

College have written extensively through books and in the College Journal, developing a completely new field of medical publications.

The Journal has changed considerably over the years under a series of distinguished editors from an initial Newsletter to what is now a highly developed monthly academic journal with research publications. Personally I found it of most interest in the intermediate years when contributions were more general and less research oriented. Other publications have included a series of Reports from General Practice, Occasional Papers and policy statements. Perhaps one of the more important was the What Sort of Doctor published in 1985 which tried to set out the way forward.

Improving the quality of medical records has been a priority over the years with the publication of simple summary cards to fit into the medical record envelope an early effort. Another innovation (in the interests of clarity and ensuring that the meat of the consultation was clearly visible and understood by others reading the notes later the pursuit of quality has been and remains its driving force) was the concept of structuring records of consultations by the use of SOAP, listing **S**ymptoms, **O**bservations, **A**ction, **P**rescription.

The College in Wales

For practical purposes the UK was divided into Faculty areas each with a degree of autonomy. Wales had two Faculties in South Wales while North Wales was linked into a Merseyside and North Wales Faculty based on Liverpool.

In 1979 Dr. Robert Harvard Davis was appointed the first Professor of General Practice in Wales. A giant of a man, physically and intellectually, he had a huge role in developing general practice education in Wales, although it must be said formal lecturing was not his strongest point. I was privileged to sit with him on many committees over the years. He chaired in 1971 the Standing Medical Advisory Committee's important Report on the Organisation of General Practice which set standards across all aspects of the effective running of general practice. An eponymous lecture set up in his honour in 1986 was the Harvard Davis lecture, hosted annually by the three Welsh faculties in turn, and he personally delivered the first one.

A move to have a separate Faculty in North Wales had been rejected in 1971 as the number of members at that time was limited to a handful. The Merseyside Faculty did arrange good lecture meetings and symposia from time to time and I attended the a few of these over the early years but the only member from North Wales who became at all involved was Dr Gwyn Thomas from Denbigh. Contact with the South Wales Faculties in the early years was virtually non-existent except on a personal basis.

After some years as the membership in North Wales grew Gwyn was active in persuading the College to allow a sub-faculty to be formed. The inaugural meeting was held on Sunday July 10th 1983 at the North Wales Medical Centre in Llandudno and consisted of a lecture by Dr Peter Thomas, curator of the Welsh Medical History Museum on "Old Medical Instruments". It was followed by an exploratory business meeting to consider setting up a N.Wales sub-Faculty of the Merseyside and North Wales Faculty whose Provost Dr. David Cooke was present together with Prof. David Metcalfe of Manchester University representing UK College Council. Both were very supportive of the concept. It was recognised by all that the geography and distances involved meant that more local arrangements were necessary in order to encourage active membership of the College. Similar problems and solutions were being considered in several other Faculties covering large areas. The members attending the meeting supported the idea and an executive sub-committee was set up with Dr Gwyn Thomas as chairman, myself as vice-chairman and Dr Huw Lloyd of Old Colwyn as secretary / treasurer. As with all meetings in North Wales finding a suitable and convenient central venue was never easy and initially meetings were held in Betws-y-Coed. In 1986 I succeeded Gwyn as Chairman and at the same time he was elected Provost of the parent Merseyside and North Wales Faculty.

The College has always been keen on its regalia and in 1986 the new sub-faculty was presented by Ciba-Geigy with a Chairman's jewel designed and made by Mrs Kathleen Makinson of Denbigh. It was cleverly designed in such a way that the "sub" in the name sub-faculty could easily be removed at a later date.

By 1987 the sub-faculty had established itself and, supported by senior member of the College Council, Drs Mollie McBride, Bill Styles and John Haesler, it applied for and was granted full Faculty status. At the 1988 Harvard Davis Lecture at Bodelwyddan the speaker, Professor Denis Pereira Gray, presented the Provost with a medallion, courtesy of Glaxo Pharmaceuticals and again made by Mrs Kathleen Makinson, to match the Chairman's jewel previously donated.

College Faculties have a Provost who is usually a senior figure with a defined formal role and who presides at the Annual General Meeting, at elections and at meetings with distinguished guest speakers, and a Chairman who oversees other matters in the Faculty. Gwyn Thomas who had previously been Provost of the Merseyside and North Wales Faculty was elected as the first North Wales Provost, perhaps uniquely becoming Provost of two different Faculties, with myself as chairman and Dennis Williams of Pwllheli as secretary.

Since in the early years the number of active senior members were few it became the norm for a while for Chairmen to move up to Provost at the end of their terms, but in 1998 Eddie Lewis from Mold, a stalwart in College meetings as in many other areas of medical organisations in N.Wales over many years and who had not previously been Faculty Chairman was honoured by being elected Provost.

Representatives of each Faculty attend the UK Council in London every two months, a very interesting and instructive exercise but very time consuming with much reading to be done and members are also often required to take part in working groups and to attend other meetings. While no-one from our Faculty has yet aspired to high office in the College our representatives have contributed considerably to its work centrally, in particular Huw Lloyd and Mike Jeffries.

The three Welsh Faculties meet at the Welsh Council, set up in 1968 and now re-named RCGP Wales, which has recently become much more pro-active and has been developing active cooperation with Welsh GPC, especially so since devolution of health matters in Wales. Dr. Roger Ramsay, first as secretary and then as Chairman has been heavily involved in Welsh Council as well as being chairman of the North Wales Medical Trust discussed later

It has to be said that Faculty meetings have, like many others in Wales, struggled over the years to attract good attendances because of distances and other commitments but this does not truly reflect the commitment to the principles of the College which members have been developing within their practices. Many members have been very active both locally and on a Welsh and UK front in developing policies and carrying them forward, and many of the apologies received at events are because the member is attending some other meeting or conference in Cardiff, London or even abroad. The time commitment is considerable, unpaid and largely unrecognised and while the numbers of active members are small the quality of contributions is very high.

On a local level the Faculty has largely concentrated on educational and research matters, although it did once in 1984 stray into the political field when it held a meeting with North Wales MPs, John Marek from Wrexham, Dafydd Wigley from Caernarfon, Sir Anthony Meyer from Flintshire and Roger Roberts the prospective candidate from Conwy.

Efforts to promote group research projects were not very successful but several members received awards for individual research papers. Peter Elliott of Denbigh presented a paper on diabetes at the Merseyside research symposiun at Chester and was given a Pfizer award for his paper on sports injuries to the Welsh Conference of Performance Review at Llandrindod, Dennis Williams of Pwllheli was given a Pfizer award for work on colonoscopy in his practice and I received one for a study of Repeat Prescribing in the practice. Robin Williams from Llanfairfechan, one of my trainees who subsequently emigrated to Australia, won both a Syntex award and a Welsh Council Prize. I had also received the Minnitt Medal at a Chester research symposium and David Williams had developed an interest in the Social Pathology of Family Life. There was work going on but only sporadically until 1984 when Dr Claire Wilkinson who had been a lecturer in the postgraduate department in Cardiff moved up to the area to live. Based on Wrexham she was given two sessions to start to develop an academic department of general practice in North Wales and to develop and encourage research, the first time there had been any paid support and experience available. The Unit has expanded with the appointment of Fellows and Lecturers in several disciplines. Now Professor, Claire continues to support and encourage research and a nucleus of six practices (three from our area, Paul Myres at Overton, Gwyn Roberts from Wrexham and Tony Roberts at Llanfaircaereinion) formed a consortium CAPRICORN (Cymru Alliance of Primary Care Orientated Research Network) to encourage collaborative research in general practice. Dr Paul Myers had previously played an important role in the Clwyd and the North Wales MAAGs as research lead by supporting research in the practices and ensuring that research was linked to audit and education. It helped that he was at the same time the CME Tutor at Wrexham. Dr Cen. Humphreys of Crickhowell reviewed and published A History of Research in General Practice in Wales

The Faculty has put on a variety of educational meetings for GPs with distinguished speakers but also saw the need to assist doctors preparing for membership, initially by the examination but more recently by undertaking the new and difficult alternative route to membership by assessment, rather than by examination. Drs Peter Elliott and Gareth Parry Jones from Caernarfon were the first to be accepted as examiners for the College entrance examination. Peter has moved away but Gareth has continued to develop post-graduate education as Senior Lecturer responsible for Summative Assessment. At one time he also edited an excellent Faculty newsletter.

In the late eighties the Faculty saw a need to encourage the educational development of the growing number of practice nurses whose needs were not otherwise catered for, certainly not by nursing administration, and helped them to set up local support groups. As an indication of their perceived needs ninety percent of all the practice nurses in North Wales attended a meeting on their Role in Health Education The Faculty provided an annual prize to encourage project work by the nurses within their practices. Clwyd FPC agreed to circulate flyers to the practice nurses but only at a cost of 10p each, an indication of a lack of support for innovation by them. Practice nurses were also encouraged to visit each others practices to see the new opportunities open to them and take ideas back. Our excellent practice nurse, Sister Zoe Haigh, was an active participant and later became recognised as a nurse mentor.

In more recent years the faculty has attempted but with limited effect to involve and support recent entrants into general practice and also to look at the needs of the increasing number of non-principals in practice

One member who has contributed immensely to the work of the College both in North Wales and nationally in the UK is Mike Jeffries who until his recent retirement was in practice in Betws-y-Coed, as a member of Council but also as an assessor and visitor overseeing doctors undertaking GP vocational training within the armed forces He also had a useful input as a member of the Trust Board at Glan Clwyd Hospital.

David Wood, John Roberts, Roger Ramsay, Dennis Williams, Huw Lloyd and DK Banerjee are amongst others who have made considerable contributions to the work and the aims of the College in Wales and their contributions are mentioned elsewhere. Mary Pendergast, a partner in my old practice in Ruabon, did sterling work as secretary to the Faculty for a number of years. Peter Saul from Wrexham in addition to work on local groups and as a postgraduate tutor has had interesting sidelines, as local radio-doctor and as media columnist, being involved in the repatriation of patients taken ill abroad, and recently as part of the consultation procedure prior to decisions on new drugs by NICE.

Younger members are coming forward to take their place and the future is bright.

The Welsh Association of Local Medical Committees

The Welsh Association of LMCs predated the Welsh GMSC and at that time provided the only opportunity for GPs in Wales to meet and discuss ideas, problems and solutions. The Chief Medical Officer for Wales would usually attend, often accompanied by Dr Graham Moses a highly respected ex-GP who was responsible for general practice at the Welsh Office, although they always discreetly made their exits or stayed away if there was any discussion that might cause embarrassment or a conflict of interest. It was an opportunity for GPs as a group and as individuals to speak with them to get a point across formally and informally. They themselves felt less constrained because they were not accompanied by their civil servants. Ministers of State would be invited as dinner guests at times. Mr Alun Jones, an accountant from the Valleys, provided efficient administrative support for many years.

The Association provided an opportunity to bring other distinguished medico-politicians to Wales, people like Keith Davidson from the Scottish GMSC and particularly Jim Cameron, GMSC Chairman, who always welcomed the chance to visit Wales and later was delighted to be asked to become Honorary Life President of the Association. Jim had a true Scotsman's love of the hard stuff, with the ability to go on well into the early hours but appear very alert and on the ball at the following morning's meeting when we lesser mortals were struggling.

In 1971 one of the major documents which the Association looked at very carefully related to Long Term Policies in General Practice which emphasised that the foundation of general practice was being undermined by the development of the new hospital specialist structure and its outreach into new fields so that hospitals might be seen as providing "the alternative general practitioner service". This was exemplified in the increasing follow-up of outpatients, by paediatricians with a declining direct demand moving into developmental paediatrics and increasing follow up of potentially abnormal cases, while the Peel Report had suggested that 100% of maternity deliveries should be in hospitals and that family planning should be an integral part of the maternity services. A draft hospital memorandum and local authority circular envisaged "therapeutic teams" in psychiatry including psychiatric nurses following patients into a community divided into catchment areas rather than based on practice areas. All these proposals posed a serious threat to the continuation of family based general practice and needed to be resisted. Arising from the discussion paper was the Convention for Referral to Hospital Outpatients developed and proposed by David Williams who was concerned as always to make clear who at any one time was clinically responsible for the care of patients after referral to secondary care services. Basically it suggested that any referral to the out-patient department should state whether the patient was being referred for consultation only, for consultation and investigation, for specialist care, or for shared care. By this convention everyone would be quite clear which doctor was clinically responsible for treating and making decisions for the patient for that particular illness.

At that time there was a tendency for almost interminable follow-up at hospital outpatients. Once referred patients were often being seen every few months by a succession of very junior doctors who did not feel they had the authority or the experience to discharge the patient and so arranged a further follow-up in a few months by which time they themselves would have moved on. This was much more in some specialties than others and was justified by some consultants because of their perceived poor care by GPs. How the situation has changed over the last few years. In many surgical departments now, and also some other specialties, the patient is discharged back to primary care often before the stitches have been removed, and with no follow up arranged. Success rates cannot be accurately judged in such circumstances. Presumably a successful operation is one in which the patient is not referred back.

While it proved impossible to introduce the concept widely at that time, the idea of a formal shared care scheme has been more widely adopted recently particularly in the medical specialties such as diabetes. The clinical responsibility for individual patients is still often very unclear to this day.

While being a useful forum and meeting place for ideas the Association had no official status and by the late sixties the need for a more formal link into the UK and GMSC structure was felt to be necessary and moves were started to have a Welsh GMSC as a sub-committee of GMSC. Scotland had had its own SGMSC subcommittee for years but the political and health service arrangements were different there and there were different Regulations to negotiate.

In due course after considerable lobbying by BMA Wales and our London representatives, aided by friends from the so-called Celtic fringes with whom alliances were often developed, and with links which had been cultivated through Welsh Association meetings, GMSC agreed to set up a Welsh subcommittee with a limited remit to deal with matters pertaining to Wales. The first meeting was held in 1971 with Dr Bill Murray Jones as chairman.

After the formation of the WGMSC the Association continued to meet periodically with a wider membership for some years but by 1979 its role was considered to have been superseded and was disbanded. Within a few years it was felt by some of us that there was still a role for the Association and it was revived. In particular it was found that at times, and because WGMSC was a sub-committee of GMSC and its minutes and actions had to be approved by the parent committee, a useful way of action for general practice in Wales could be blocked by a wrecker in London or referred back for further consideration resulting in delay. Since England and Wales operated on an identical contract and terms of service obviously there was the sensible view that arrangements for practice within the UK or at least within England and Wales should be uniform, but at times relatively local solutions could be worked out without prejudicing this concept.

A somewhat similar bipolar arrangement was developed later between the WGMSC and the Advisory Sub-committee in General Practice of the Welsh Medical Committee. The membership of both was very similar, with one or two politically necessary variations, and with Miss Rosemary Roberts acting as secretary to both so they were able to meet as one group and discuss consultation documents and other matters together, although it must be said the way the minutes were written did at times vary depending where and to whom they were to be sent.

The Welsh Association continues to meet at least annually for a weekend Conference and at other times discussions are held either formally or informally between members as necessary. With the devolution of powers to the Welsh Assembly particularly in the Health and Social Services field opportunities to develop specifically Welsh answers to problems are possible. The Conference provides a wider opportunity to debate issues and formulate local policies than is possible during formal WGMSC meetings with long agendas, as well as allowing doctors from across Wales to meet each other.

Welsh General Medical Services Committee

Wales has always had two seats on GMSC (the General Medical Services Committee - the BMAs GPs committee) in London and in spite of the great difference in numbers of doctors in the two parts of Wales it has always been accepted that one should be from the South and one from the North. This has always been amicably arranged so that formal elections have not been necessary. On only one occasion do I recall that a third nomination was put up from South Wales, an attempt to change the local representative rather than to have two members from the South, and an election was necessary but the outcome was the same, most of the South Wales doctors honouring the tradition. There was also one seat on GMSC for a Welsh representative elected by the BMA ARM and this was for some years my personal route to the committee. There was for years no official Welsh GPs committee, and the absence had been covered by the Welsh Association of LMCs, whose history has been already detailed.

In 1970 Wales was given its own GMSC Wales (later re-named WGMSC) as a sub-committee of GMSC with limited powers and with all major decisions having to be ratified by the central committee. The treasurer in London kept a very watchful eye on any suggestions which might prove expensive. Dr G. (Bill) Murray Jones of Caerphilly was elected the founder chairman. This was at a time when devolution for Wales was on the political agenda for the first time and one of its early major tasks was to consider the discussion document and the health implications. In the end after a national referendum devolution did not happen at that time.

The secretariat for WGMSC was provided by BMA Wales, at first by Dr Maldwyn Cattell the BMA Welsh Secretary and later for many years in the capable hands of Miss Rosemary Roberts. She also looked after the Consultants and the Public Health Committees and so had an encyclopaedic knowledge of all that was going on medico-politically in Wales. She was invaluable to new chairmen finding their feet and referred to members as "her boys" and made sure they toed the line. She was ably assisted for some years by Kath Pope.

The start coincided with a major reorganisation of the NHS with its subsequent problems. In both 1974 and 1980 the administrative structure in Wales was undergoing one of its frequent reorganisations with the formation of new counties and the creation of new Health Authorities.

In addition the committee had to be active in the development of the new GP Vocational training structures. It produced the significant Reports discussed later, on Health Education, on Audit by Peer Review and on Prescribing Costs in Wales.

For a long time it had been recognised that Wales had a serious problem of chronic illness and social deprivation and, at the request of Dr Gareth Crompton, the Chief Medical Officer for Wales, the committee as one of its early actions set up a working party which I was pleased to chair on Economies and Priorities in the NHS. It highlighted potential areas for improvement, many of which have gradually and with much effort been achieved over the last twenty-five years.

Dr David Williams of Holywell, already a negotiator in London became chairman in 1975, followed in 1981 by Dr Bryan Davies, a jovial and well respected fixer GP from Maerdy in the Rhondda. Bryan Davies and John Lynch had seats on GMSC in London from the Welsh regional elections and David was there by election from the Annual Conference of LMCs. WGMSC did not initially have a seat on GMSC for its chairman as of right and to make sure the Welsh chairman was a member of GMSC required some initiative and organisation at times. It was not until 1985 that the Welsh chairman was granted an automatic seat at GMSC.

In February 1981, following on the sudden and tragic death of Dr Maldwyn Cattell, Rosemary Roberts acted up as Welsh Secretary for two years as well as continuing as committee secretary. She was followed briefly by Mr Roger Doherty.

Dr. Bryan Davies was appointed as BMA Welsh Secretary in 1984 and as a consequence I was elected Chairman of WGMSC sooner than expected. With the agreement of GMSC I was allowed to attend their meetings as an observer until I could be elected unopposed via the Welsh seat at the Annual Representative Meeting (the ARM) in July. I continued to attend the ARM each year in order to be re-elected until 1995 when I was ready to leave GMSC and when my seat was required for Dr Greg Graham from Pontypool. Greg has continued as a member there since then, in addition to his chairmanship of the Advisory sub-committee of the Welsh Medical Committee and a spell as chair of the Welsh Association. (In Wales one has to be prepared to wear several hats at the same time).

I must say that the ARM, while an integral and vital part of the BMA organisation, was for most of the time probably the least interesting body I attended over the years. The GP matters were usually cut and dried having been sorted out in previous fora but having to get the cachet of BMA approval, and the general subjects like smoking, public health matters and ethical motions which attracted the media attention were interesting only at times. Only occasionally did we get real fireworks.

The Welsh Association and WGMSC held a joint dinner in 1980 at the (as it turned out later, temporary) disbanding of the Association and at which Dr John Ball the newly elected chairman of GMSC was the chief guest. John always had a soft spot for Wales, he had a cottage and fishing rights near Dolgellau in mid-Wales. Over many years one of the highlights of our annual week-end conferences held at Llandrindod Wells was a "state of the nation" address by Dr. Norman Ellis, the BMA secretary to the GMSC where we were introduced to the inner thinking about the medico-political issues of the day.

At this time the first timid steps towards the introduction of audit were being taken and the First Annual Clinical Review Day organised by Dr Derek Llewelyn, the Regional Adviser in General Practice, and actively supported by WGMSC, was held at Llandrindod Wells in 1983. The history of audit in Wales is dealt with later.

WGMSC always aimed to be pro-active and in 1981 set up a working party on Health Education chaired by Dr Hubert Jones from Port Talbot, a significant pillar in Welsh medical politics whose talents were sadly lost by his early death. Hubert taught me a good lesson at the Welsh table at the Annual Conference dinner at the Park Lane Hotel, tip early rather than at the end. He slipped the waiter a fiver and the wine bottles kept arriving at our table.

Issues concerning the interface between hospitals, consultants and GP recurred regularly on agenda over the years and was part of the thinking behind the David Williams "Convention governing referral to outpatients" which he had first introduced at the Welsh Association in 1971. Its attempt to define clearly who had clinical responsibility for a patient at any one time was vitally important for both patients and doctors. It was a good example of the advantage of the Welsh Association over the WGMSC when it came to putting forward new ideas. Had it appeared on the agenda of the latter it would have appeared in the minutes, with the risk that it might be found unacceptable in GMSC in London, whereas from the Association it could be circulated around LMCs in Wales and used in local discussions and initiatives.

Over the years the WGMSC produced a number of working party reports which on re-reading now are still pertinent and had many of the suggestions been taken up the service to patients would have benefitted. By attaching these as appendices to the minutes and annual reports they received a wider circulation and were well received.

Prescribing for hospital outpatients was another regular agenda issue although the position had been made quite specific in government guidance in 1969, repeated in 1980 and again in 1987, that "there should be no attempt by health authorities to arrange that patients are referred to their general practitioner for prescribing, or that that the prescriptions (from the hospital) should not be for a lesser period than is needed to cover the time until the hospital doctor is likely to see the patient again - either for financial reasons or on the contention that a general practitioner has a continuing responsibility for all his patients". Quite specifically clear but management over the years have consistently failed to bring this to the attention of their doctors and to see that they adhered to the government guidelines. As a result patients have had to make unnecessary visits to their GP and he has had to provide an unnecessary consultation. From a purely legal standpoint unless the GP satisfied himself by seeing and examining the patient that the prescription was justified he could at some time in the future face a complaint of inadequate care, a note from a hospital doctor might not be sufficient. At one time if the prescription was dispensed at the hospital there was no prescription charge payable by the patient whereas if the prescription was taken to a pharmacy one was levied. GPs regularly over the years and to this day have brought this to attention but the position remains unchanged. The role and responsibilities of GPs and the legal constraints under which they work have never been understood by the secondary care services

Community Hospitals were another recurring issue with considerable dissatisfaction amongst GPs about the minimal level of payment for working in them and the contractual terms, although in fact few GPs could recall ever being given a contract. There was doubt as to which Complaints Procedure applied to GPs working in them and at times doctors were at double jeopardy from both the GP and hospital disciplinary procedures since it was usually the GP`s own registered patient who was also being cared for in a hospital bed. Unfortunately negotiations on community hospitals were the remit of the Consultant committees rather than GMSC and little progress could be made. By 1984 we had clarified with Welsh Office that GPs would not be dealt with under the hospital procedures.

A major discussion issue following a working group in 1980 was that of the underprivileged areas in the South Wales valleys and which was later expanded at GMSC level to include other so-called deprived areas, mainly urban. This is discussed at length in a later chapter.

Welsh Office were over the years active in producing a series of policies and strategies about health issues, especially on health improvements and prevention, on Health Gain areas, and on setting targets. Targets are not new and the contents are still much the same. What is new is that targets now have a much tighter time-scale and there are more penalties for not achieving them. All these required detailed responses from WGMSC.

One of the major frustrations in trying to develop services within general practice has been that arrangements and agreements arrived at in one area after hours of discussion between doctors and managers and after much referring back were not accepted by other health authorities with similar issues to resolve, also that at local levels agreed arrangements were sometimes later unilaterally withdrawn without discussion or even warning.

Membership of WGMSC also meant the need to represent it on other

Welsh committees and working groups. I spent many very interesting years on the Sub-committee for General Practice of the Standing Committee for Welsh Postgraduate Education, dealing with both vocational training and continuing education for established doctors as discussed elsewhere and where it was often difficult to defend the pragmatic GMSC view against the might of the academics and RCGP members.

Welsh GMSC also had representation on the Welsh Medical Committee, the statutory advisory committee to the Secretary of State, and I spent some eight very interesting years on this. Here again GPs were in a minority amongst the academics from the Medical School and representatives of the other branches of the profession, but we did manage to make substantial contributions. It was from this committee that the working party on Community hospitals, discussed later, was set up

In 1988 I was succeeded as chairman by Dr Bryn John from Neath, one of the up and coming younger generation and who was instantly recognisable by his completely bald pate, long before such were fashionable. Bryn has since gone on to involvement in many spheres in Wales including chairmanship of BMA Welsh Council and became the first GP to chair the Welsh Medical Committee. He was honoured by the award by the BMA of the Associations Medal at the ARM in 2005.

Bryn was succeeded in 1993 by Dr. Owen P. Jones a GP from Llanberis in Gwynedd, known to all as O.P., ex-army and a different character altogether and he in turn in 1997 by Dr. Tony Calland from Gwent who has subsequently gone on to become a successful chairman of BMA Welsh Council and a negotiator at GMSC. He has recently taken the chair of the very important and high profile position of Chairman of the BMA Ethics Committee. Part of his practice extended over the border into England and this did not always go down well with some of the South Wales representatives

Dr Gruff Jones from Holywell would normally have become the next chairman but by this time and following on from devolution the requirements on the chairman made it difficult for anyone from the north to carry them out (in addition to London GPC and local LMC commitments) and Dr Andrew Dearden from Cardiff took over in 1999 and remains in the chair at present. Other North Wales LMC members who have become prominent in the last few years are Dr Jay Nankani who as Chairman of the GP Forum of the International Doctors Association has a seat on GPC in London and as a consequence is also on Welsh WPC., and Dr Jonathan Jones.

The General Medical Services Committee

The GMSC, or to give its full title the General Medical Services Committee (more recently renamed as the General Practitioners Committee or GPC), is the premier GP committee and is responsible for negotiating on all GP matters. Its counterpoint for consultant affairs is the Central Consultants ands Specialists Committee (CCSC).

While both operate within a BMA structure neither are strictly BMA subcommittees and both have a degree of autonomy. In particular and very importantly it is not necessary for all members to be members of the BMA, although most are, and as such it is recognised by Government as representing all GPs within the NHS. Within its membership of some sixty members it has representatives of the smaller Medical Practitioners Union (the MPU) admitted in 1951 at the time of one of the early crises in the new NHS, the hospital specialists, dentists, and doctors in training grades and of the Postgraduate Deans. It also has cross-representation from the RCGP and this has become increasingly important over recent years. It meets on the first Thursday of every month and this day takes precedence over everything else in the calendar, meetings lasting from 10.00am until often 6.00pm., a marathon for any chairman.

For North Wales members this either meant an evening train and an overnight stay on Wednesday night or a 6.0am start for myself from Colwyn Bay station and a dash from Euston where I arrived at 10.01a.m so that I missed only the first few minutes of the meeting. Luckily BMA House in Tavistock Square is only some 300 yards from Euston. Arriving at the meeting on time was very important as the first major agenda item was the Chairman's report on events and negotiations since the last meeting, followed by members questions to the chair, often very searching, and the whole lasting an hour or more. A full formal agenda followed for the rest of the day. Immediately after lunch was the time for chairmen to present sub-committee minutes for debate and ratification. As chairman of the Education sub-committee an early lesson learnt from my predecessor's mistakes and discomfort was to make sure the minutes were written carefully and words scrutinised and made clear. If there was any confusion it gave the opportunity for wreckers to refer the matter back for further discussion and clarification, quoting the Dr. John Marks` aphorism "Words mean what words say", and resulting in considerable delay as subcommittees usually met only twice or at most three times a year.

Proceedings were always formal with speakers who wished to speak in a debate putting in speaker slips. This in itself was a bit of a lottery, time constraints sometimes meant one did not always have a chance to speak but also one never knew at which stage of the debate one would be called. On occasion if one wanted only to make an observation on a matter of detail one might be called very early in the debate before the major points had been aired, leaving one feeling slightly stupid. Speakers were only allowed three minutes and a system of green, amber and red lights indicated two minutes and then time up. At which time the speaker had to finish a sentence and sit down,unless the committee felt and agreed that more time should be allowed him or her to complete a point. Being a less than confident public speaker with a quiet voice I never felt too happy at speaking at the main committee and always felt my best work was done in the sub-committees and working groups.

The majority of members tended to stay on GMSC for many years and this was in fact essential to build up a personal expertise and a herd memory of what had gone before. Also the time commitment was such that practices had to make special arrangements to cover absences, sometimes involving taking on a further partner or additional appointments locally, which could not easily be switched on and off. In my case I was lucky to be able to take a 24-hour retirement at age sixty and work part-time in the practice for the last four years when I was most involved centrally.

I arrived at GMSC suddenly and unexpectedly in 1984. As previously described, as a result of the sudden death of Dr. Maldwyn Catell, the well respected BMA Welsh Secretary, Dr Bryan Davies was appointed the new Welsh Secretary in February 1984 and had to resign from GMSC, leaving me as WGMSC-chairman co-opted to take his place.

Initially I found GMSC quite intimidating even though I knew many of the members from their visits to Wales and from the Conference of LMCs. Agendas were long and complex and it was necessary to read the papers carefully beforehand as well as being aware of what had gone on previously. While the whole atmosphere of the GMSC was friendly and cooperative there were a number of cliques, wreckers and spoilers and it was necessary to know who one's friends were and to have allies to rescue you if ambushed. I was on GMSC for ten years in all, on top of my WGMSC experience, and at the end still felt somewhat unsure at times

My personal contribution, apart from overseeing Welsh interests, was in the field of education and I enjoyed chairing the sub-committee for three years and being involved in the very early discussions on the re-accreditation of doctors, or revalidation as it was first referred to. As discussed in detail later I continued my interest in vocational training and became a member and later chairman of the JCPTGP

The major players were the negotiators, the chairman and four others elected by the committee annually but who tended to remain in office for some years. The commitment was huge, at least two days a week in London and often one or two other whole or part-days as well, together with travel to all parts of the UK to address local committees and rank-and-file GPs, especially at times of crisis and difficult negotiations. The profession owes a great debt to all those who undertake the very onerous job of negotiators, and to their families for their support.

North Wales has contributed its share in the negotiating arena and in recent years both David Williams and John Lynch served as negotiators and as vice-chairmen for a number of years. David would probably have become GMSC chairman but the extent of the commitment at one stage was too much for the well-being of his practice and he had to resign in 1982 in order to attend to a problem in the practice and to tactfully ease a partner out, returning to the committee in 1985 until his retirement in 1989.

In the last few years two South Wales GPs, Tony Calland and Andrew Dearden, have played active parts as negotiators in London and in Cardiff. Over the years negotiators have frequently come under fire for not achieving all the profession had demanded but negotiating has been defined as "the art of the possible and the achievable" while at the same time laying down markers for the future.

David on one journey home related his account of one particular negotiating session with senior civil servants. There was one point which GMSC did not expect to achieve but when this was reached the other side conceded immediately. In private discussion afterwards seeking the reason for the capitulation the civil servants said " We owed you one because on a previous occasion when we had made an error and were in trouble with the Minister you got us off the hook". In such ways are battles won.

In 1990 just after the new contract was introduced John Lynch stood for the chairmanship and was expected to take over but was felt by some members to have been too closely associated with the ideas and policies of the outgoing chairman Michael Wilson and in the vote lost out to Ian Bogle from Liverpool. One of the pitfalls for any chairman was that there were usually at least two ex-chairmen still sitting on the committee and ready to throw a spanner in, not unlike the position of new Prime Ministers.

Apart from responding to various consultation papers and initiatives GMSC produced two very important documents during my time. The first was" General Practice- A British Success", written because of a feeling that the contribution of general practice over the years was not fully appreciated and to set out its achievements as an additional negotiating tool.

The second, "Defining Core Services in general practice - Reclaiming professional control" in 1996 and the follow-up "Core Services - Taking the Initiative" was an attempt to define what the basic or core services which GPs should provide were and more importantly what services GPs were not expected to undertake without special local negotiation. It was becoming increasingly necessary because work was being dumped back to GPs from hospitals and other clinics without any consultation, communication or additional resources. Much of this was at a local hospital level making it difficult for individual doctors to say no without some official backing. Guidance from the LMCs was being ignored.

Although one only saw some members once a month a considerable club atmosphere developed. Like all clubs it had to have a club tie, and true to tradition some years ago and before my time a working party was set up to design one. The tie consisted of a plain maroon or plain navy tie with a single motif of a two-headed cockerel with twisted neck balancing on a weathervane. It was a tie which when worn caused many people to ask what it was, and perhaps a full description from the tongue-in-cheek working party report is appropriate.

The Club tie. This design presents the cock of Aesculapius in a novel form, for in Aesculapius` day cockerels only had one head. The two heads of the bird presently displayed (regardant sinister and dexter) symbolise by the convolutions of their respective necks the complexity of the issues with which the committee is frequently faced - or alternatively, the complexity which the Committee will frequently introduce into consideration of a subject of relative simplicity. This bird speaking in two directions simultaneously manifests another of the features of the Committees activity - a constant desire to obtain the best of both worlds ; perhaps the most notable example of which is repeatedly crowing about the unique status of independent contractors, whilst at the same time seeking to obtain from the Health Departments as many as possible of the advantages of the salaried employee. To preserve poise in such circumstances is a rare feat and this is symbolised by the bird perched in the form of a weather vane on its point of vantage. The compass points which bear the initials of the Committee symbolise also the ability to maintain this posture despite all blasts of opinion from whatever point of the compass they may originate. In other words the GMSC stands four-square and firm despite the varied assaults of administrators, politicians, public and sometimes of other sections of the medical profession. At the same time the bird reserves the right, at any time, to be synchronously both revolutionary and stationary, without prejudice.

Meetings were held at headquarters at BMA House, Tavistock Square, an impressive building designed by Edwin Lutyens but which has no residential accommodation. A number of us if we were in London overnight would stay at the Royal Society of Medicine (the RSM) at No.1 Wimpole Street, just off Oxford Street. It gave an opportunity to see and mix with doctors from other specialties staying there. It also gave an opportunity to walk over together to BMA House, perhaps discuss items from the agenda, and at the same time get a breath of fresh air and clear one's head before the all-day meeting. If I was down in London in time, which did not often happen as I often travelled after evening surgery, there was the opportunity to meet up with some of the Scottish contingent, usually at a small restaurant near the British Museum, officially El Castelletto but later dubbed El Cost-a-lotto

John Lynch who was in London far more frequently at one time used to catch trains from either Crewe or Runcorn to give more choice but over the years lost three cars stolen from the station car-parks and gave up.

It was at the RSM that a major tragedy occurred when John who had failed to arrive at the meeting was found in his room having suffered a major stroke during the night. He was admitted to University College Hospital near to BMA House and all day the committee in a sense of shock and distress heard regular bulletins on his condition. Thankfully he survived but with a major speech impediment which was a great loss to John who was a great talker and debater. He has battled bravely and actively with his disability ever since. His loss to medical politics at GMSC and in Wales has been immense.

All in all my time on GMSC was a very stimulating and a happy period of ten years and one which in spite of its huge commitment I would hate to have missed.

The Welsh Medical Committee

The Welsh Medical Committee (WMC) is arguably the most important and influential medical committee within Wales and has a remit to advise the Secretary of State on all matters medical. It has a very powerful membership made up of representatives from academia, the Medical School and the Postgraduate Departments, assorted Professors, from the Consultants, General Practitioner and Public Health Medicine Welsh committees, together with representation from those in training grades. Additionally it has representation from each of the District Medical Committees. The Chief Medical Officer, his (or later her) deputy and usually another assistant are in attendance to hear the discussion and give any necessary guidance on current thinking both in Wales and of his counterparts in the UK. Altogether a very daunting arena to enter and one where one needed to take time to find one's feet and understand some of the internal politics of the South Wales scene and the rivalry between Cardiff and Swansea before becoming too vociferous. I became a member representing WGMSC in 1980 and in all spent some ten years on WMC.

The Chief Medical Officer at the time was Dr Gareth Crompton, with whom I had worked as a member of Gwynedd Area Medical Committee in the mid-seventies which was a help, while his deputy Dr Deirdre Hine, who later returned as the CMO, has recently completed her year as President of the BMA.

The chairman was Dr Lyn Rees with David Williams as deputy chairman. It was unfortunate that David, because of his negotiating commitments in London, was unable to take the chair in due course and become the first GP chairman of WMC. Several years later Dr. Harry Edwards, an anaesthetist from Bangor was elected chairman and I was in line in seniority amongst the GP members to become vice-chairman but this would have meant two officers from North Wales at the same time which was not very practical. Additionally since the chairman normally stayed for four years his deputy would require to be there for at least eight years to complete his time in the chair and I was unlikely to be there that long. Another WGMSC member, Dr Bryn John from Neath, was elected and in time became the first GP chairman, a position which he carried out with considerable success.

When Bryn completed his term the chair was taken by another member from North Wales, Mr David Thomas, the Obstetrician from Ysbyty Glan Clwyd, and subsequently Dr Jane Wood, the geriatrician from Glan Clwyd took over. The time commitment from North Wales is huge, with the need to meet up both formally and informally with those in the Welsh Office and others from many different spheres, and has increased immensely since devolution of responsibility for health to the Assembly.

Welsh Medical Committee had a number of advisory subcommittees including one for general practice. The membership of the sub-committee proved to be little different from that of WGMSC, with one or two additions, and since both committees often had very similar agendas and discussed the same consultation documents it was decided to hold meetings in tandem although the minutes would be written differently depending on where they were to be presented.

One of the major issues at the time was that of community hospitals, one which still remains unresolved because of differing approaches and different concepts across Wales. Guidance was sought by Welsh Office from WMC which decided to set up a multi- specialty working group to produce a report and I was asked to chair this. The other members were Dr. Sandy Cavenagh from the Brecon practice who had long experience in the Community Hospitals Association of UK, Dr. Gareth Hughes, consultant geriatrician from Aberystwyth, Mr Aled Williams consultant obstetrician from Wrexham, and Dr Alan Spence, a community physician from Powys. We spent a year holding our meetings in a number of community hospitals across Wales and were able to reach a consensus and produce a report without any difficulty. However presentation of the report to the committee ran into difficulties and controversy because of one feature. Amongst over a hundred recommendations we had mentioned that occasionally a child might be admitted into a community hospital, perhaps because he or she needed observation for say a bout of asthma which could not be conveniently done in an isolated home miles out in the country. This really upset the paediatricians who rolled out the big guns to block the report and as a result it was never formally adopted for presentation to the Secretary of State. Apart from this single aspect the report was very received and copies of it were requested from many quarters including from England, to such an extent that several reprint runs had to be made informally within the Welsh Office. The lesson I learned from this was that one needs to be very careful in drafting and that anything likely to be controversial needs to be played down or omitted so as not to lose everything.

By the mid nineties District Medical Committees which were the only place where consultant and general practitioner representatives met formally and whose representatives into the Welsh Medical Committee were a vital part of the input from those working on the ground in the Districts, were functioning less than effectively in many Districts, largely because the Health Authorities either were not consulting them or were consulting too late and ignoring advice given to them. Doctors felt they were wasting their time and some committees had ceased to meet. Dr Deirdre Hine who by this time had returned to Welsh Office as Chief Medical Officer after a very successful launch of the Breast Test Wales screening programme made considerable efforts to revive them. The

North Wales DMC which survived longer than most went into limbo with the demise of the Health Authority and the setting up of Local Health Boards in 1996 but has been resurrected in 2005. With the replacement of one Authority by six Boards (LHBs) in North Wales there is a need for a group with a wide geographical remit and a place where consultants and general practitioners meet to discuss policies. The Assembly government have now accepted the need for such a representative committee structure and this is in process of being set up. Only time will tell how effectively they operate this time.

The Medical Practices Committee

Before and in the early days of the Health Service there was considerable inequality in the distribution of general practitioners around Britain with many doctors obviously favouring the more affluent areas in the south and the leafy shires. At this time the majority of practices were single-handed or with at most two or three partners. Pre-NHS a free-market mechanism was the usual way practices changed hands but when it became unlawful to sell the goodwill of the practice the situation changed

Aiming to ensure a more even distribution a Medical Practices Committee (the MPC) was set up as a statutory committee under the NHS Act 1946. The profession opposed the arrangement initially and the early medical members, who themselves had been against it, had a difficult time relating to their colleagues.

The MPC consisted of a chairman and eight members, the chairman was until the last years always a GP, there were six other GP members and two lay members, usually one was a lawyer.

Members were appointed by the Minister after nomination by GMSC who attempted to get reasonable representation from all parts of the UK except Scotland which had its own MPC. In 1984 there was a move from the Annual Conference to have members elected on a regional basis. GMSC set up a working group chaired by Dr David Pickersgill of Norfolk and on which I represented Wales to review the working of the MPC and to consider regional elections. It was noted that no other members within the European Community (as it then was) had any geographical controls relating to establishment in general practice. The working group rejected the call for regional elections but produced a number of constructive suggestions for improved arrangements centrally and at the local vacancy committees.

There was always a representative from Wales on the MPC and the profession owes a great debt to those who served so diligently. The amount of work for many years, particularly in the early years when there were many more single handed practices to decide upon was vast and occupied Wednesday and Thursday every week throughout the year. There was a massive amount of reading matter to study with each application. From North Wales Dr Graham Williams from Holyhead used to travel down to London every week on the Tuesday night sleeper and return on the Thursday evening. For his successor Dr Gilbert Clark from Porthcawl in South Wales the night train was unnecessary as one could travel to London in the morning, albeit with a very early start. Dr John Griffiths from Brynsiencyn took on the onerous task in 1994 and served until 2000 when he was followed by Dr Greg Graham from Pontypool.

For many years after the start of the Health Service in 1948 the MPC busied themselves trying to even out the distribution of doctors across the UK, taking all factors into account. The MPC set criteria about list sizes, with appropriate variation for rurality and other factors, against which applications to enter or set up a practice were judged. Areas were classified as Open where any doctor could set up a plate and start a practice, Intermediate where the approval of the MPC had to be given, and Closed or Restricted areas where no additional doctors were allowed to move in.

Special criteria were necessary for parts of Scotland because of remoteness and the islands of the Hebrides. On occasion a practice might have only a few hundred patients with these scattered over several islands and the concept of Inducement practices was introduced with special funding arrangements. These doctors had on occasion to deal with emergencies far beyond the scope of GPs elsewhere. Hospital admissions and even outpatient appointments were difficult, but access has been much improved in recent years by the use of helicopters. While some parts of Wales appear isolated and remote, nowhere is more than two hours by road from a District General Hospital and nowhere is comparable with the smaller Scottish islands.

In the early days of the NHS there were a large number of small single handed practices but the number has decreased markedly over the years as most doctors found it more convenient to work in partnerships. Some doctors were single-handed because they preferred to work that way, others were by force of geographical circumstances. I particularly remember Dr Beresford who for years provided services for the whole of the Ceiriog valley with no-one to cover time off. In spite of this he managed to be a prominent personality in the LMC and the BMA.

All appointments to single handed practice appointment were the responsibility of the MPC who after checking with the Executive Council (who were required to consult with the LMC) that the list sizes in that particular area justified a replacement confirmed that a vacancy existed and could be advertised. The actual appointment interviews were carried out locally by the Executive Council (later the Family Practitioners Committee and later still the Family Health Services Committee). After the local selection had taken place the MPC approved the decision unless an appeal had been made, in which case it reviewed the decision and allowed or rejected the appeal. With partnership vacancies the MPC would decide whether a replacement partner could be appointed but the selection of the partner was left to the practice with the appointment subsequently ratified by the MPC.

The appeal procedure tended to take some weeks. Sometimes if the vacancy was as a result of sudden death or if the outgoing practitioner did not wish to stay on until a successor was appointed there was a lengthy interim period when the practice had to be run by the Executive Council with a locum or locums. Many of the appeals had no justifiable basis and were sometimes malicious.

I was personally involved in such a situation. In 1959 I had applied for a single handed vacancy in Benllech on Anglesey which attracted a number of applicants and after due process the practice was given to an older doctor from Darwen in Lancashire, a non-Welsh speaker. This created a major outcry by local residents as the island was still very Welsh-speaking at that time and a further hearing was held in London. I must admit I was not a strong candidate, young, unmarried and with only thirteen months of practice experience, twelve months of which were as a trainee, but I was a Welsh-speaker. One other applicant was another Welsh-speaker, Dr W. Parry-Jones from Llangefni six miles away, who proposed to join the practice with his existing one, and bring in his son Owen, a school contemporary of mine in Llangefni, and who was doing National Service at the time. His application was successful and the arrangement subsequently worked well.

It was generally the case that when a doctor retired at least ten per cent of the list moved on to another practice and if there was a long delay this percentage was considerably higher, sometimes leaving the incoming doctor with an uneconomic list size. Reasons for change of doctor included loyalty to outgoing doctor until his or her retirement, families who had moved out of practice area but remained registered with their known doctor until some crisis arrived which necessitated immediate change to a local doctor, both partners in a relationship wishing to be with the same doctor, and joining a new practice more convenient to their home or work.

Another major factor distorting list sizes in the earlier years were "ghost " patients, still registered at the practice but who had either died, gone abroad, duplicated names particularly in ethnic areas, or registered with another GP elsewhere but the administrative systems had been inadequate to keep track in all cases. As the admistration in the FPC improved with computerisation then the number of ghosts dropped considerably, although they were still much more active in some areas than others. Having many ghost patients in an Executive Council area did as a consequence lead to a diminution in the average cost of prescribing. At one count Gwynedd had less than 1% of ghosts while some urban areas with high mobility in their populations had more than 30%

With more and more women entering general practice and wishing to work part-time, and with other doctors becoming so involved in representative work on various bodies locally and nationally, the MPC were frequently asked for an extra half-time partner. In later years the new concept of job-share doctors developed, two doctors agreeing to work as equivalent to a full-time doctor and sharing responsibility for the work between themselves. Now it is not only women doctors who wish to job share, sometimes it is a husband and wife partnership, at others it may be a male doctor who wishes to pursue another interest either within or outside the health service.

At one stage there was a move driven by Clwyd FPC to ask for a separate Welsh MPC but by this time the workload had diminished to a significant degree. A Welsh meeting each week could not be justified and meeting less frequently would have resulted in delay and inconvenience to doctors so the suggestion was resisted. However since devolution Welsh practice vacancies and applications to modify doctor's contractual hours have been dealt with by a Welsh Medical Vacancies Committee. Following on from the new contract introduced in 2004 where the contract is now between the Local Health Board and the practice rather than with individual doctors perhaps no central arrangements are necessary.

Back in 1971 Dr Julian Tudor Hart who was working in a dead-end valley at Glyncorrwg in one of the most deprived areas in South Wales, and remembering that most people knew of Isaac Newton's Inverse Square Law even if few remembered what it said, had formulated his Inverse Care Law which set out the position in our society that communities in the most need of good care were the least likely to get it, and where civilisation was subordinated to the market economy. Regrettably in spite of lofty aims and various government initiatives over the years the situation remains true in many areas today. A more positive view has recently been named the Positive Care Law which states that unqualified people and informal carers provide unpaid care to their relatives and friends and their communities which is almost completely appropriate to needs.

While in the early years some success in redistribution of doctors was achieved by the MPC, by the seventies progress had virtually ceased and recent publications suggest that by 2003 the mal-distribution was worse than in 1974.

The Medical Practices Committee has now been disbanded but whether the politicians who decide such matters were aware of this or whether the decision was based on political dogma is debatable.

Pay disputes and resignation issues

Unhappiness about remuneration within the NHS, and indeed before then for GPs during the Insurance Act days, has surfaced regularly, and has been a source of considerable stress and dispute right from the start.

Doctors were very disillusioned by the way the NHS had turned out in regard to their conditions of work and their pay, both in the amount and in the way the global sum was divided up. As far back as 1949 doctors were very dissatisfied with their financial position and general practitioners complained that their status had fallen compared with their hospital colleagues and with other professions. On occasions because of intransigence on the part of governments and their failure to respond to what were perceived as legitimate fears this dissatisfaction has reached fever point. Calls for resignation of GPs en masse from the NHS have arisen and on occasion have gone far down the line.

It is interesting to note that awarded pay rises have been held back on many occasions "in the interests of the national economy", the first time way back in 1918 and again in 1941, both because of wartime, and later Review Body awards were fairly regularly deferred or phased in, causing recurring disputes with the government of the day. In 1950 it was resolved that preparations for general practitioners to terminate their contracts should be made and this was to go to a Special Conference of GPs in March 1951. By then however Aneurin Bevan, the Minister for Health who had introduced the Health Service, had resigned and his successor agreed there was a case for review. Progress was slow and arrangements were made to collect resignations unless arbitration was agreed to. This pressure resulted in the Mr Justice Dankwerts Review which after a hearing lasting only three days was very favourable and led to a substantial betterment factor of 100% for 1952.

Problems continued and further unsuccessful negotiations in 1956 with the then Minister of Health, Mr Vosper, led in early 1957 to him announcing that a Royal Commission would be set up under Sir Harry Pilkington to "consider the remuneration of the Medical and Dental professions".

The second significant major development at the same time was the setting up of a Joint Working Party chaired by a senior civil servant, Sir Bruce Fraser, "to consider the report and recommendations of the Annis Gillie Committee, together with any other matters relevant to the work of the general practitioner in the National Health Service".

On the day following the announcement of the Royal Commission the GMSC (the GP central committee) decided not to co-operate with it and to recommend that general practitioners be advised to tender their resignations. Over the following weeks and after meetings and heated discussions around the country the GMSC chairman Dr Talbot Rogers expressed his personal view that they should agree to cooperate. Following on from a special meeting of the GMSC which showed a serious difference of opinion between the chairman and his committee Dr Rogers resigned and Dr A.B Davies was elected to the chair. A Special Conference was called. On the very morning of the Conference Dr Solomon Wand, the respected former and first chairman of GMSC and at the time the Chairman of BMA Council, shook GMSC by advising that because of assurances given to him by Sir Harry Pilkington he now supported co-operation with the Commission. In a close vote by twenty-four votes to twenty-two GMSC agreed to recommend cooperation to the Conference that day. Representatives who had arrived at the conference mandated to support non-cooperation were stunned and after a noisy debate refused to approve the change in tactics and deferred consideration to another conference the following month, at which after further heated debates in LMCs around the country they agreed to cooperation.

Payment for general practitioners within the NHS was on the basis of a capitation fee for each registered patient out of which all practice expenses were to be met. The infamous "pool" system was in operation. Briefly this meant that there was a global sum or pool of remuneration fixed for the following year and calculated from the total number of GPs working in the NHS, together with the total sum of their allowable expenses retrospectively agreed by the inland revenue. This "pool" was subsequently divided into capitation fees for each patient and fees for certain other services such as immunisation. Since the total number of doctors, and of items of service carried out and the practice expenses from Inland Revenue returns could not be known for some time a sum on account was paid with a balancing amount two years later.When the total figure was eventually known and since the Pool was a pre-ordained fixed amount there was usually either an under or an overpayment which then had to be clawed back the following year. On one particular year, largely because of the poliomyelitis epidemic and massive immunisation programme by GPs with the newly available vaccine, there was a large overpayment and the fees for the following year were reduced to bring the total into the Pool calculated figure. This created massive disquiet and unrest and a demand for change.

An excellent letter to the Editor of the Sunday Tmes in February 1965 set out how a similar system would work if applied to MPs.

It was into this atmosphere in the early sixties that I came into medical politics for the first time through the Denbighshire and Flintshire Local Medical Committee.

The Royal Commission reported in early 1960 with a reasonable increase for GPs, and with new proposals for merit awards for GPs and for the establishment of a Standing Review Body to consider future professional remuneration for doctors and dentists. Government and Conference accepted the "package deal "but only on the understanding that separate discussion should take place on differential payments, or as they were labelled merit awards.

The Review Body in its first Report in February 1963 recommended a 14% increase in medical and dental remuneration which was acceptable to the hospital staff but because of the way it was calculated many GPs received far less than they expected, leading to much bitterness. Since there was at the time the further issue of the considerable differential between the earnings of GPs and of consultants and of the existing consultant merit awards the Review Body offer of differential payments within the GP pay structure only aggravated feelings.

The ARM in Oxford in 1963, the first one I attended as a representative of the Wrexham BMA Division, agreed "That the Representative Body instructs Council to ensure that discussions between the GMSC and the Joint Consultants Committee proceed with the greatest possible speed so that the differential between the remuneration of general practitioners and consultants be placed before the Review Body for its consideration".

The perceived differential between the pay (and as a result the pensions) of GPs and consultants has been one of the main points of friction between the two crafts over the years and has usually been in the consultants` favour. Consultant pensions have been related to their final salary whereas GP pensions have been based on their earnings in each year and added up over forty years. This might have been acceptable in times of low or nil inflation but proved to be very unsatisfactory when inflation took off. After considerable negotiation by the BMA Superannuation Committee a new dynamising factor was introduced Every year a factor would be agreed by which a GPs income in each particular year would be brought up to present day equivalent before being used to calculate the pension and this has proved acceptable.

A major medico-political crisis arose over this GP/consultant pay differential. Evidence to the Review Body was always presented by a BMA delegation consisting of an equal number of GP and consultant members and the evidence it gave was not allowed to be published. The GMSC planning committee produced a claim for an increase in pay on two issues, the basic case and the differential, but the full committee removed a large chunk of it because it might alienate the consultants, and the draft was then further amended by the consultants committees. The GMSC chairman, Dr A.B.Davies, suggested in the December 1963 Council meeting, without the full authority of his committee, that the differences were so narrow that they could be amended by a small group of officers. Council also agreed that an extra general practitioner should be appointed to the evidence committee. After a vote Dr Ivor Jones, an activist from the North-east of England with a lot of support in the country failed to be elected. The following GMSC meeting in January 1964 heard that the Review Body had agreed to consider the case for a pay increase, to accept the extra general practitioner on the evidence committee, and to allow the profession's evidence to be published. This last was a significant development as it allowed the rank and file doctors to see exactly what was being put forward on their behalf. (It was many years later when the government finally agreed that its` evidence would also be made available). The Review Body significantly asked the government to obtain statistics about the career earnings of general practitioners and hospital doctors, supporting those who had argued that they were relevant to the arguments.

A Special Conference in March insisted that additional evidence be included to show that recruitment to practice had been adversely affected by the poor financial prospects including poor pensions, and that paragraphs from the Porritt Report and the Annis Gillie Report referring to the difference in career earnings be included in the evidence. Late in the day Conference rejected a motion of no confidence in the delegation to meet the Review Body, but after a challenge to his ruling, the chairman allowed a debate on the motion "that Dr Ivor Jones be asked to be a member of the deputation to the Review Body" and this was carried, although there is doubt as to whether a quorum was present at the time.

Dr A.B Davies took this as a vote of no confidence in the GMSC and of himself as chairman and resigned from the chair and the committee, together with his deputy chairmanship of the Representative Body. Two GMSC chairman lost in seven years, unprecedented although none have felt the need to resign since then. At the following GMSC meeting with the Chairman of the BMA Representative Body Dr Ronald Gibson in the chair discussion took place as to whether the whole committee should accept responsibility and resign along with Dr Davies. After arguments both ways the motion was withdrawn and Dr J.C.(Jim) Cameron was elected chairman. A Special Representative Meeting held in March rejected a motion "that this Association has no confidence in the General Medical Services Committee " and it also agreed that Dr. Ivor Jones accompany the joint Evidence Committee.

All the inter-craft and constitutional differences highlighted over the approach to the Review Body resulted in a motion to the Annual Conference suggesting "that the GMSC should be completely autonomous and answerable only to Conference". It was defeated, as was another that the GMSC should have the right of direct access to the Review Body. The Annual Conference resolved that general practitioner earnings "should be assessed solely in relation to general medical services provided to patients on their lists."

In the 60's and early 70's the BMA negotiation machinery was frequently in dispute with government and on occasions called for all GPs to submit to them undated resignation forms. So unhappy were GPs and so effective was the organisation that in 1965 over 90% of GPs, myself included, sent in their forms (a total of 17,800 resignations were sent in to the Guild). In a previous resignation crisis as far back as 1922 over 94% of the panel doctors submitted their undated resignations of withdrawal threats have always had to be considered seriously. The result of this brinkmanship was an early resolution of many of the problems within a new contract in 1966.

Withdrawal from the NHS would have meant direct patient contributions to the cost of care and treatment including drugs, and very often the cost of the drugs might far outstrip the cost of consultations. Details of a private GP insurance scheme run by doctors were developed and costed with Dr Ivor Jones amongst the proposers and was very seriously considered by the profession. In the early years there were still many doctors who had had pre-NHS practical experience of book-keeping and fee collection, and many patients who had experienced this. As years went by these doctors left practice and younger doctors were much less happy dealing with cash payments. Indeed many doctors still feel embarrassed to ask for fees which they can legitimately claim from the patient for services outside the NHS and often the patient will be told to see the receptionist to make payment. A further factor was that the drugs available were becoming more numerous and effective, but out of the range of patients in poorer areas. Doctors working a private system would possibly be faced with having to consider using older or less effective drugs which the patient might be able to afford rather than the best available option.

An illustration of this drug cost problem arose in my early years. In the more affluent area of Colwyn Bay (as in many other areas around the country) there had developed out of the pre-NHS private patients what were known as "semi-private" patients who paid for the convenience of often unnecessary visits or consultations but had their drugs prescribed under the NHS. Strictly illegal of course and this provided considerable ethical, moral and practical problems with senior partners for us younger doctors joining practices where this arrangement went on. On arrival at the home of some of these patients the silver tea service ritually appeared and much social chit-chat took place before perhaps a chest was listened to or a blood pressure taken.

The initially very effective sanction of threatened resignation gradually became a less effective weapon as fewer and fewer doctors had any experience in working in a private pre-NHS system, and as more and more became tied into expensive premises then the risks of resignation and the fervour for it and a return to some sort of private service diminished.

The existence of a Review Body and the considerably improved communication and negotiating channels between the profession and government has meant that things have never quite reached the same point again, although sticking points and phasing of awards by government have led to much tub-thumping with calls for resignation. Certainly resignation from the NHS en masse has not been seriously contemplated in recent years

Later a less drastic but probably very effective sanction was proposed, namely refusal to issue medical certificates of incapacity, which would have caused administrative chaos without unduly harming patients. The issues surrounding certification will be considered later.

Part of the pay award in 1960 was the offer of an additional £500,000 a year for the introduction of differential payments in recognition of distinguished general practice (the so-called Merit awards) which led to much controversy. The concept of payments for quality (which was not defined) was unacceptable to many doctors as they had seen the problems and disquiet that similar merit awards made in secret had given rise to within the hospital consultant body. The consultant awards of graded A+ to C additional, substantial and secret payments were introduced at the beginning of the NHS and were considered by many to be the way in which the consultants in the Royal Colleges were bought into acceptance of the proposals against the opposition of the BMA. Nye Bevan was reported as saying he "had stuffed their mouths with silver". These consultant merit awards continue in existence although much of the secrecy surrounding them has been reduced and there is now greater local input.

Following on the report of the Review Body the Conference passed a motion by a large majority "that this conference opposes the introduction of merit awards for general practitioners". The following year it voted by 106 votes to 100 that "conference accepts the principle of differential payments in remuneration of general practitioners" but only as a reference to the GMSC. A working party report was submitted without comment to the next Conference, which passed the motion "that this conference rejects the principle of differential payments" by 99 votes to 70.

GMSC and the College had a major difference of opinion on special payments or merit awards. The College were keen to introduce payments recognising quality whereas GMSC were very aware of the problems perceived in the Consultant Merit awards scheme and did not wish to go down the same road. By 1963 a proposed scheme had been developed within GMSC which was again decisively rejected by Conference, although it is true some representatives would have accepted a different scheme.While it was recognised that some practices operated at a higher level than others the worry was about who would set the standards and who would make the decisions. Certainly at that time there were no accepted criteria and there was considerable anxiety about the views of the RCGP. The proposals and the principle were again not accepted and the money was lost.

The issue of differential payments or Merit awards resurfaced in early 1967. The Doctors and Dentists Review Body had set aside an additional two million pounds to be used specifically for this purpose. A GMSC working party had been set up in Jan 1966 to examine the proposals and had submitted a draft scheme to ministers, receiving a censure by Denbigh and Flintshire LMC amongst others for doing so. At a special meeting of local GPs which I attended in March 1967 the report was rejected in its entirety, thirty-six against, none for.

While rumblings in favour of some sort of rewards for "merit" occurred over the years the issue of merit awards never resurfaced and nothing concrete was agreed until the 2004 contract which introduced QOF (Quality and Outcome Framework) points for practices to aim for. The difference is that all doctors are now qualifying for these, some more than others, whereas the old proposals would have seen them limited to far fewer doctors. Significantly QOF points earned over and above the expected level do not reduce the amount available elsewhere in the pay structure and is "new money". Many proposals within both general practice and in the hospital service have faltered or failed over the years because no "new money" was identified. The standard of care which was already present in practices was demonstrated by the expectation by the government that the average GP practice would be able to claim 700 to 800 out of a possible 1050 whereas the average figure claimed for 2005-6 turned out to be 958.7 (91.3%) giving GPs substantially higher income than government anticipated.

The Review Body, the DDRB, has continued to report annually. While nominally independent of government its deliberations and findings in recent years very frequently seem to reflect very closely government guidelines on pay policy and a failure to address the concerns of the profession. This has frequently led to calls from some LMCs to withdraw from the Review Body system. It has however avoided the problem of direct negotiation on pay with governments and its findings have never been such as to cause serious discussion about resignation, which for the reasons already alluded to would now be much more difficult to do.

Private practice and the pay beds issue

Labour's original intention was the setting up of a full-time salaried service, nationalising the doctors. The BMA and the consultants leaders in particular resisted and Nye Bevan was forced to concede at the very last minute that private medicine could co-exist and continue within the NHS hospitals. Failure to do so would have jeopardised the service before birth but it did not go down well with the Labour party. Many of the consultants` leaders were teaching hospital based with considerable private practice in Harley Street and elsewhere. Aneurin Bevan who was advised by Lord Moran, President of the Royal College of Physicians, the one who once infamously described GPs as "doctors who had fallen off the consultant ladder", later claimed he had "stuffed their (the consultants) mouths with silver"

From the start there were accusations that the arrangements were not satisfactory, that consultants were pressurising patients to go private and building up waiting lists to increase private work, and that NHS equipment was being used for private work without charge.

By 1972 demands for the arrangement to be abolished were surfacing in parliament. The designated private beds in hospitals, the so-called pay-beds, came in for criticism and targeting. In fact they totalled only 4500 in the whole NHS, most were only achieving 50% occupancy, and they accounted for only 1% of patients treated each year. Nevertheless they gave rise to major confrontations, both with the consultants and with the health unions, NUPE (the National Union of Public Employees) and COHSE (the Confederation of Health Service Employees). Ward staff from nurses to cleaners resented having to provide special care and attention to patients in private wards with only the consultant reaping the benefit. The unions found that the most effective action in their disputes was to target pay-beds, while the public resented the fact that some could jump the queue to an NHS bed by paying a consultant privately for an initial consultation.

The other issue at the same time was the negotiations for a new consultant contract which now become part of an industrialized world of labour relations. The consultants were very angry, they wanted to be able to undertake more private practice than was allowed under their contract not less and appeared close to taking action.

Private practice for GPs had virtually disappeared with the onset of the NHS except in the most affluent areas. The only purely private practice I have been aware of was that of two sisters, Drs Rosentyl and Bryneilin Griffiths, who had qualified in 1928 and had run a private practice in Cardiff. At the start of the NHS they opted not to join the new health service and intended to retire but under considerable pressure from their patients they decided to stay on and continue to practice privately. Most practices joined the NHS but retained some private patients.

Prior to the start of the NHS in 1948 five possible grades of general practice patient were recognised, the very poor on the Parish, the Club associated with various Friendly Societies, the Lloyd George National Insurance panel, the poor private, and the well-off private. The last group often benefited from using the front surgery and waiting room while others entered and waited separately. Not all groups were represented in every practice.

I do not recall any private patients in Ruabon and when I moved to Penrhyn Bay in 1967 I inherited perhaps a dozen. This number was more of an irritant than a money-spinner, the fairly low fees charged in order to retain them did not justify the effort. Gradually the number dropped, sometimes by death, others said that did not mind my fees but that the cost of drugs on private prescriptions was becoming too high.

Although the issue was purely a consultant one in negotiating terms GPs had an interest on behalf of their patients but also because success against one part of the profession can have spin-offs and repercussions on another part at a later date. The GP committees spent considerable time discussing the private practice issues.

Over the lifetime of the NHS the attitude of Government to private medical care has fluctuated markedly depending on political dogma. In larger conurbations there have been separate Private Hospitals or wings of an NHS hospital with separate staff. The demand in N.Wales was never big enough to justify this and the larger hospitals had private beds alongside NHS ones, usually in side-wards, and with the same nursing and support staff. This never went down well with staff as the only ones to benefit from the private status were the consultants while paying patients understandably expected special attention and services from the nursing and other staff. At various times the number of private beds allowed by Government and the conditions attached to their use has been very restrictive and at present no private beds are available in any of the North Wales DGHs.

Porritt in his report attached the greatest importance to the patient's right to seek private medical advice and the preservation of private practice. He stated that the private bed provision both within the NHS and outside was grossly inadequate. The daily cost to the patient for a private bed was always very high, a calculation being made from the total costs of running the hospital divided by the number of beds. Patients were paying for services not relevant to them and no allowance was being made for the fact that they were saving costs to the NHS.

There was a third way, the so-called Amenity Beds, whereby for a very reasonable charge a side-ward could be allocated when there was no medical or nursing reason for this, just purely a wish for privacy, on the understanding that the ward might be taken back if needed on clinical grounds for an ill patient. These have also disappeared and the question of privacy remains a major issue for patients right across the social scale. Even more so since the concept of mixed -sex wards was introduced, causing great embarrassment at times especially to older patients. Although now no longer officially permitted they still exist and patients still find themselves mixing in wards with the opposite sex.

Mrs Barbara Castle, an old-fashioned socialist known as the Red Queen, was the Secretary of State for Health and Social Security at the time with Dr David Owen as Minister for Health. She has stated in her memoirs that her aim was not to outlaw private practice if patients wished it but to separate it from the NHS and to limit the freedom of consultants to come and go as they pleased leaving their over-worked junior doctors to carry the burden. The juniors themselves were getting very restless and militant. She also said she wished to improve the contract for those doctors working full-time for the NHS, often in areas and in specialities such as geriatrics and psychiatry where the opportunity for private practice did not exist and to increase the total number of consultants to ease the juniors workload but that the consultants did not want more rivals for their private practices. In addition she wished to see the merit awards scheme modified.

The Hospital Consultants and Specialists Association and which claimed to represent half of all consultants had been formed to 1948. It began to press for more radical action. Many of these consultants were from the district general hospitals in the periphery who felt that the BMA was dominated by teaching hospital and Royal College officers. Consultant and GP Conferences and the BMA Annual Representative Meetings were very interesting and stormy at this time.

After bitter and protracted negotiations led by the formidable BMA negotiator and surgeon Mr Anthony Grabham the consultants finally climbed down in 1975 after a substantial increase in their NHS salary recommended by the Review Body. They agreed to drop the idea of a completely new contract and to work on modifying the existing one.

The settling of the contract issue itself did not solve the pay-beds impasse. Barbara Castle wanted to allow them to continue at their existing level but to avoid expensively trained NHS staff being lured away any extensions to private facilities around NHS hospitals would have to be approved by her. She failed to get the support of the Prime Minister Harold Wilson and his Cabinet on this and after long and secret negotiations a compromise was reached whereby 1000 of the 4500 existing private beds would go immediately and the remainder would be phased out by a Health Services Board including two trade union members and an independent chairman using agreed strict criteria. Mrs Thatcher abolished the Board as one of her first acts on becoming Prime Minister.

Locally in North Wales the total number of pay-beds was never high and were scattered between six or seven hospitals, some were cut and the rest remained but problems with the unions and staff action continued. Since they were not in separate units or wards sometimes the beds were occupied by private patients, at other times by NHS patients and this did not help staff attitudes. Private patients themselves were at times very unhappy about the care they received and it was into this climate that the North Wales Medical Centre, discussed later, was opened to provide private facilities in 1978.

A new consultant contract has recently been introduced, juniors hours of work have been regulated with strict restrictions imposed on their duty periods under European directives. A new postgraduate consultant training programme has been introduced. It is too early to judge how well these changes will work, how attitudes will change in relation to private practice and what problems they will bring.

The North Wales Medical Centre and the Medical Trust

This private hospital of sixty-one beds in Llandudno has had a very interesting history. It was for some years the only private in-patient facility in North Wales although more recently BUPA have opened a hospital at Wrexham.

When I first started in general practice the private practice service was largely provided by Welsh consultants based on Liverpool, the best known being Dr Emyr Wyn Jones, the cardiologist, and Mr Hywel Hughes, a general surgeon. If patients wished in-patient care they were admitted into private nursing homes in Liverpool.

To return to the North Wales Medical Centre and its beginning. There was in the West Shore in Llandudno a small private nursing home where consultants admitted patients for treatment, all the other nursing homes admitted patients treated by GPs on the NHS. Most of these private patients were under the care of Dr Oliver Galpin, Consultant Physician at Llandudno, and Dr D.A.Jones, known to all as Dafydd Alun, a consultant Psychiatrist at the North Wales Hospital, Denbigh, which is discussed elsewhere. Patients with psychiatric problems of depression or alcohol abuse at that time did not wish the stigma of association with Denbigh as it was generally known.

Llandudno, like many other seaside resorts, had always had a number of convalescent homes run either by Local Authorities in England or by organisations such as Friendly Societies and Trade Unions. A period of convalescence in pleasant surroundings with nursing support was very popular and indeed very necessary for many of the illnesses of the time, especially for patients from deprived backgrounds. By the early 1970`s the need for these had dropped considerably and some were being closed, although some are still active in the area today.

The Lady Forrester Home in Queens Road, Llandudno, a fine purpose-built building in fifteen acres of grounds and with sea-views of Llandudno Bay, was one of these and in 1978 was to go on the market. Llandudno Town Council were interested in taking it on but in an act of immense bravery, some at the time thought foolhardiness, the West Shore Nursing Home owners had the vision of developing a North Wales Medical Centre with a much wider remit than presently available to them and stepped in very quickly to purchase the property under the noses of the Town Council. Having done so they then had the task of setting up a charitable Trust and selling the concept both to the profession in North Wales and to potential patients. Neither proved easy in the short term and the financial viability remained very insecure for some years.

Over fifty doctors were founding members of the charitable Trust, both consultants and GPs. Having the local GPs involved and the fact that they contributed a very nominal amount of capital (£100 if I recall correctly) was helpful to the fledgling Centre indicating to the public and to potential financiers that it had their support. Some twenty GPs from the local practices in Llandudno, Penrhyn Bay and Conway were persuaded to provide out of hours care, a routine evening visit and then emergency cover as needed and this worked well for a number of years until a resident doctor was appointed.

Initially the patients admitted were mainly medical and psychiatric and Dr D.A. in particular worked strenuously to seek out and admit patients from far and wide across England and Wales. It was comparatively easy to develop outpatient consulting facilities but further expansion required the development of surgical facilities and the building of theatres to a high standard. It took some considerable time for surgeons, many of whom were based in Bangor or Bodelwyddan and often lived even further away, to develop the confidence to use the facilities regularly for anything other than minor surgery. This was of course before the building of the A55 and the Conwy Tunnel and travel times could be very long.

In 1985 the Medical Centre was able to build a number of sheltered homes within the grounds. Financing remained a problem and eventually in 1987 the Centre was sold to a development company but continued to develop as a first class facility in an area where previously there was none. The range of treatments offered continued to expand. The Centre over the last few years provided a base for much NHS Waiting List Initiative work to be carried out. Unfortunately new owners who took over in 2005 have decided that it was no longer financially viable and after a short consultation period the Centre was closed.

A North Wales Medical Trust was set up at the time of the original sale in1988, utilising in part monies which consultants and GPs had put into the centre, and with the stated aims of providing administrative support services to organisations in the field of medical education and research. The trust operates from Tyldesley House in Craig-y-don, Llandudno, where a variety of office and seminar room accommodation is available and it is where the N.Wales RCGP now has its base. The current chairman of the Trust is Dr Roger Ramsay who has for many years provided stalwart service for the College, as Faculty secretary and also as secretary and then chairman of the Welsh College Council.

The Welsh Hospital Recognition Committee scheme which in liaison with the specialist Royal Colleges oversees the recognition by the RCGP of the suitability of hospital posts for GP vocational training is based there, organised by one of my former practice partners, Dr Bridget Osborne. Wearing another hat she also has responsibility for responding to the needs of the increasing number of non-principals, salaried GPs and locums, under the umbrella of Meddwl.

Support for Educational Continuing Professional Development within the Conwy and Denbighshire LHB areas, under the supervision of the coordinator Dr Huw Lloyd, is also available. Medical student placements within local practices, an increasingly important part of undergraduate training, has been organised in partnership with the University of Liverpool Faculty of Medicine. The Trust has also provided Hafan Wen, a purpose built Treatment and Detoxification unit at the hospital in Wrexham.

Amongst other activities the Trust provides administrative assistance to the charity North Wales Medical Aid to Tamil Nadu set up in 1999 under the chairmanship of the Archbishop of Wales, the Most Reverend Alwyn Rice-Jones. This charity has set up medical clinics which provide health support to Tamil Nadu, an area in South East India. Dr Vizwanathan, a consultant psychiatrist at the North Wales Hospital left for the village in 1999 and returns there frequently. The Trust provided a mobile clinic to serve outlying villages. Friends of the charity was set up in 1990. The Health Care Studies department of the local Llandrillo College during 1994 started visits to establish a health education programme in the villages and in 1996 District 18 of Inner Wheel raised funds to develop a child development centre in the area. The whole project has taken off and the work was given an international award in 1999.

The Administration of the NHS

It may help readers of these recollections to understand the context of events if a section on the administrative set-up of the various health authorities and of the hospitals is included at this point although many of the issues and areas of interest arising from them are discussed under other headings. Even those of us who have lived through the various changes have difficulty at times in recollecting them accurately and the dates at which they happened and certainly have difficulty in understanding the reasons behind them.

Throughout the NHS the administration of hospitals has been separate and distinct from that of the independent contactor professions, the doctors, dentists, chemists and opticians. The 1948 NHS Act saw the amalgamation of municipal and voluntary hospitals together with the asylums and colonies for mental defectives into one hospital service.In my early days hospitals were overseen by the Welsh Regional Hospitals Board and were run locally by Hospital Management Committees in Wrexham, Rhyl and Bangor but the real management was in the hands of the Medical Superintendents and the matrons. The names of Mr R.S "Bob" Ninian at Wrexham, later followed by the pathologist Dr Lionel Wise, Dr JHO Roberts at the North Wales Hospital Denbigh, and Dr "Bill" Biagi at Llangwyfan are the ones I was most familiar with, all great characters and innovators in their differing ways, and the hospitals ran efficiently.

The GP and other independent contractor services were overseen by the Executive Councils set up in 1948, one for Denbighshire and Flintshire in the east and three separate ones for Anglesey, Caernarfon and for Merioneth in the north-west. Their main role was in the registration of practices and of patients with them, administering doctor's contracts and acting as paymasters. There was little input by them into the way doctors ran their practices provided they adhered to their contracted Terms of Service, which were defined vaguely but in effect all-inclusively as providing such services as other general practitioners normally provided, terminology which gave rise to many arguments and disagreements over the years as will be discussed later. Doctors contracts were to provide services to the patients on their registered list twenty-four hours a day throughout the year as well as providing care in emergency to patients not on their lists. The concept of a registered list of patients was unique to the NHS and was not found anywhere else in the world. The Executive Councils administered using the Statement of Fees and Allowances, the GP bible known as the Red Book, which was a loose-leaf binder with irregular updates. It is true to say that in many practices the updates were not regularly filed, and in many cases completely ignored until problems arose. The wording of the individual Statements was however crucially important and one of the duties of the

GMSC negotiators and of its sub-committee chairmen was to go through each amendment with a tooth-comb before it was approved and issued.

Up until then there had been considerable fragmentation of care between various agencies, a situation which has gradually and to some extent only reduced over the following years. General practitioners had always considered themselves as family doctors providing necessary care on demand to the patients registered with them, and without much specific thought to the health of the community or population as a whole. This was always considered to be the responsibility of the Medical Officer of Health, often an ex-GP, who was employed by local government and had responsibility for issues such as water, sewerage, schools and factories as well as immunisation and various health clinics.

As practices started to develop their role and as these additional services became introduced into the payment structure more and more of this work was taken over by GPs and many clinics closed. This was not without its downside in some respects particularly in family planning and cervical smear clinics, removing patient choice where the absence of a female doctor, a Catholic GP with religious objections, or where close family or social relationships existed within their practice, created anxieties and difficulties for some. Another unfortunate practical consequence of fewer clinics in family planning and cervical cytology was the reduction in opportunities for hands-on training outside the practice for new doctors and for retraining for established ones.

In 1947 the Welsh Regional Hospital Board in its Review of Proposed Developments had identified the need for as many as fourteen District General Hospitals supported by GP hospitals and long-stay units and one university hospital. Following "A review of the Medical Services in Great Britain (the Porritt Report) and the 1968 green paper The Administrative Structure of the Medical and Related Services in England and Wales published by Mr Kenneth Robinson, the Hospital and Specialist Services, family services and public health doctors, who now came to be called community health physicians, were in 1974 brought together. Local Government restructuring in Wales created eight new counties from the fifteen old ones and with a new Area Health Authority co-terminous with each. North Wales saw the creation of Gwynedd from the counties of Anglesey, Caernarfon and Merioneth, and of Clwyd from the counties of Denbighshire and Flintshire.

For the first time in 1974 general practitioners were brought to some degree into the organisational and management structure of hospital services, previously hospital management committees had often had a token GP representative on the board. The new Health Authorities oversaw and funded services provided by the various hospitals and in the community, together with the Contractor services. The independent contractors continued to be administered separately by new Family Practitioner Committees which replaced the Executive Councils but which maintained much the same functions. While technically sub-committees of the Health Authorities in practice they remained relatively autonomous. Bringing the public health functions within the Health Authority was a major change and heralded the start of more community based thinking, although responsibility for some of the environmental health issues such as water and sewerage remained with the local government who usually employed the Authority public health physicians on a part-time basis.

The new structure saw the setting up in 1974 of Area Medical Committees (AMCs) with equal numbers of consultants and general practitioners and with the Community Health Physician in attendance to provide a forum for advice to and to comment on proposals by the Authority. At the same time Area Management Teams (A.M.T.s) were set up with the Chairman of the Authority, the Chief Executive, the Treasurer, the Chief Nursing Officer (probably another first), the Public Health physician, together with the Chairman and vice-chairman of the AMC (a consultant and a GP) meeting weekly and giving clinicians a place at high table, although it must be said that often a consensus had been reached amongst the Chief Officers on many issues before matters were brought to the Team. It was a good concept but one which was unfortunately lost again in the 1980 reorganisations.

The Gwynedd Area Team consisted of the Authority Chairman Mr Jack Berry from Dolgarrog, the general manager Bob Freeman and the treasurer Bill Owen. Together with the first clinicians Dr Hubert Jones a radiologist from Bangor and a powerful personality, and Dr Graham Williams, a senior GP from Holyhead, who resigned within a few months because of ill health. I was elected in his place giving me my first real taste and input into medical politics and administration, a taste which led on to many further involvements over the next twenty five years. The public health member was the young and enthusiastic Dr Gareth Crompton from Anglesey who later went on to become a very successful Chief Medical Officer for Wales while Mr David Jones, the Chief Nursing Officer, later went on to become Chief Executive to the English Nursing, Midwifery and Health Visiting Board in London and later became a Board member of Glan Clwyd Trust so it was a powerful team. Dr Cedric Davies succeeded Gareth when he moved to the Welsh Office in Cardiff while Mr Hywel Oliver replaced Hubert Jones on the team and later as a member of the Authority.

Clwyd Health Authority at first had two administrative Districts, Clwyd North based on the Rhyl hospitals and Clwyd South based on Wrexham hospitals. It had the old Flintshire Medical Officer of Health Dr Wyn Roberts in charge with Dr David T.Jones as its community physician responsible for medical manpower and planning. David later became CAMO (Chief Administrative Medical Officer) in 1978. In 1986 he went on to become deputy manager of the Authority and then General Manager the following year on the retirement of Mr Don Cope. Following on David's retirement he was appointed a Professor in the developing School of Health Care Studies at the University in Bangor. Later still he spent time in Bahrain in a collaboration between the Arab State and Clwyd Health Authority and, together with Dr Bruce Lervy of Swansea, in Hong Kong setting up a computer system for the health services.

David T. Jones had a clear vision of the very important role of community hospitals as support fot the specialist hospitals and this resulted in the Authority developing and updating them in Clwyd at a time when they were being neglected in other areas. He had a particular vision of developing new hospitals to replace those in Mold and Holywell. The Mold hospital was built years ago, building the Holywell only started in 2006. David had spent some time as a GP and was an enthusiastic supporter of the potential contributions of GPs and in recognition of his support he was awarded Honorary Membership of the College at the instigation of the North Wales Faculty.

The creation of Health Authorities in 1974 provided an opportunity to start to reorganise the provision of care provided in various clinics such as infant welfare clinics previously run by local authorities, antenatal clinics run by local authorities with an input from consultant obstetricians, and cervical smear clinics and family planning clinics run by the Family Planning Association. These had originally been set up to provide a service which was not generally being provided by general practitioners in all areas and particularly in the larger centres of population. Many clinics operated in very poor facilities and in particular many antenatal clinics were very busy and impersonal with heavily pregnant women with their stockings around their ankles queuing to be weighed and then often waiting patiently for the hospital doctor to arrive. Clinic attendances on occasions led to considerable conflicts of interest with GPs, and frequently led to problems because of poor or absent communication and conflicting advice. Nothing changes.

In 1980 Sir Roy Griffiths, the chairman of Sainsburys, produced a report which demonstrated that the move to consensus management introduced in 1974 was not working (although it was working well in Gwynedd) and which started to move the NHS from administration to management. He stated pithily that "If Florence Nightingale were carrying her lamp through the corridors of the NHS today she would almost certainly be searching for the people in charge" and called for every health authority and hospital to have a general manager with commercial style boards and devolution of responsibility to unit level.

1980-81 saw the replacement of the Area Health Authorities by the District Health Authorities, again two for North Wales at the time when the new District

General Hospitals envisaged in the Hospital Plan were being built. Bodelwyddan DGH was the first replacing the acute services provided at the Rhyl Alexandra Hospital, the War Memorial Hospital in Rhyl and Colwyn Bay Hospital while as part of the plan Llangwyfan Hospital closed in 1981. Abergele Hospital and St Asaph Hospital remained open although some services were moved to the DGH. Ysbyty Gwynedd which replaced the old C&A Hospital and St. Davids Hospitals in Bangor was opened in 1984. While the DGH at Wrexham developed in stages over a number of years on the old Maelor Hospital site rather than having a new build.

GPs as a group had little direct contact with the Health Authority chairmen but for the record the Clwyd chairmen in order were Lord Kenyon, Dr Emyr Wyn Jones, Mr Michael Griffiths, and then Mrs Ann Roberts whose father, Dr Ifor Davies from Cerrig-y-drudion was the secretary of the Denbighshire and Flintshire LMC when I first joined.

The hospitals and the community services were re-organised into two directly managed units under the Health Authority but in the early nineties they were permitted to apply for Trust status and to become independent of, but funded through, the Health Authority. In 1991 Clwyd Health Authority created the Clwyd North District Hospital NHS Trust which resulted in major organisational changes to the hospital management with the creation of a Trust Board advised by the Trust Management Team and its Clinical Directors who were the heads of each department. It became the Conwy and Denbighshire NHS Trust in 1999. Similar trusts were created at Wrexham and at Bangor.

The Clwyd Health Authority had two GP members, Dr Eddie Lewis and Dr Gruff Jones while two consultants, Dr Gordon Row from Bodelwyddan and Mr Aled Williams from Wrexham were appointed. Dr Eleri Edwards also served for some years on the Authority, and on many other committees throughout Wales and made major contributions. Following the 1991 reorganisation the medical representation on the health authorities was reduced to one with Dr Gruff Jones being appointed by the Secretary of State and serving until the Authority was scrapped.

The Gwynedd chairmen in turn from 1974 were Mr Jack Berry, Mr Idris Davies 1976-82, Mrs Noreen Edwards 1982 to 92, and Mr Graham Hulse from 1992 until the merger into the North Wales Health Authority in 1996, while the managers, later named chief executives, from 1974 were Mr Bob Freeman,and then Mr Huw Thomas until the two authorities were merged into the North Wales Health Authority in 1990 with Mr Brian Jones as Chief Executive. The North-west Wales Trust chief executives from 1991 on were Mr Barry Shingles, Mr Keith Thompson and currently Mr Martin Jones. GP medical members on the Authority from 1974 on were Dr Iolo Griffiths, followed by Dr Rob Howarth while Mr Hywel Oliver was the consultant member. When the two District Health Authorities were amalgamated medical representation on the Authority was reduced to one but the Chair and vice-chair of the District Medical Committee were allowed to attend as observers and could speak at the discretion of the Chair.

We were lucky in North Wales in that the first Chairman of the new North Wales Health Authority was a GP, Arthur Kenrick, the only one appointed in Wales. He had previously been secretary of the Gwynedd LMC and later chairman of the Gwynedd FHSA and was aware of the whole scene but of necessity had to "go native" in some respects and adopt civil service speak in his new position. The Authority did appoint a part-time Medical Adviser, Dr Wally Murfin from Tywyn,who was proving very effective until his illness and his tragically early death in 2001.

The numerous reorganisations have taken their toll on the confidence and morale of NHS workers who aresuffering from "reorganisational fatigue" particularly within the hospital service. Some consultants quote ten reorganisations, internal and external within eleven years. A period of stability is urgently required.

The Independent Contractors

The independent contractor services remained under the Gwynedd and the Clwyd FPCs which became autonomous and independent of the Health Authorities in the 1980 reorganisation. Within the hospital administration Clwyd H.A. were probably more responsive to GPs views than Gwynedd whereas within the contractor services GPs in Gwynedd were the happier with their administrators.

Coinciding with the 1990 contract we saw the formation of Family Health Services Authorities (FHSAs) to replace the Family Practitioner Committees (the FPCs), again one each for Gwynedd and Clwyd. This resulted in a further reduction in the representation and direct input in management by the independent contractors, there now being only one GP member appointed by the Secretary of State rather than the six nominated by the LMC on the old FPC. and previously on the Executive Councils. In Gwynedd Dr Ian Roberts of Bala was our representative and the FHSA also had a medical chairman, Dr Arthur Kenrick.

Clwyd FPC had Dr BD Chowdhury as chairman, followed by Dr Bob Jones of Rhyl. Later Mr Tom Jones, a local farmer and county councillor, was appointed with Dr Eddie Lewis as the vice-chairman and he continued until the change to Local Health Boards in 1996. Dr Peter Wykes of Denbigh replaced Dr Lewis as the medical member on his retirement.

GPs in the north-west counties have always felt very fortunate in having a succession of very approachable and helpful administrators. The old Executive Councils had Mr Eric Frobisher in Caernarfon, Mr Alec Hughes in Anglesey and Mr Eric Hughes in Merioneth. Following the 1974 amalgamation Alec Hughes was appointed Gwynedd FHSA Administrator, later succeeded by Mr John Llewelyn Jones and in 1985 by Mr Arfon Thomas who continued in post until the FHSAs were replaced by Local Health Boards in 1996. Their Chairmen, Mrs Florence Treen who chaired the FPC for some sixteen years from 1974, and Dr Arthur Kenrick who succeeded her both contributed considerably to what was over the years a harmonious working relationship with no major disagreements.

In the eastern counties the administrators were Mr Tudor Williams when I first started, followed shortly afterwards by Mr Hugh Tunnah, and then by Mrs Jennifer Edge (who later became Mrs Jackson). When the FHSA was formed in 1990 one of a new breed of administrator, with no previous experience within the NHS, took over in the shape of Major General Christopher Last and he served until the two FHSAs were merged under Mr Arfon Thomas in 1996. Although my personal involvement was more with Gwynedd it is safe to say that there were from time to time more friction between doctors and the Clwyd administration, some over major issues, some over nit-picking interference over minor issues. Certainly in the past there were continual and long-running disagreements between Dr Chowdhury and the chairman Mr Tom Jones and other non-medical members.

1996 saw the next major reorganisation, the creation of a single Health Authority for North Wales, one of five in Wales and a single FHSA. Mr Arfon Thomas was appointed general manager. It is interesting to note the progression in titles over the years from Clerk to the Executive Councils, to Administrators of FPCs, to General Manager of FHSAs and to Chief Executive of the Local Health Boards.

I think it is safe to say that, in spite of some inevitable problems, GPs perception of the services provided across North Wales and relationships with the various authorities over the years has been better than in some other parts of Wales.

Local Health Boards

The North Wales Health Authority remained in existence until the creation of Local Health Boards (LHBs) proposed in 1996, six for North Wales replacing a single Health Authority and the FHSA. (In England they were known as Primary Care Trusts or PCTs). In all twenty two LHBs were created in Wales, mirroring the twenty-two newly created local authorities, replacing the previous five Authorities, against the advice of the BMA, WGMSC, the consultant's committees and the Local Medical Committees. Six was too many for North Wales. At worst we would have been happier with three Health Boards in North Wales roughly corresponding to the three Hospital Trusts. Administrative costs have escalated following the establishment of LHBs and events since suggest that both administratively and financially six was too many. There is a view that the next reorganisation will not be far away and changes have already taken place in England

The stated aim was to bring organisation and control closer to the people and to make them co-terminous with the County Councils. The latter had for many years wanted, unsuccessfully, to have control of health services but the profession had always resisted this. In the new Health Boards there was much closer working and cross representation but the two still remained separate.

With so many new Boards being created there was a shortage of NHS-experienced administrators to run them and difficulty in finding experienced chairmen and medical members to sit on them. The new Chief Executives came from a variety of previous posts. Three LHBs in North Wales appointed GP chairmen, one a pharmacist, one a nurse and one a former local authority executive. I would personally very much liked to have had the opportunity to be involved as a member, and possibly as chairman, in the development of the new LHB scene in my practice area of Conwy where none of the GP members wished to take on the chair but by then I had recently retired from practice and was out of time by a couple of months. Informal lobbying on my behalf at WAG was unsuccessful.

The three North Wales Hospitals Trusts previously overseen by the North Wales Health Authority became directly accountable to Welsh Assembly Government (WAG) but services from them were to be commissioned by the Local Health Boards. To those of us in general practice it appeared that the Hospital Trusts had always been too powerful for the Health Authority as commissioners and had been able to conjure up additional monies for their new needs while at the same time withdrawing services without consultation. They had also in practice, over many years and without censure, ignored Welsh Office guidance on good practice, particularly in the fields of prescribing, certification and patient discharge arrangements. They continue to do so. Six North Wales Local Health Boards were dealing with three Trusts with considerable overlap between their catchment areas. While the Boards have recognised the problems and, encouraged by the LMC, have endeavoured to adopt similar policies across North Wales there remains much duplication.

As a result the commissioning process appears to be failing and withdrawal of services provided by the Trusts to general practice is continuing at an alarming rate.

There has been a strong feeling amongst GPs as a group that the Trusts` concept of efficiency savings seems to be to transfer services to the budgets of other organisations such as the LHB`s and to GPs. In old GP contract 70% of the costs of the ancillary staff, receptionists and nurses were reimbursed by the FPC, now all of this was transferred to the global sum, so 100% of any additional staff employed to take on the extra work has to be taken from the practice profits.

While the LMC has been pressing the LHBs to reduce funding to the Trusts for services withdrawn this appears impossible to do because the commissioning in the past has not been detailed enough to identify specific amounts,

Strictly speaking LHB's commission services from Trusts and pay them for these services. The LHB's and to be fair to them, the FPCs before them, seem not to have the necessary data or experience nor the desire to monitor the contracts and to withdraw cash for services not performed or those withdrawn by the Trusts

The Trusts are already in considerable over-spend situations and claim that they do not have any money to pay back.

Much time and resources have been expended and much frustration has been caused over the years by repeated administrative changes which are often viewed as being unnecessary and flawed before they are introduced. It is of interest that Lloyd George, when proposing the new National Insurance system in 1910, said that there were too many councils and wished to see them replaced by larger councils with burgomasters.

During all these changes a game of musical chairs seems to have been played, the only difference according to one cynic is that when the music stops another chair is added.

The whole structure of healthcare in the UK has uniquely for many years been based on the general practitioner/family doctor as the custodian of the interests of the patient and with the only continuing medical record, extending theoretically from the cradle or on occasion before birth to the grave, passing to a new doctor on moving home or practices and containing a complete medical history. This has so far survived through the many changes and reorganisations, although as will be discussed later the many recent changes with a variety of different agencies providing care independently of each other makes it likely that records will be fragmented and incomplete.

The Hospitals of North Wales

Prior to the reorganisation starting from the construction of the DGHs from 1980 onwards hospital services were provided from a variety of sites of varying age and suitability. Even twelve months after the setting up of the NHS the hospital service was found to be costing far more than anticipated and Aneurin Bevan had to go back to the Treasury to ask for supplementary estimates. The situation remains unchanged today.

In the area of north Clwyd, the hospitals providing specialist services were one in Colwyn Bay, two in Rhyl, one in St. Asaph, one in Holywell, the old sanatoria in Abergele and Llangwyfan, and the Mental Hospital at Denbigh. In many cases departments were split between two or more sites leading to problems in staffing cover, particularly perhaps in anaesthesia, and other difficulties. Changes over the years have been aimed at centralising services as far as possible. In additional there were cottage or community hospitals in Denbigh, Holywell, Ruthin and Prestatyn

The Royal Alexandra at Rhyl had been nominated as the administrative base at the start of the NHS. Building had been started in 1884, with extensions in 1902 and 1908 and it covered medicine, surgery, dermatology and paediatrics. The War Memorial Hospital in Rhyl was opened in 1923 and in the early years most of the surgery was done there, mainly by visiting surgeons from Liverpool. In 1948 it became the centre for orthopaedics and the main accident unit until the opening of the DGH in 1980.

St Asaph Hospital was formerly an old Poor Law workhouse but in 1948 beds were provided for surgery, medicine, obstetrics and gynaecology and later for ENT, oral surgery and ophthalmology. In 1959 it was renamed the H.M.Stanley Hospital after the African explorer who spent years of his childhood in the workhouse there. Some of the poor law inmates were still there until 1960. In 1980 medicine, oral surgery and ENT moved to Glan Clwyd, and obstetrics and gynaecology followed in 1992. Geriatrics and ophthalmology remain there together with the recently developed St Kentigern Hospice and the administrative headquarters of the Welsh Ambulance Trust.

Abergele Hospital was opened in 1912 and completed in 1931 initially by Manchester City Corporation as a sanatorium for children with tuberculosis and this included some surgery. The arrival of the internationally known surgical pioneer Mr Ivor Lewis who moved back to North Wales from London, was the start of major thoracic surgery. As the need for this service declined beds were progressively closed. Rheumatology beds were opened and the orthopaedic unit was moved there from the War Memorial Hospital. The layout intended for the fresh air treatment of tuberculosis makes it difficult to run cost-effectively and its long term future has been under discussion for many years. It is scheduled for closure under the Review of Acute Services now under consultation.

Colwyn Bay Hospital is discussed again later as it changed from an acute unit to a GP community hospital in 1981. Built by public subscription at the turn of the century as the cottage hospital, it was renamed the Colwyn Bay and West Denbighshire Hospital in 1925. It had originally had medical beds and surgery provided by GP surgeons and anaesthetists but in 1961 it became part of the acute surgery service with Mr Owen Daniel and Mr Maurice Jonathan carrying out surgery there and at the Royal Alex. Mrs Noreen Edwards, later chairman of Gwynedd Health Authority had been matron of the hospital some years previously.

In the Vale of Clwyd within a few miles of Denbigh there was another large hospital, Llangwyfan, originally proposed in 1910 as the King Edward Memorial Sanatorium and extended during the second World War. Two sanatoria were built in Wales, the other being at Talgarth in Mid-Wales and developed at a time when treatment was largely based on bed rest and exposure to fresh air. Wards had open balconies and no windows. At first men were treated at Talgarth and women and children at Llangwyfan. Thoracic surgery for lung conditions especially tuberculosis was regularly undertaken by Mr Hugh Morriston-Davies who in 1922 performed the first thoracoplasty outside London, by Mr Hugh Reid and by Mr Ivor Lewis. Mr Howell Hughes also operated there from 1939 until its closure.

My first recollections of it was at the time when it was being run down as a sanatorium and was increasingly being used for other medical cases particularly for the elderly and for some surgery. I well recall Dr Bill Biagi who was the Medical Superintendent from 1951 until its closure and was prominent in BMA circles and chairman of BMA Welsh Council from 1973 to 76. The hospital, which is close to where I now live, was recommended for closure in the Heaf Report in 1965 but was not finally closed until 1981. It was sold by Welsh Office and then resold two days later for almost double the price. Care Concern Ruthin set up a village there for mentally handicapped people over sixteen with a mission to provide a sheltered environment in which they could develop skills, self-management and "a sense of personal worth".

North-west Wales had the Caernarfonshire and Anglesey Hospital and St Davids Hospital in Bangor, replaced by the Ysbyty Gwynedd DGH at Penrhosgarnedd (with St Davids moving to the site later) with smaller hospitals in Llandudno, Conwy, Caernarfon, the Stanley Hospital in Holyhead, Valley and Llangefni. The western end was served by community hospitals at Pwllheli, Penrhyndeudraeth, Dolgellau, Tywyn, and Blaenau Ffestiniog.

Bryn-y-Neuadd, the large hospital at Llanfairfechan for patients with mental handicap as they were described at the time served a much wider area. A very similar scenario has been played out there as had happened in Denbigh. The Hospital housed nearly 200 patients at its peak, but the hospital has gradually been reduced in size by discharging patients into the local community or if possible back to their original communities and families. Patients had originally come from a large area including many from England and the remaining hard-core of patients who required more intensive and therefore much more expensive supervision and care have been difficult to relocate with their original local authorities reluctant to assume responsibility for them. Some fifty patients remain and it is unlikely that these will ever be discharged. Part of the extensive hospital grounds have now been taken over to provide a medium secure psychiatric unit, Ty Llewelyn, a development which certainly at the outset was not widely welcomed by the local community. There is no doubt that both the North Wales Hospital and Bryn-y-Neuadd have over the years contributed greatly to the local economy in terms of employment and services and their closure has been a great loss to the communities.

Our practice at Penrhyn Bay used mainly Llandudno hospital or else the Clwyd hospitals, partly because I had used them during my time in Prestatyn and because we were associated with the vocational training scheme at Glan Clwyd and the Postgraduate Centre was there. Also at that time travel to Glan Clwyd was easier than to Bangor.

Llandudno Hospital was part of the Bangor group and when I started in Penrhyn Bay it was a very active and in many ways self-sufficient hospital with two general surgeons of the old school, Mr McInroy and Mr Ken Hallstead Smith, who dealt with most things which came to them including major trauma. At that time before the new A55 road and the tunnel under the Conwy river were built travel across the old Telford bridge and through the towns of Conwy, Penmaenmawr and Llanfairfechan was slow and often dead slow. As a result patients were referred to the Denbighshire hospitals and emergency ambulances found it easier to take patients to Rhyl rather than to Bangor. Dr Oliver Galpin the consultant physician had been appointed two years before I moved to the area, previously medical consultant care was provided by Dr Donald Makinson based in the C.& A. at Bangor and who later moved to Cardiff as Postgraduate Dean in the University. Dr Glyn Penrhyn Jones appointed as the first consultant geriatrician at Bangor in 1959 covered the elderly beds at Llandudno until his untimely death in 1973 which was a great loss to his speciality. Dr Lyn Vaterlaws was appointed as the second physician in 1981. There was a paediatric ward which took surgical cases and children who were not too ill or were having routine operations such as tonsillectomies and also gynaecology beds although both these specialties were covered by consultants from Bangor. Midwifery deliveries were still being carried out by GPs at the

Oxford Road maternity unit but this closed fairly soon after I arrived in Penrhyn Bay and I used it very little. Our practice admitted to the Nant-y-glyn maternity unit at Colwyn Bay where I also provided cover for Dr Kenneth Evans who held the post of clinical assistant and was responsible for the patients of doctors who, usually because of distance, did not wish to attend their patients in the unit. Gradually over the years the services at Llandudno hospital have been reduced and the gynaecology and paediatric wards were closed. A geriatric unit was opened under the care of Dr Beulah Simpson who was later joined by Dr O`Bairn. The accident unit has probably justifiably been downgraded to a minor injuries unit but still deals with a significant workload and provides a useful service to visitors to the town and its hinterland.

Over the years there has been tension between Llandudno based consultants trying to maintain and develop services at the hospital and those who were Bangor based and who saw merit in centralising services and who were supported by the views of the Royal Colleges responsible for recognising posts as suitable for junior doctor training and by the Trust management seeking economies. The local population has always been very supportive of keeping and developing the hospital and it must be remembered that Llandudno and its hinterland which stretches up the Conwy valley and as far as Blaenau Ffestiniog forms a major part of the population of North-west Wales. Indeed it has been said that in the1974 boundary reconfiguration Llandudno would have become part of Clwyd except that it would have left Gwynedd as a very small economic unit of dubious viability. Suggestions have been put forward from time to time over the years that GP beds might be provided on the Llandudno Hospital site but have never been seriously taken up as there was no enthusiasm for the idea from the Llandudno GP practices.

When I started at Penrhyn Bay there was a small hospital at Groesynydd which was used as a longer stay unit but this closed soon afterwards. The Conwy Hospital sited in the old workhouse provided beds for the long-stay and the slow rehabilitation beds of the geriatric unit. Long discussions took place about possible ways of rebuilding or replacing it by some sort of community hospital but proved fruitless and it was closed

The Wrexham area and North-east Wales had the War Memorial which had medical and surgical beds and an Accident unit while the Maelor Hospital had surgical and medical beds. The Maelor incorporated the old Croesnewydd hospital across the road which when I worked there in 1955 had the paediatric unit, the obstetrics and gynaecology unit and the isolation wards which at that time housed poliomyelitis patients including several in the so-called iron-lungs. The War Memorial Hospital closed in 1986 as the new Maelor DGH was opened in stages and which continues to grow. In addition there were long-stay units at Trefalyn, at Dobs Hill and at Meadowslea. Community hospitals existed only at

Chirk and at Llangollen. There was also a small hospital at Penley which cared for an ageing group of Polish expatriates.

Rationalisation of services across North Wales has taken place gradually over the last fifty years, as and when these could be agreed on and finance made available. Clwyd in the 1976 under the Chief Administrative Medical officer Dr David Jones made a firm policy to base services on the two district hospitals at Bodelwyddan and Wrexham but with a strong emphasis on the expansion and development of its community hospitals, whereas Gwynedd in spite of several working groups which have looked at the topic has been much less enthusiastic about developing its outlying community units. Community hospitals are discussed in detail later.

Hospital beds and the patients within them are an expensive commodity and various ideas have been developed over the last decades to reduce these. The Welsh Health Planning Forum in 1991 wrote that "a proportion of patients in hospital do not require nursing or medical supervision but are "residing" in the hospital awaiting tests and treatment or recovering from some event and many could benefit equally from less expensive accommodation". The concept of patients hotels situated close to the hospital as had been introduced in Scandinavia was studied but was never developed in Wales.

Increasingly diagnostic tests ordered by GPs and by consultants have been carried out as outpatients but some patients still spend too much time in hospital waiting for tests and results. Surgical advances have meant both shorter stays and admission on a day-case basis and have allowed better use of fewer beds. Long term hospital stays have virtually disappeared with discharge to nursing and residential homes or into the community. There remains however considerable misuse of beds because of delays in organisational or financial arrangements for discharge to these alternatives.

Management within hospitals are continually looking for ways to reduce the number of beds and close wards or to convert some into five-day wards dealing with day case surgery only. While this does not at present appear to be affecting services unduly there is considerable anxiety as to how they might cope should an epidemic occur. "Winter pressures" lead to red alerts on admissions.

Many of the changes have been introduced without full consultation with general practice and primary care which have to have to take on the additional workload. Nor have the reasons behind changes been adequately explained to the community. Further changes have recently been out for consultation, based on three major hospital sites only and with the centralisation of certain specialties on one site. Economies of scale together with the requirements for the recognition by the Royal Colleges for the training of junior doctors, essential to attract staff, make this likely in at least some of the specialties and their sub-specialties.

The Penrhyn Bay Practice

Perhaps now is the time to return to my personal narrative.

After seven years in Ruabon I felt the need for a change and experienced the Medical Practices Committee at work again. In December 1966 I applied for a vacancy at Penrhyn Bay, Llandudno, which arose as a result of the single-handed GP, Dr. Lumsden Smith, suffering a heart attack and deciding to retire. The appointment process took its course and I was appointed in mid-February, subject to appeal which did not materialise, and was required to take up the post on April 1st 1967.

The whole process from the heart attack to my taking up the post was three and a half months during which the practice was looked after by locums so I experienced the usual drop in list size as previously described. Over-visiting by one's predecessor, as already described in the Ruabon practice, gives rise to problems for the new doctor who invariably wishes to introduce new ideas and working methods, and for patients on top of their natural anxiety about losing a trusted doctor and old friend. Dr. Lumsden Smith was a gregarious outgoing character who was a great story collector and raconteur and he used to make many home visits, said by some to be a way of getting away from his boisterous children at home. Considerable tact was required at times in the early months.

Dr Lumsden Smith used to live in the centre of the Penrhyn Bay village, although not over the surgery which was a small lock-up in a semi-detached house. He did not have a good relationship with the FPC at Caernarfon and was unwilling to sell or rent his existing surgery to any successor. So there we were with six weeks to find new surgery premises, obtain planning permission for change of use, purchase it and get it operational. This quite apart from finding somewhere to live, and at the same time I was working my notice at Ruabon.

I managed to persuade the local chemist who was shortly to retire that he should sell me his semi-detached house in the centre of the village, but of course he also had to find somewhere to go and move out, which he did on March 31st. I duly held my first surgery on April 1st, which by luck was a Saturday so we only had a morning surgery to cover and then had the weekend to sort ourselves out including transferring the medical records from his old surgery.

The house had a front room which we converted into a waiting room, a room at the rear as consulting room and a kitchen which was in due course partitioned off into an entrance via the rear door and a reception area. One did not need much in the way of office space in those days.

I was also lucky to be able to take on Valerie, his receptionist, only eighteen but who had been there a couple of years and was invaluable during the transfer process and for several years after. Good reception and office staff are invaluable, often insufficiently appreciated, and need to be retained. We were very lucky to have a number of excellent staff over the years and the practice has been a friendly and happy one over the years.

The practice area covered Penrhyn Bay in Caernarfonshire and Rhos-on-sea in Denbighshire, the county border being only half a mile from the surgery. Unfortunately it did mean that administratively one had to deal with two FPCs and send claims to both. In the early years of the Health Service one would have had to use different prescription pads for the two areas but luckily this requirement had by then been negotiated away. We did have to deal with two lots of District Nurses and Health Visitors, as well as two different Social Services departments with differing policies and views. Since it was not infrequent for patients to move to live across the border this did lead to considerable lack of continuity of care at times. Some years later we informally negotiated for our district nurse to cross into Denbighshire but after a while someone in authority found out and the arrangement was stopped.

My wife and I found the house we were looking for, but it was across the county border in Rhos-on-sea. This did not go down at all well with some, and one elderly lady berated me at great length about living so far away. The distance from home to surgery was just over a mile. Again how things have changed since then, with many doctors now living many miles or long travelling times from their work, sometimes until recently only staying within the practice area overnight when on call. Certainly to my knowledge some years ago there was a doctor practicing in Birmingham who commuted daily from London.

Dr Lumsden Smith did all his own on night and weekend on-call, not at all unusual at that time. While researching the possible move from Ruabon I met up with Dr. Nigel Thomas who I had known previously and who was in the three man practice of Drs. Evans, Wainwright and Thomas in Colwyn Bay and after discussions they agreed to forming a four-doctor rota for nights and weekends and also agreed to cover emergencies in my practice during its half-day. I was very grateful for this and it is very doubtful whether I would have moved without this arrangement.

Obviously there were considerable differences practicing as a single-handed doctor rather than as junior partner in a group, but having the availability of an out of hours rota meant that the advantages far outweighed any disadvantages. For a start there was only a single surgery and a single set of medical records. I could organise the practice arrangements to suit myself and no-one changed a patients treatment when I was not looking.

It happened that at exactly the time I took over the practice a major housing estate was being started across the road from the surgery. This had two effects over the next few years, the practice grew but it also meant that a number of younger families came on to the list. Penrhyn Bay had always been very much a residential retirement area and also to some extent because my predecessor had been nearing retirement the list was very heavily loaded towards an older age group. Such retirement areas have been referred to as God's waiting room. This demographic weighting had a considerable influence on my future interests in the care of the elderly. It did however remain heavily weighted towards the elderly to the time I left. The list had 40% of its patients aged 65 or over and 22% over 75, by far the highest ratio in Welsh practices. A doctor from Porthcawl in the South Wales retirement area once bemoaned his 22% of elderly but soon quietened when I gave him our figures. Luckily considering their ages they were a reasonably healthy and active group, although one which wanted attention and their needs attended to. .

By 1973 the practice had grown just too busy and needed a part-time partner. I took on Dr Anne Neville, known to all as Dil, a local Chemist's daughter married to a local dentist and this arrangement worked well for a while.

By now we had outgrown the surgery at Glanymor Road and a large property with garden was bought and converted into a state of the art surgery with two consulting rooms each with a separate examination room, a nurse's treatment room and a room for a Health Visitor, as well as a large office space. Upstairs was converted into a spacious flat. The whole was being financed by myself, at a time of high inflation when borrowing rates were twenty percent p.a. and unfortunately the flat took a long time to sell.

By this time we had been accepted as a vocational training practice and our first trainee Dr Patrick Edwards, who returned later to become a partner, started for six months in 1975.

In early 1977 a small practice at Deganwy three miles away became available. Dr Jack Bell, who ran the practice in partnership with Drs Dennis Wharton, Muriel Hughes, and Robert Rouse at Colwyn Bay some six miles away, had a heart attack and died some time later. After experiencing difficulties in trying to recruit a suitable replacement partner they decided to give up the Deganwy branch of the practice and concentrate on Colwyn Bay. The Deganwy practice was not considered by the Caernarfonshire FPC to be viable as a stand-alone entity and was advertised locally to the Conwy, Llandudno and Penrhyn Bay practices.

With some reservations from my partner Dr Neville we applied and in due course were selected in January 1977 to take it on and the intention was to take in another doctor who was shortly to complete vocational training in South Wales. However at the last minute and for a genuine reason he decided to go to a different practice in North Wales. My former trainee Paddy Edwards was willing to come to join us but he would not complete his training until the end of July. The second bombshell arrived in March just after we took over the practice. Dr Neville gave in her notice as she and her husband Chris were going to emigrate to New Zealand. (In the end they only got as far as Southern England). With one partner leaving, a replacement not available until August, a third partner required, and the new Deganwy branch to hold together with the help of whatever locums I could find life was hectic to say the least for the next few months.

The expansion had been partly triggered by the wish to add a third partner and Dr Elwyn Parry who was also just completing vocational training also joined on August 1st. Two new partners on the same day. It did mean however that a one and a half partner practice had increased to a three man set-up with the addition only of enough patients to finance a half-time partner so there was a considerable shortfall in the early years. This was partly compensated for by Dr Edwards taking on two clinical assistant sessions in Rheumatology at Glan Clwyd Hospital and I was able to obtain two sessions at the geriatric day hospital in Llandudno. One of the problems of a capitation based remuneration system is that adding a partner within a small practice is not financially as easy as in a larger group. In addition and following the tragically early and sudden death of Dr Emyr James from a Llandudno practice we took on the police work described later.

Clinical assistant sessions are an interesting area of hospital medicine, providing support for consultants at a time when they are unable to justify (or to finance) a full-time hospital registrar. They have usually been filled by GPs or by married women who like the strictly limited time commitment. Contractual terms were always inadequate, lowly paid and posts could be terminated at a months notice, even after many years. Clinical assistants were also employed to cover care in consultant, usually geriatric, beds in the peripheral hospitals and in some instances to cover maternity beds. Dr Kenneth Evans was the clinical assistant at the Colwyn Bay maternity unit at Nant-y-glyn covering patients of GPs who did not themselves wish to undertake deliveries there.

Having survived the difficult transition the practice settled down well and flourished and all ran smoothly. Three years later in !980 Elwyn, having previously gained a science degree before turning to medicine, decided to get something out of his system and left to work in pharmaceutical industry research in Cambridge. He subsequently returned to practice in North Wales at Penygroes. Dr Rod Gilmore came to join us in 1980 and he and Paddy Edwards remain in the practice today.

We had also been on the move at the Deganwy end of the practice. The three-storey premises belonging to the previous practice were never satisfactory and I stalled over buying these for a long while looking for a suitable alternative but eventually had to buy. To increase space we had to move to the second floor as well. Eventually in 1990 a large single storey bungalow which we had previously earmarked as a potential surgery came on the market and a further period of planning, building and moving started. We finally moved in 1991.and now had two consulting rooms, allowing a trainee to consult in tandem, a good office and a nurse's suite, and a kitchen together with an overnight room and shower room for trainees on call. We were very happy with the move and so far it has remained of adequate size.

By this time we had needed an additional partner and Dr Bridget Osborne came to work as a part-time partner in 1998 but had to give up working when she had her third child. She returned to work some time later in another local practice, together with undertaking valuable work through the North Wales Medical Trust with junior doctors training arrangements.

When Bridget indicated she wished to leave in 1990 I happened to meet up in the local supermarket with Dr Wendy Brigg, who had previously done some locum work for me and was now working in a Conwy practice. I asked whether she knew of any women doctors living locally who might be available as a replacement. The following day she rang my partner and indicated she would be interested in joining us as a part-time partner. Thankfully no need for prolonged advertising and interviews.

The arrangement worked well and when I myself wished to go half-time on my 60th birthday she moved up to working full-time. At that time regulations allowed GPs to take "24-hour retirement", take an NHS pension and return to the NHS list the following day. This suited me well as at the time my medico-political commitments were considerable and it provided more doctor hours for the practice.

This 24-hour retirement arrangement was popular with many doctors wishing to reduce their workload and perhaps their out-of-hours work. The regulations were subsequently changed making doctors retire for at least a month rather than a day and without the certainty that the FHSA would reinstate them on the list. The situation has changed again with the 2004 contract where the contract is between the LHBs and the practice rather than with individual doctors.

By 1989 we had, like many other practices, again outgrown our premises at Penrhyn Bay and a new surgery was built on a greenfield site right in the centre of the village. Each time we were very fortunate to be able to obtain new premises very centrally and close to our previous ones and after considerable delay we moved in 1993. How long these premises will last remains to be seen but already an extension with an additional consulting room has been added, and a further extension of four rooms is being negotiated. The continual need for upgrading of all practice premises is not so much as a result of massive increase in patient numbers as in the increase in the services offered on site and the increasing number of nursing and administrative staff needed to cope with this. Another factor is the need for space to accommodate those in training including medical students, registrar GPs and nurses.

I continued to work part-time until October 1996 when I finally retired. From what I have heard since I think I had the best years to be in general practice, although perhaps not the most lucrative ones.

Surgery Premises

In the early years of the 20th Century when the concept of State involvement in Health Care and Welfare Services was being developed, leading on to the National Assistance Act of 1911 introduced by Prime Minister David Lloyd George, the concept of Health Centres bringing all community services under one roof was first mooted, the first attempt at the one-stop shop scenario now being actively touted and championed. The important report by Lord Dawson of Penn, the Dawson Report presented to Parliament in 1920, set out a framework for health-care provision in the UK. At that time hospital provision was quite different and embryonic. Hospital care was provided in Voluntary Hospitals and Borough Hospitals or in private hospitals and nursing homes. One of his proposals was for the development of Primary Health Centres providing general practitioner and nursing services with the aid of visiting consultants and specialists. Serving a group of these primary centres were to be Secondary Health Centres with beds and dealing with cases of more difficulty and requiring specialist treatment, the treatment being provided by specialists or by GPs acting in a consulting capacity. Like most reports only parts were adopted and those randomly in different areas.

General practitioners traditionally worked from their own premises, often part of their homes with a consulting room and a dispensary and staffed by their wives or housekeepers, or from a small lock-up surgery provided by themselves. Most were single-handed, sometimes with an assistant. This type of practice was well portrayed in the popular TV series Dr Finley's Casebook in the late sixties. Formerly the practice premises which were sold off at retirement formed part of the doctor's pension fund. General practitioners have since the outset of the Health Service valued highly and fought to retain their independent contractor service contract and the right to run their practices as it suited their neighbourhood and themselves within a loose general framework set down by the service.

The 1946 NHS Act required Health Authorities to build health centres. While some Authorities, particularly in the larger conurbations, developed a number of Health Centres, without beds but with G.Ps, there were only a very limited number developed in North Wales. Those GPs who did work in them were often frustrated because they had little control of their working environment and changes to the premises to suit changing work patterns were dependent on finance being made available within the Authority. Community services have always come below hospitals in the pecking order when finance and priorities have been concerned.

Most GPs provided and financed the premises and their staff. Financing of private surgery premises has changed over the years. In the early days GPs not practicing in health centres were entirely responsible for providing and equipping their own surgeries and the health authority would reimburse the doctors according to a District Valuer's rental assessment, which never appeared generous and frequently gave rise to dispute. The other services including the nurses and the community health doctors, both of whom initially were employed by and came under the control of the County Councils, worked from purpose built clinics or in other rented facilities and even from their homes.

The number of single-handed practices has dropped markedly in most areas over the years. It was only in the fifties and sixties that larger partnerships started to form, needing bigger premises. Improvement grants were introduced. A survey of what was common practice and an indication of what was coming to be accepted as good practice in 1954 can be seen in Stephen Taylor's book Good General Practice. Practices are now much larger and they tend to conform to the norm in their area As a result individuality has often been lost. More staff have been employed, record and computer systems have enlarged, and more hands-on work has been carried out on the premises. Consequently there has developed the need for additional rooms for more nurses, doctors in training, administrative staff and others using the surgery. Space has been a recurring problem for all practices.

Not many completely new premises were built in the early years, many practices finding it more practical to add an extension to their existing premises. The 1966 Contract introduced the concept of cost-rent payments for new-build premises built to approved specifications and budgets and which was in fact an interest-free loan on the capital involved. On completion a cost-rent based on current interest rates was calculated on the total approved cost. Practices had the option of either taking a fixed rate or a variable rate repayment. With the high interest rates in the eighties a decision on this was a significant gamble.

For those practices wishing to buy an existing property and convert to a surgery, as we wished to do at Penrhyn Bay, or to extend their existing premises rather than build from new the cost rent arrangements did not apply. Doctors had to apply for an improvement grant and stick with the Valuer's recommendation. The injustice of this later led to the hybrid cost rent scheme whereby any completely new-build parts were eligible for cost rent payments while the parts which were already existing and were updated had the improvement grant.

Restrictions on the number of rooms and the sizes allowed were set down in the Red Book often resulting in premises being designed down to a schedule and a price and which did not necessarily reflect the true needs of the practice. The regulations did not allow for any forward planning to cover an expected expansion of patient numbers or of an additional partner. Nor did they make allowance for the developments taking place in general practice with increased services being provided on-site way ahead of schedule changes. The additional space needs of training practices, both for a separate consulting room and for library and teaching facilities were not considered. Thus many new premises built were inadequate from the start.

The capital values of surgeries were becoming very high. Problems now arose when incoming partners, particularly the increasing numbers of part-timers and salaried partners, did not wish to take on the leaving doctor's share and the remaining equity partners had to take it on. Fixing a value on premises has been notoriously difficult as many are not of value as anything other than a surgery or for its site value.It was necessary to ensure that no element of "goodwill" was included. Certainly now if doctors wish to invest in property they might gain better returns investing in the commercial property bond markets.

Much tighter control, budgetary and otherwise, from the administration from the LHBs and their control of new surgery provision and developments limits the actions of the practice. As premises have needed to be enlarged building costs have escalated and many practices have been encouraged to develop under the government's Private Finance Initiatives (P.F.I.s). These are however coming under increasing scrutiny particularly within the hospital service for the substantially higher costs incurred over the longer-term. Local Health Boards are now starting to pressurise neighbouring practices to agree to share new premises which also provide other health care resources, not always to the convenience of patients. The advantages of the independent contractor contract. now seem much less attractive.

On an individual basis I have already described the premises in the Ruabon practice and now on moving to Penrhyn Bay, the previous doctor's surgery was not available but in any case inadequate and I faced an urgent dilemma to find one. Over the years there I developed and moved into three new premises, plus two in Deganwy.

By 1975 at the time when the practice consisted of myself and Dr Anne Neville working part-time and with doctors starting their vocational training within the practice we had outgrown the surgery at 6 Glan-y-mor Road and were looking for larger premises. I was fortunate to find a large detached property some 50 yards away on the corner of Penrhyn Isaf Road and St. Davids Road with sufficient land for parking at the rear. Dr Neville was not interested in purchasing a share in the premises so I had to finance it alone. The property was too large for our present needs and I was only eligible for an improvement grant so the development had to be a downstairs surgery and a very large self-contained flat above. At that time mortgage lending rates were in the region of 20% p.a. but rental values on flats were not high so keeping the upstairs would have been uneconomic. The flat had to be sold off, a process which because of the interest rates took some considerable time and a lot of bridging payments to the Bank. Had I been able to keep the upstairs for some years we could have incorporated it into the surgery later and avoided the need for a further new build in 1993 when we again outgrew the premises and moved to Trafford Road. Here again we were lucky to be able to buy a plot right in the centre of the village. There were now three partners together with a steady stream of trainees from the V.T scheme as well as an increased need for space for our practice and attached nurses. We were able to design a property with much of the office space upstairs. We also managed to find space to allow a physiotherapist and an osteopath to work on the premises but again it was too small before we moved in. When we came to building this third new surgery in Penrhyn Bay I knew I was within a couple of years of retirement so I opted not to be part-owner of the property but to pay an appropriate nominal rent to the other partners/owners. This surgery has already had one extension built on and a further four room extension is planned, if finance can be agreed.

In addition to the Penrhyn Bay surgery into which we moved in 1975 we took over the Deganwy practice in 1977. The existing lock-up premises used by the previous practice was a three storey semi-detached house near the centre of the village, with quite inadequate facilities, basically a waiting room and a consulting room. I was able to rent this for a few months while at the same time desperately but unsuccessfully seeking alternative accommodation in the right place. In the end purchase had to be made by the practice and we made do as best we could. Some years later in 1990 a large bungalow which I had had my eyes on as a possible surgery came on the market and we were able to undertake an excellent cost-rent scheme. By this time Paddy Edwards and Rod Gilmore were there to share the work and costs with me. At least all this time we were in Gwynedd and our dealings were with the Gwynedd FPC who were both cooperative and efficient.

Some eighteen practices working in the Clwyd FPC area were not so fortunate and became embroiled in the cost-rent fiasco in late nineties and which still had not been fully resolved in 2006. Many practices in Clwyd were applying to build under the cost-rent scheme and submitted detailed plans and costings based on the Red Book criteria, all discussed in detail with the Clwyd FPC officers and approved. The misinterpretation of the strict parameters of the Red Book in the Clwyd FHSA area led to incorrect approvals being given to practices to proceed Only considerably later was it discovered that the criteria had not been accurately reflected in the cost calculations. In one case approval had been given for a £1million pound build whereas it should have been restricted to £850,000. Building plans would have been modified if the problem had come to light earlier but it was now too late to make corrections as the money was now tied up in bricks and mortar and in daily use by patients. The annual cost-rent payments subsequent to completion in some cases resulted in so-called "overpayments" which when discovered lead to a reduction in future payments and a request to practices to repay what allegedly had been overpaid. For some practices the amounts were relatively small but in some were massive. In some cases partners had retired or moved on in the interim and considerable anxiety resulted for many doctors. Long and detailed negotiations involving BMA lawyers and others over a number of years resulted in reduction or cancelling of the error in some practices but the issue has still not been closed for others. In other fields much larger amounts are written off by authorities.

Following on the collapse of property values in the nineties many practices across the U.K. found themselves in a state of negative equity which gave rise to problems when partners had to be bought out of their share in the premises on retirement, and in assessing the value of shares to be bought by incoming partners. A new situation was also arising with the number of doctors who did not see a particular practice as a lifetime commitment and of the increase of part-time partners, men and women, who did not wish to commit themselves to investing in surgery property.

Later because sufficient capital funds were not available within the health service the concept of building through Private Finance Initiatives (PFIs) was introduced for both secondary care and GP surgery developments. Private developers were contracted to build, maintain and lease premises to the NHS over long periods, allowing developments to occur but at considerable extra long-term cost to the NHS. Many practices have over the years run branch surgeries, some dating from the time when transport was not so universally available, some when new major housing estates were being built, and some like ours from takeovers or amalgamation of practices. Many of these have now served their purpose and are inadequate for today's needs and practices are applying for permission to close them to allow the practice to provide a centralised service, a move often opposed by local communities although attendances have diminished and only very limited services can be provided at them. Woodrow Wilson is quoted as saying "If you want to make enemies, try to change something".

In our case both premises provided a full twice a day surgery service and there was no thought of closing either. Running on two major sites does however have considerable additional medical nursing and administrative manpower and financial implications which are not recognised within the regulations. A number of North Wales practices have this problem which we have not been able to resolve satisfactorily.

Why have all these premises changes been necessary in Penrhyn Bay, and in most other GP practices? The answer is in the number of people working in them and what is carried out there, rather than a great increase in patient numbers. Probably the biggest problem within general practice at present is that of the inadequate space in the premises and often the impossibility of expanding them within the present sites. In addition to the increase in the number of partners, each requiring a consulting room, there is often the need for space to accommodate doctors in training, registrars and increasingly now medical students, practice nurses, attached district nurses and health visitors, social workers and counsellors. The latest government suggestion for adding to the list are visiting specialists and advisers on state benefits. All of these will require additional waiting areas and administrative staff to run their appointments and support them. Most existing sites could not cope.

While one solution may be to centralise all in one large "health centre "first proposed by Lord Dawson in 1920 this would only be acceptable in urban conurbations. In North Wales centralisation and closure of surgeries in many towns would not be acceptable to the public or to the doctors. While amalgamation of small and inadequate surgeries on to one site may be a good idea in some urban areas and some South Wales valleys, in North Wales the majority of practice premises are of good quality, although admittedly too small, and well sited to serve their communities.

In latter years the concept of an estates strategy within the NHS has been introduced and this now extends to GP premises. The restrictions, budgetary and administrative, of this has meant that long delays have been introduced and that premises which have been in a planning stage by practices for years have now been stopped. Pressure, sometimes subtle, sometimes bullying, is being applied to practices to agree to move against their wishes into shared premises which are unlikely to be built for years. In the interim many practices find themselves unable to fulfil their obligations under Disability legislation amongst others because of this lack of funding. Local LHBs share the concerns of GPs and the LMC but a change of thinking at Assembly and Regional levels appears necessary if the potential for primary care to take on many of the services now provided by the secondary care services is to be fulfilled.

Medical records

Part of the reason for the increasing need for space within the surgery premises has been tied up with the storage and handling of medical records. The first National Insurance Act in 1911 setting up an embryonic Health Service included the introduction of a medical record envelope record, five inches wide by seven long. It has persisted largely unchanged until now. Originally made of reinforced linen it was later reduced to stiffened paper and is still in regular use in some practices although in many practices it has been superseded by A4 size records and now in most by computerised records. The only major change to the medical envelope over many years was the addition of a gusset to accommodate the fat files which became much commoner as communication from secondary care became more frequent. Hospitals have continued to send out reports on paper which does not fit easily into the envelopes. Letters from consultants and hospitals have varied very considerably in shape and size, with no consistency. All required at least one fold and most two or even three, private reports on high quality paper taking up even more space. At one time we attempted to persuade hospitals to send reports in memo form without the big headings with the hospital administrative details taking up a large amount of the paper. Considerable savings could have been made on hospital budgets. Many practices adopted the use of guillotines to try to reduce the size before filing but this was time consuming and not always easy.

Even in the new computerised records the old past correspondence and record cards needed to be stored as part of the overall record as the newer systems generally did not deal adequately with past history details. Many attempts have been made by practices to edit and destroy old reports and test results to reduce bulk, a time-consuming procedure which it is not easy to delegate, especially as medico-legally cases can in some circumstances be brought many years later. Obstetric records need to be retained for 25 years, records relating to persons under 18 should be retained until the age of 25 or eight years after the last entry. Records of mentally disordered persons need to be kept for 20 years after no further care is necessary. All other personal care health records should be retained for eight years after the conclusion of the treatment, while the minimum time for a person who has died is also eight years. These difficulties resulted in records becoming even bulkier and more difficult to take out and stuff back into the old type record envelopes.

Microfiche records have been used in archives in other circumstances elsewhere for many years although there has never been any suggestion that they might be introduced into general medical practice.

In the earlier pre-NHS days the records were of a very simple nature, patients and their families were less mobile and were generally well known to the doctors in the practices, many of which were single-handed. Referrals to hospital and specialist care were very infrequent because specialists were largely based in the larger conurbations and often had to be paid for privately. Even in the 1950`s there were specialists such as the surgeon Mr Hywel Hughes and the cardiologist Dr Emyr Wyn Jones who worked in Liverpool and were called in to see patients in their homes in N.Wales as required and, except for the wealthy, only in extreme emergency or difficulty. The consultation was so memorable, with the GP present and traditionally discussing the case immediately afterwards as hands were washed and before the verdict was given to the patient and relatives, that there was really no need for written communication.

The pharmacopoeia at this time was also so restricted, mainly digitalis, purgatives and a selection of simple medicines dispensed in the surgery from a series of Winchester bottles. The main need was to remember what colour the last medicine was and whether it satisfied the patient. Faith in the bottle was all important to recovery.

The other important role of the medical record pre-NHS was to indicate, often only by a tick, a C or a V, that a consultation or visit had been made and therefore potentially chargeable.

The use of A4 size records similar to those in hospital practice was introduced in the seventies allowing potentially better access to past history, reports and investigations. At the same time attempts were made by the College of GPs to devise structured recording with summary sheets recording significant past events, and structured consultation recording based on SOAP, (Symptoms, Objective findings, Advice, Prescription) but with average consultations at that time lasting three to four minutes one had to be very methodical and obsessive to adhere regularly to the protocols.

Since the A4 record itself at that time cost the government about £1 each and there were 50 million records in the UK to be changed, the new records were only made available in Wales to practices on special request. That cost did not of course include the considerable time to transfer data from one record to another which the GP had to finance. In our practice we decided that the only practical solution was to start by using A4 envelopes only for newborn babies without any previous history and build from there. Another problem was the storage of the larger records, new and bulkier cabinets being needed. Storage space in most surgeries was at a premium. There was also the feeling in 1979 that the new fangled silicon chip would make written records unnecessary. Perhaps we are now starting to see the beginning of this. A4 never really took off in many practices and a position developed where as patients moved practice a mixture of old-style, A4 (with old envelopes pushed in) and later computerised records became intermixed.

The whole change from Lloyd George envelopes through A4 to computerised records has been characterised by a lack of central direction and policy, and because records move with the patient individual practices have found difficulty in achieving their ideal solution.

Some very special letters are occasionally found on reading old notes. They would certainly not pass the test of political correctness today. One obstetrician noted for his wit once sent our practice a letter about a patient of somewhat uncertain morals who he was seeing with a pregnancy or a miscarriage for the umpteenth time. He wrote only

> *Dear Doctor*
>> *Jo Goode*
>> *says she would*
>> *like to be good*
>> *I wish she would*
>> *She really should.*
>>> *Yours*
>>> *Owen Jones*

Coming across this letter in her records some time later with the patient sitting across the desk required a considerable effort not to smile. Today he would probably be suspended. Another letter from the same doctor who had seen a fifty year old Italian lady with an abdominal swelling thought to be fibroids but who was in fact pregnant wrote

>> *Mrs De Pesta*
>> *had a fiesta*
>> *in her siesta*
>>> *Yours*

Many statements in letters which today would be considered derogatory did give one a sense of how the consultation had gone and whether it had been a dysfunctional one. There has recently been a spate of correspondence in medical circles about the use of terms such as "this pleasant lady" and whether the practice should stop. The Access to Health Records Act of 1990_allowing the patient the right to see their records has put a stop to such comments, but has also stopped doctors adding speculative but often very useful thoughts or information (often strictly confidential) about other family members or relationships as an aide-memoire in a patient's record.

The working of the Act has in itself caused many problems for doctors and for reception staff because patients have been led to believe that they can see their records on demand and immediately. Solicitors have been guilty of requesting complete records as a "fishing exercise" rather than information about the issue in question and have not always ensured that the patient has given true informed consent to disclosure.

Quite apart from the actual words written the problem of inadequate communication letters from hospital to GP, and in the other direction, has for many years been a source of much frustration, of wasted time and it must be said of medical errors or potential errors and shows no signs of being solved. Indeed in many ways it is now much worse with many patients having admissions and even surgery never having a discharge summary written about them. Lack of secretarial time or change in the junior doctors contracts have been cited as reasons. Consultants themselves claim that delays in sending out reports are frequently the result of secretarial shortage and many are resorting to including the date the report was dictated as well as the date the letter is typed.

It is surprising that with more complex treatment regimes and in an increasingly litigious society no one in authority seems to feel there is a need to act across the board. Examples of illegible discharge notes or prescription copies are frequent, and others do not always contain the necessary and correct patient identification. information. Letters were unfortunately still being sent out to patients long deceased causing distress to families or to doctors who have long retired from a practice. Hospitals in responding say that the letter from GPs on admission is also inadequate, but usually much information has been communicated over the phone while arranging an emergency admission. The problem now is that the information is given to a different person, not always a doctor, from the one who actually sees the patient. By definition almost, emergency admission letters are written in difficult circumstances, often not by the regular doctor, and without the medical records to hand. Perhaps patient held records or at least a summary, but only if carried at all times, would be a step forward. Any patient-held record which may be one way forward must of course be kept up to date or otherwise it may be potentially dangerous.

As more and more practices move to computerised paper records the need to extend the present pathology and x-ray reporting on-line to discharge and consultation records must be a priority. It will then be possible for authorised persons to link-in to both the hospital laboratory and the practice computer at all times.

With the development of new out-of-hours arrangements and the encouragement of patients to use NHS Direct and with out-of-hours arrangements sometimes covering periods of days at a time, the need for access to patient records becomes more necessary. Of course the issues of confidentiality then become even more complex. What appears strange is that there has never over many years been any attempt by government or health authorities to involve patients and their representatives in any discussion of the whole problem of medical records, their content, who has access to them and for what purpose. Strangely although the GMSC and the GPC have frequently drawn the issues to the attention of the public their representative organisations have been slow to respond and appear to have been less worried about the issue than have the profession. Recent legislation in the Access to Records Act and the Data Protection Act and more recently in the Freedom of Information Act has complicated the day to day running of the practice for doctors and for the whole team While their seems no problem of access to notes and computer records for practice employed staff who have been trained in the intricacies of the Acts including exemptions a more difficult situation exists for access by Trust-employed staff such as district nurses and health visitors who may be unknown to the practice. These may well need to access details but ideally they should also be able to input data to provide a complete patient record.

The need for strict confidentiality is even more essential in rural areas where there is only one practice to choose from and where staff may be handling information about their families and friends.

In my experience families do not always appreciate the confidentiality issue and are sometimes very surprised when one refuses to answer their questions. Husbands may casually but legitimately ask about their spouse, usually if one knows the family one knows their attitudes and when to discuss, at times one is specifically asked not to tell the spouse and this can cause problems. Occasionally one needs to consider whether information provided should be include in the records or not. Reception staff are frequently rung for test results and some practices have rules that these can only be given to the patients themselves. This as one knows well from similar requirements in other fields where the Data Protection Act is quoted can be very irritating. In all these situations commonsense and practicality has to come in and all must work within sensible but flexible guidelines. Unfortunately current trends are for laying down strict guidelines on everything, with their inherent difficulties.

Further anxieties are arising when non-medical administrative staff from the health authority wish to see medical records, on occasions to check claims for possible fraud. A consultation paper on this issue has given rise to strong criticism from both the Faculty of Occupational Health and from the Medical Defence bodies, and safeguards will need to be written in.

The issues of confidentiality can be summarised in a quotation from one of the Defence Bodies " If patients cannot be sure that their information will be kept confidential, they may be reluctant to give doctors the information they need to provide good care "

A new problem is arising from the development of walk-in clinics available to patients unable to attend their own practices, perhaps because of commuting or their working patterns. If such clinics deal only with minor illness and emergencies then good communication afterwards can deal with the problem, but if these clinics start to provide a continuing follow-up of chronic illness then the incompleteness of available records will be a potential hazard. The strength of British general practice has been based on being the only holders of the complete medical history.

General practice as we have known it with the GP acting as gatekeeper to services and holding the only complete record of a patients medical history and care is under threat by the plethora of different providers of health care developing separate pathways. There is a move to a central national record, or partial record, although there appears to be a limited amount which will be available on this, while detailed records continue to be still kept locally. There are still major discussions required about whether this is acceptable to the public, what is held where and in particular who, and under what circumstances, will have access to the record.

Only time will tell how these issues will pan out.

Computerisation in practices

It seems so long ago that we started to introduce computers into general practice, the first discussions were about 1981, and for many years there was no active encouragement by government for practices to computerise. Things were allowed to develop piecemeal by enthusiasts in various practices across the country, sometimes with the assistance of commercial firms. The Department of Health had sponsored the Exeter system which recorded consultations for the first time, and in 1982 another government sponsored scheme Micros for GPs put computers into 150 selected practices

A major advance took place in 1987 when two major companies, VAMP and Meditel, offered free computer systems and training to practices in exchange for a commitment over a number of years to accurately record all consultations, diagnoses and prescriptions, providing information on incidence and prevalence not at that time available elsewhere and of considerable marketing value. Data was extracted by the firms every three months entirely anonymously and confidentially. A number of North Wales practices took up the offer including ours in Penrhyn Bay. We opted for the VAMP system but there was little to choose between them. Luckily my partners were all keen and enthusiastic to pursue the project but I know some practices where problems arose because one or more partners refused to cooperate or were less than diligent in entering data. Obviously much of the data outside the consultation would be entered by reception staff and again some were capable of learning the new skills while others had to be taken away from this area and re-deployed elsewhere. User groups were established for both doctors and staff for mutual support but also to provide feedback to the firms. for system development

This cooperation with the industry continued until the nineties. By 1993 there were 50 commercial systems to choose from. and 8500 practices had some system in place. During this time no central departmental guidelines or specifications for computer systems were laid down.

The Arthur Anderson Report in the late eighties studied the Family Practitioner Services administration and their use of computers but did nor look into general practice systems except in their communication with the FPC. It expected that practices would select and operate their own systems. One of its recommendations was the introduction of new personal NHS numbers to be used throughout the health service. We are just about there now. It also discussed the extended role of the pharmacist and pharmacy held records, another concept developing over the last few years, but to be really effective this would require patients to register and use one pharmacy exclusively and this has never been proposed.

To enter data into computers and particularly to allow easy extraction of data an acceptable coding system is necessary. Hospital disease coding has for years been based on an ICD (International Coding of Disease) system but this was quite useless as a recording system for general practice where many consultations were for conditions never seen in specialist practice and many more came into the Not Yet Diagnosed category and where symptoms rather than a diagnosis had to be entered. Dr James Read a general practitioner began to develop his own code which was later purchased by the NHS and which has gradually been improved and expanded. Unfortunately new detailed codes are not being developed rapidly enough to allow for accurately recording details the government require for targets.

One of the major advantages of computerisation now is the transfer of pathology and x-ray results on-line from hospitals, resulting in quicker receipt but also meaning that results do not have to be typed in from paper reports with the possibility of error. It has become so much easier to check against previous results to assess progress. Unfortunately the system is not yet sufficiently advanced to allow all tests done by hospital doctors in outpatients or inpatients to be sent to the GP, giving an incomplete record and very often leading to unnecessary duplication, added inconvenience to patients and considerable avoidable cost. Hospital consultants locally still cannot access laboratory results electronically but have to ring the laboratory.

A view often expressed by patients when computers entered the consulting room was that that their doctor was continually looking at the computer screen instead of at them and listening. This was indeed very true especially so if doctor was not very confident or competent with the computer system or, as was usually the case, a poor typist. Unless one is very careful a wrong code will be entered and present the patient with a completely new illness.

Depending on the layout of the desk and consulting room patients could sometimes view the screen and read what was being entered. In the early days certainly many doctors did not like this but in the new era of openness and transparency this is no longer seen as such a problem. Doctors are more careful now of what they write and avoid the snide comments previously seen.

The setting of targets in areas such as smears and immunisation has certainly focussed attention on completeness of recording and the new 2004 contract with its various quality issues has reinforced this.

While computerisation in general practice is still in its developmental stage there is no doubt it is light years ahead of any hospital computerisation. Where that exists it tends to be Department based and not linked into a complete patient record. A major disadvantage remained that much of the patient's past history had not been adequately transferred to the computer record although the main significant problems may have been recorded, and the old paper records have needed to be kept easily available. A further problem at the outset was that the computerised information had to be printed out on to paper and sent to a new practice when a patient moved. If the new practice was computerised the information then needed to be re-entered. When a patient moved practices the old doctor did not know where the new practice with which a patient was registering was and could not check on the state of computerisation within it. Having records on computer does create problems at times when solicitors seek information and where only information relevant to the enquiry needs to be sent. Sometimes the record can include confidential information about another person. Previously it was easier to photocopy only a relevant entry or letter. Obviously the situation changes rapidly but a much more effective system could have been developed if more central steer had been given to computer development from the start rather than leaving it to commercial sources.

In the late eighties the COMCARE- Community Care Computer System, was introduced for the use of district nurses and other community workers. Apart from giving a master index and information about all patients/clients under care and naming those involved in the care it recorded management rather than clinical information and did not appear to be of much use to our nurses.

In 1992 our practice started to use the early hand-held computers produced by Psion for carrying information and later in 1993 we experimented with using our rudimentary Nokia mobile phones to link in to our practice computer records from a patients home, helpful at times but the information accessible was very limited.

The next obvious development in record keeping may well be some sort of patient-held credit-card sized computer record, carrying major problems together with prescribing data. This concept will be no doubt fall foul of personal liberty guardians in the same way as the proposed personal identity cards. This is not an entirely new concept in Wales. Back in the late seventies a pilot scheme was run between the Pricing Authority in Cardiff and a pharmacist (a Mr. Strawbridge if I recall correctly) in Pontypridd where all the medication and repeat prescriptions were recorded on a credit-card carried by patients. This experiment was apparently quite successful but the cost if generally introduced would have been about £5 per card, a significant sum at that time if extrapolated to all patients in Wales, and the scheme never saw the light of day. It may be time for it to arise phoenix-like from the ashes as the potential benefits and also savings are considerable.

Having a computer on the desk and with immediate access to the internet and the secure NHS intranet, means that today's doctor can immediately access the latest clinical information about any condition or treatment, and can also print out any appropriate leaflets for the patient. The Government believes that with its concept of a single computerised system covering the UK it will be possible for a doctor also to access any hospital in the country to check waiting times and make appointments, the Choose and Book system, but most doctors remain very sceptical about this at least in the next few years. The pilots in England are already two years behind schedule and three times over budget. Consultation times will have to be increased and much work and finance will have to be put in before such ideas are practical.

Wales is tackling the problem of access to medical records in a more practical way, in bite-size chunks and by developing systems in cooperation with users including patient groups. One of the obvious needs was for doctors to be able to access clinical information and medication history in the emergency care situation out of hours. Since ninety per cent of attendances involve local people attending local hospitals there is no need for a national database. A system has been developed and successfully introduced in Gwent and will shortly become available in North Wales. The safeguards introduced resulted in only thirty-seven patients out of a total of six hundred thousand opting out. Other interface areas are being developed.

GPs and the LMC require an enthusiast to be continually monitoring new developments both nationally and within local hospitals making sure they are acceptable and practical. The LMC locally is leaning increasingly on Dr Dafydd Morris to do this for them.

Practice Nursing

In earlier years practices did not employ their own nursing staff working on the premises, anything done there in the way of dressings and injections was done by the doctor personally. Sometimes these tasks were even carried out during home visits. There were the district nurses employed by the local authority health department under the Medical Officer of Health who worked in patients homes, sometimes from their own homes or from a clinic. They were sometimes contacted directly by patients or neighbours, at others they carried out work at the request of the GP or hospital. In some areas the two met from time to time, in other areas particularly in the towns doctor and nurse rarely met. Each nurse had a patch or district to cover, irrespective of which GP was looking after the patient and there could be twenty or more doctors on a patch.

As practices evolved and premises improved some district nurses started to do part of their work such as dressings and routine injections in the surgery which was often mutually convenient for patient and nurse. Gradually bureaucracy took charge and rules were laid down by their employers as to what they could or could not do, and when. They might also be withdrawn from the surgery without notice to cover absences elsewhere or to attend a course or meeting, leaving the work to be done by the GP. On one occasion I recall the reason for a nurse's non-appearance was that she had to be fitted for a new uniform. This led to frustration amongst GPs and to the direct employment of a nurse by practices, even though this was at a considerable expense. Practices moved at different speeds depending on the local situation and whether they had suitable accommodation or not. By 1974 the district nurses were employed by the Health Authorities and later by the Hospital Trusts, who took differing viewpoints on whether their nurses could provide services within the surgery or not. Nurses themselves also had their own ideas as to whether they wanted to do this and whether they thought this was part of their work or not, and a very piecemeal situation existed across the same districts.

With improved patient transport and improved facilities and equipment much of the work carried out at home could now be better done at a surgery. The nursing workload within the home changed markedly as patients came out of hospital in a much better state than in the past and required much less follow up care. The workload within the surgery increased substantially when vaccinations and injections were taken over from the infant welfare clinics, when patients preferred to attend at a time suitable to them rather than wait at home for the nurse to attend for removal of stitches and dressings, and when regular routine checks on blood pressure and urine became commonplace. Even if dressings were done by the district nurse it was necessary from time to time to inspect progress and redress wounds and in particular chronic varicose ulcers and to reassess treatment. The early practice nurses were frequently considered as being the doctor "handmaiden", carrying out simple tasks at the direction of the doctor. In 1988 there were relatively few of them, five years later a census showed that there were fifteen thousand, and the number has increased considerably since then.

In recent years the practice nurse has taken on much more advanced roles carrying out much of the work previously done, or not done, by the doctor. With the extended role absences need to be covered by someone of equal skills and knowledge. Obviously a nursing presence is not possible in branch surgeries and perhaps this is another reason for closing them.

In 1994 the UKCC put forward a definition of the role "As one of the specific areas for specialist community health care nursing, general practice nurses provide care for individuals and groups within the practice populations, demonstrating a wide spectrum of professional activity. This range of intervention potentially includes the provision of care with the nurse as the first point of contact to undifferentiated patients and clients; initiation of health teaching; routine health checks and screening programmes to all age groups; provision of counselling and psychological assessment; management of chronic diseases and the maintenance of patient care programmes and health promotion activities. This role may contribute to the wider public health function". A quantum leap from the early nurse who just did dressings.

Before practice nurses became more numerous and widely established they felt isolated and with no colleague support. Although they belonged to the Royal College of Nursing they felt this did not provide for their needs and wished for some local organisation to support them. With the support of the LMC and the N.Wales RCGP Faculty they formed two groups, one in the West and one in the East. The Faculty presented a prize annually for the best practice work project submitted. It was also involved in setting up a practice nurse training school in Wrexham, the first in Wales.

At the same time the GMSC and the RCGP centrally and LMCs locally were working to develop primary health care teams, to get a team of health professionals with a continuous membership based on a practice, working from one base at the surgery and sharing the same patient list. While this would seem to be a sensible working relationship many difficulties were encountered along the way, usually by middle management but sometimes from individuals who did not wish to change their ways.

Practice nursing developed at different speeds in different practices, some initially employed a nurse at a fairly low grade to do relatively simple tasks and often the nurse did not wish to expand her role. Other nurses saw a much more progressive and challenging role, started to go on specialist courses such as asthma, diabetes, hypertension and the taking of cervical smears, and gradually took on more responsibility for the care of these patients. They also took responsibility for the annual influenza vaccination programmes and for the increasing demand for travel advice and immunisations. Patients often appreciated this as the nurses had longer appointment slots than the GP and more time to explain in detail. Similar developments were taking place within some hospital departments, in particular in ophthalmology, accident and emergency, and medical clinics and the new grade of nurse practitioner was introduced.

We at the Penrhyn Bay surgery employed our first practice nurse in 1980. Mrs Hilary Squires was already a highly experienced nurse in several fields and she started to develop an extended role very early on.we were very fortunate to take on a succession of excellent nurses, a succession only because they moved away from the area, and this made for better patient care but also an opportunity for the doctor to pass over unpopular jobs, and at times unpopular patients as well.

The new role which they were undertaking meant that they were frequently required to interrupt the doctor to get prescriptions signed. After considerable pressure the concept of nurse prescribing was introduced following the Crown Report in 1989. Only a limited range of items were initially included in the Nurse Prescribers' Formulary and Drug Tariff, although this will no doubt expand gradually. Unfortunately the legislation as written stated that the only nurses allowed to prescribe were those with a District Nursing or a Health Visiting qualification which excluded the great majority of practice nurses.

The increasing role of the practice nurse meant that there was a huge gap if she was away, and so more than one nurse was required. There was also the need for induction and continuing training of new practice nurses and, with the enthusiastic support of the FHSA, some established nurses were appointed mentors. It was the first time that nurses had been taught by those who had practical experience of working in a practice.

District nurses attend patients as required in residential homes but are not allowed into registered nursing homes who are required to have their own nurses to cover their needs. However there were occasions when the Nursing Homes would welcome the practice nurse in to discuss the practices` policy on night sedation, on incontinence, and other issues and this was informally encouraged to mutual benefit.

In a service situation where certain procedures such as immunisation and influenza vaccinations attracted a fee and procedures like cervical smears attracted target payments the nurse could contribute considerably to the practice income. In some practices the district nurses objected to giving flu vaccinations in the home because of this, forgetting that the practice nurse by doing dressings was helping their workload. Nursing management were loathe to recognise this.

Patient demand for same-day access to a doctor is not always possible and practices are now using a practice nurse working to agreed protocols to see, advise and treat minor and self-limiting illnesses, referring to the doctor when appropriate.

An important document produced in 1998 by a working party of RCGP Welsh Council, the WGMSC and the Welsh Practice Nurses Association and chaired by Dr Huw Lloyd gave considerable guidance on roles and responsibilities. It also suggested possible new options for contractual relationships. The expanding role of the practice nurse is making some doctors realise that they should share in the increased income which they are generating. With the new 2004 arrangements where the contract is between the LHB and the practice rather than with individual doctors as in the past this may lead to practice nurses, or Sisters as they are increasingly being called, becoming profit-sharing partners.

The Primary Health Care Team

GPs have over the years worked closely as and when required with district nurses, midwives and health visitors, sometimes more effectively than others, personalities and differing employment status playing important parts in the relationships.the concept of developing a team has been around since before 1986, has taken a long time to formally establish at local levels and has given rise to much discussion and differences of opinion. Even the definition of the team has been argued over.

One of the aims has been to provide a better service for patients through effective team working and to reduce the need to attend hospital clinics and follow-up.

The Government published "Primary Health Care-an Agenda for Discussion together in England with the Cumberlege report "Neighbourhood Nursing-a Focus for Care. Even though health matters had not at that time been devolved to Wales the Welsh Office commissioned the Edwards Report " Nursing in the Community" which was published at the same time in 1988 to reflect the different communities in Wales.

Our report in Wales, written by an widely experienced nurse, was considered a better way forward than the English document and was widely welcomed. Mrs Noreen Edwards had been matron of our local maternity unit at Colwyn Bay, our local hospital, chairman of the Gwynedd Health Authority for ten years as well as having held the chair of the Royal College of Nursing and she had a good grasp of the Welsh scene.

While Neighbourhood Nursing suggested that the effectiveness of the PHCT needed to be improved it also proposed that community nursing services should be planned on a geographical neighbourhood basis. The latter proposal may have been appropriate to inner city areas with poorly developed practices but not to other areas. The Social Services Select Committee of the House of Commons while giving it a cautious welcome expressed a hope that it would not be implemented rigidly.

Many documents and papers have been produced about the structure and work of the PHCT, complicated at times because sometimes they refer to Primary Health Care and sometimes (occasionally in the same sentence) to Primary Care which involves a much wider spectrum of interests which include social services but also other local authority provided services

Other members of the nursing team with work bordering on the practice nurse are the district midwives, the health visitors and more recently the community psychiatric nurses, all of whom work with patients in the community. Sometimes nursing management insisted that they be patch -based looking after patients of many doctors, at other times they were practice based but because they were health authority rather than practice employed they were subject to movement, absences or withdrawal without notice.

Health visitors in particular were often much more elusive and certainly in the earlier days when they were running infant welfare clinics with a public health doctor they were often competing with the doctor for the child and advice was not coordinated and sometimes conflicting.

It now seems to be generally accepted that there is an inner core team of doctors, practice nurses, community (previously district) nurses, health visitors and perhaps midwives although some midwives see themselves as working completely independently of other professionals except when they wish to involve them. Others who belong to an outer orbit and may because of scarcity work a neighbourhood and relate to a number of teams are social workers, psychiatric nurses, psychiatric social workers and counsellors, and school nurses.

One of the most important objectives needs to be that everyone's role and responsibilities within the team should be discussed and agreed, together with the establishment of effective communication channels.

Development has been hindered at times because of the different contractual employment status of members of the team, some employed by doctors and indirectly funded by Health Authorities, some employed by the Trusts and some by local authorities. I recall discussions at GMSC level back in the eighties about the possibility of district nurses being employed by GPs but this was thought not to be advisable or practicable, one of the reasons being the potential financial risk to the doctors arising from the high sickness and injury rate of district nurses with bad backs at that time. Heavy lifting is not as prevalent as it then was and in fact it is often the carers who do the heavy lifting many times a day, the task literally falling on the backs of carers.

District midwives were more numerous in my early years of practice and home deliveries were common. Much of antenatal care had been traditionally run by hospital specialists in weekly or monthly clinics, sometimes in village halls, and some of which were referred to by patients as cattle markets. Everyone attended at the same time, were weighed and had their urine tested. They then sat around in dressing gowns with their stockings rolled down to their ankles to wait for the doctor to arrive, which could often be an hour or so late if hospital commitments or road traffic caused a delay. In the late fifties some doctors started to sit the diploma examination in obstetrics, the D.Obst RCOG, and the Diploma in Child Health, the DCH, and with better premises felt they could provide a better and more convenient and patient-friendly system within the surgery. Again there was at times competition for patients as attendance numbers were important to the clinics.

I sat and passed the obstetrics Diploma in 1960 and the fact that I held this led to quite unfounded rumours which seemed to erupt from time to time in Ruabon, and years later in Penrhyn Bay, that I was leaving to become a hospital specialist. On one occasion a lady who I did not immediately recognise came up to me in the street and thanked me most profusely for the excellent care I had given to her daughter who had just had a baby. I gratefully accepted the plaudits but was still unsure who her daughter was. A few days later I discovered that a new obstetrician had started at Wrexham Hospital, that his name was Arnold Humphreys, and that it was he who deserved the praise. Hospitals then as now were slow to let GPs know about new consultant appointments. Often the only notification received was a card from the consultant indicating that he was available for private consultations. Arnold and I had something else in common apart from the name, we both drove Kharmann Ghia conversions of the old Volkswagen Beetle.

Home deliveries as well as deliveries in the GP maternity unit at Llangollen Hospital six miles away from Ruabon were still reasonably common and gave me considerable pleasure and satisfaction as well as anxieties and panics at times. There was an obstetric flying squad based at Wrexham but most of the time one had to deal with one's own emergencies which included haemorrhages and the use of obstetric forceps. At such times it is vital to have a cool and experienced midwife and we were very fortunate in Ruabon to have such a paragon in Sister Parrish. There has been much talk of team development and bonding over the last few years, but there is nothing comparable to the bonding which occurs while sitting with a nurse and a patient in labour or in the process of dying.

In later years the midwives would carry out clinics in the surgery but all deliveries were out of our hands in the specialist unit. Home deliveries became rare but a few expectant mothers would insist against advice on being delivered at home. Midwives were in danger of being frustrated and de-skilled and a "domino" system was developed allowing the district midwife to go into the specialist unit with the mother in labour and deliver her there. Mother and baby would normally be home some six hours later. Recently home deliveries have been increasing again and last year 3.5% of births occurred at home, up from 2.5% the previous year.

Community psychiatric nurses were a new breed of nurse, thin on the ground and working initially mainly with the consultants. Their ability to change drugs and dosage without reference to a doctor gave rise to some conflict at times because the GP was legally responsible for any medication he issued prescriptions for. More recently they have become much more team based as much of psychiatry has become primarily a GP field of responsibility but recruitment and retention remains a problem. They are still too thin on the ground.

Perhaps one of the more helpful members of the extended team are the Macmillan nurses who provide valuable support to patients and their families suffering from potentially fatal illnesses. We were particularly fortunate for some years to have Mrs Margaret Cooper working on our patch in Penrhyn Bay and Rhos-on-sea and we found her assistance invaluable. Since many people immediately associated the name Macmillan nurse with terminal care and would immediately start to get upset and panicky it was usually better to introduce her, or for her to introduce herself, initially in a different way and allow a relationship to develop and for the concept of hospice care to be raised in due time. We were fortunate in my later years that the St Davids Hospice was developed at Llandudno and others opened at St Asaph and at Wrexham. Their role and development is discussed later.

Social workers have always been on the fringe of the team, they originally started as the lady almoners working in the hospitals. Later psychiatric social workers and those employed in the Children's Officers departments worked only within their specialties. The Seebohm Inquiry in 1968 changed all that by introducing the concept of generic social workers who were generalists and employed by local authorities under a Director of Social Services. This was a disaster as far as we in practice were concerned. I recall an occasion when my urgent request for someone to attend a psychiatrically acutely disturbed patient brandishing a knife in an isolated garden with a view to urgent admission under a Section order resulted in a social worker attending who had until recently dealt only with children, who had never seen a disturbed patient and did not understand the legal procedures for admission. The young police constable who also attended was no better. Certainly for years after we felt severely the loss of our very effective and cooperative mental welfare officer with his contacts with the psychiatric hospital.

For some years many of the social workers were not formally trained or qualified although this gradually changed, not always for the better, when they took degrees at Colleges. In the end and for a relatively short time we did have a very helpful and sensible social worker as part of the team - but she retired.

Confidentiality of information about patients has been a particular anxiety amongst doctors, both at local and at central levels. Problems arose because of the relationship of social workers with their employers. While doctors would often share information with the social worker in confidence on a "need to know basis" very often the outcome of their subsequent visits would not be fed back.

At national level Departments of Health and of Social Services have been amalgamated but no re-organisation has taken the bull by the horns and brought the NHS and social services locally under the same umbrella. Fundamental organisational and attitude problems persist and so prevent them becoming full members of the Primary Care Team.

A vital part of the team are the practice administrative staff who now undertake considerable work to support the whole team including the attached staff. Receptionists have had a bad press as the dragon at the gate preventing access to the doctor but the ways they work are according to policies laid down by the team. Regrettably in recent years they have been receiving significantly more verbal abuse, and in places actual physical abuse while carrying out their duties. The increase in abuse of health care staff at all levels by patients and often their relatives or friends and in all situations continues to cause worry

The team continues to get bigger gets bigger, with the potential danger that organisation can become fragmented unless everyone's role is clearly defined and communication is good. The days when a doctor's wife could step in to cover absences have long gone. Practice managers are now almost more important than the doctors in the successful running of a practice.

Relationships with professional colleagues

Contact and dialogue with the other caring professions, dentists, pharmacists, opticians, physiotherapists and others have been surprisingly infrequent, sporadic and unstructured except on a personal level. In some cases this has been because of their commercial and private practice status, in others because of different employment status. In many cases contacts only occur, usually at the instigation of GPs, because of some local difficulties or problems.

Even on a UK or all-Wales level there have been few standing arrangements. At local level the Executive Councils and their successors were required to have statutory Local Dental Committees and Local Optical Committees which had to be consulted but there was little contact between them. There was a place for a dental representative on the Executive Councils but not for the opticians. Of the six GP members one had to be reserved for an ophthalmic medical practitioner, a doctor (often but not always a consultant ophthalmologist) who also did eye-testing, but over the years it proved difficult to fill this spot on a regular basis. They would sometimes attend for a few meetings, find there was little of relevance to them and disappear. This did however leave the GPs one short (5 to 6) compared with the lay members. Mr Edward Lyons, the eye consultant from St Asaph, did attend the Denbighshire and Flintshire LMC and its successors regularly for many years since meetings were held on Sunday afternoons and he was a valuable member who also brought other hospital problems to our attention.

Contacts with pharmacists have been discussed elsewhere within the narrative and it must be emphasised that close relationships with the local pharmacies make for better practice.

Although dental problems arose fairly frequently there was no regular contact with the Local Dental Committee (the LDC) even though there were frequent complaints by individual doctors raised at the LMC about dental practices in their area. Complaints often centred on the unavailability of dentists out of hours to deal with dental abscesses and with toothache which was not considered an emergency by dentists but certainly was by patients who rang the doctor. Another problem was that the dental practice was often a considerable distance from the patient's home while the GP was closer. Many patients did not have a dentist anyway. As charges were introduced into NHS dentistry and this changed from being mainly an NHS service to one which was largely private it was also cheaper for patients to contact the free GP service.

An interesting item in the GP remuneration structure was the availability of a fee for the arrest of dental haemorrhage, a fee which I claimed regularly while at Ruabon where it was not unusual for patients to have a total dental clearance with subsequent bleeding gums out of hours. Many of these patients had been unable to afford any dental care before the NHS and their teeth were in very poor condition. With improved dental care and the reduction of extractions I do not recall ever having to claim a fee in recent years, even though it remained in the fee structure.

The health authorities have tried hard but often unsuccessfully over the years to improve the NHS dental service in North Wales with various incentive schemes. They have now started to develop contracted services with large national commercial companies, at considerable cost. Whether these will provide an effective service and where the dentists come from remains to be seen.

Physiotherapists have always been in short supply within the NHS and many battles have had to be fought to get direct access by GPs to them. Referral had to be made to a consultant first, resulting in considerable delay while the benefits of physiotherapy were usually best achieved by early access and treatment. One in five consultations in practice are for musculo-skeletal conditions, an area where physiotherapy is often the treatment of choice Similar restrictions applied to access to simple aids to recovery including crutches and splints which were usually required immediately. In earlier years physiotherapists were not allowed by their professional body to accept patients except by referral by a doctor, again resulting in delays. This was often circumvented in practice by developing understanding with physiotherapists who one knew and trusted. Since 1978 they have been recognised as autonomous practitioners professionally responsible for diagnosing and treating patients. The NHS still does not allow direct access to physiotherapists outside hospitals but pilot trials are very belatedly about to start in England.

As a consequence treatment by osteopaths and chiropractors was common but as these were at that time unqualified and unregistered doctors were not allowed to associate with or refer patients to them. We had a very sensible and useful osteopath, Mr Alwyn Hutton, in Penrhyn Bay when I went there first and found informal communication between us worked to everyone's benefit. Later Mr Keith Greenhalgh provided a very useful service to patients in the area.

The best health care is provided by allowing access to the most appropriate care worker whether within the NHS or outside and by good communication between them.

The Consultation

The Consultation is the fundamental core of the doctor-patient relationship, defined many years ago in 1960 by Sir James Spence as…"the occasion when, in the intimacy of the consulting room, a patient who is ill, or believes himself to be ill, seeks the advice of a doctor whom he trusts", and is the key to all good and successful relationships. Consultation skills never figured in any formal training during my medical school days, and one learnt by listening to one's seniors during hospital posts. Certainly not all of the consultants were good role models, and many would not be considered politically correct in today's climate. At that time patients lying in their beds and surrounded by the consultant, registrar, houseman, Sister, junior nurse, and a group of students were largely ignored as persons as opposed to as cases, with discussion of their symptoms and possible diagnoses and prognoses carried out within earshot. Many patients were left unnecessarily anxious because of words heard or misheard during these sessions and were often too frightened to ask questions afterwards.

Moving into practice with its one-to-one consultation was a completely new situation requiring a different approach. One of the fundamental differences was that this was now an on-going relationship, hopefully continuing for years, where trust had to be earned and established. A situation where a breakdown in communication could lead to medical mistakes as well as to losing a family from the list and consequent loss of practice income.

Trust was a very necessary part of a doctors armamentarium at a time when therapies were less effective and outcomes were depressingly less favourable. Decisions and advice were usually accepted unquestioningly. "Trust me, I'm a doctor " is a saying much parodied now but is the basis of on-going relationships, and similarly the aphorism "listen to the patient, he is telling you the diagnosis " is one not to be forgotten. In medical school if one was given a 30-minute long-case in an examination the advice was to spend twenty-five minutes taking the full history and five minutes making an examination to confirm the diagnosis you had already made. It would be nice if one had thirty minute consultations in practice although often of course much information about the patient is already known.

George Bernard Shaw wrote that "a medical degree is no substitute for clairvoyance. We can never eliminate the insecurity of medical uncertainty which is precisely why we need trust" while Blau writing in the College Journal stated "the doctor who fails to have a placebo effect on his patients should become a pathologist or an anaesthetist,.. or in simple English, if the patient does not feel better for your consultation you are in the wrong game".

Many of the changes which have occurred in medical care and in the style of consultation over the years and which are discussed later have to be looked at with this in mind. At present, and in spite of all the adverse publicity about individual cases and scandals and new attitudes, public opinion polls still show GPs as having the highest trust ratio of all professions.

It was in the early seventies that the art of the consultation was first analysed and discussed by Balint and others. A group had been set up by Michael Balint, a psychologist, in 1966 and the results were collated and published in 1973 in a very readable book Six Minutes for the Patient. Other publications at the same time such as Games People Play by Eric Byrne which explored ploys that people adopt to react to and to control situations in fields wider than purely medical, and The Consultation - an approach to learning and teaching by Pendleton 1984 added further to the increasing interest in the study of consultation techniques.

At about the same time in 1976 Dr Patrick Byrne, later appointed by Manchester University as the first ever Professor of General Practice, together with Barrie Long, published their work " Doctors talking to patients." It identified that most doctors appeared to have achieved set routines of interviewing patients, and that few of them demonstrated the capacity for variations of normal style and performance to meet the needs of those patients whose problems did not fit into an organic disease pattern.

Acceptance of the new concepts took time. While of considerable academic interest and leading to gradual change most doctors at the time were struggling to cope with patients being rushed through at an average of three minutes each. If one takes into account the time for patients to come in, sit down, perhaps remove a coat, pass the usual pleasantries and then reverse this on leaving at the end of the consultation, very little actual time was left for clinical matters. In such circumstances an increase in average consultation times from three to four minutes represents a virtual doubling in effective time. Many consultations at the time were of course quickies, the patient and his or her history already known, and involving only the issue of a repeat prescription or a medical certificate. Many patients especially in working class areas resented the suggestion that they needed to be examined.

Not having heard much of these new ideas I was attracted by an advert in 1982 for a course on Behaviour in the Consultation and spent three very interesting days in Essex. Course members were expected to tape-record a series of surgery consultations over a week and these were to be studied and dissected by the doctor and then by the group, a rather harrowing experience. Barrie Long took the course and Paddy Byrne also dropped in.

In those early days while the need for confidentiality was well established there was no thought of getting consent from patient to record the consultation, the fact that the recorder was the only one who knew the identity of the patient and that the discussion was taking place far from home seemed to make everything acceptable. Techniques such as reflecting questions or answers and the use of silent pauses to encourage the patient to open up were previously unknown to most doctors. During these sessions I learnt quite a lot about myself and my consulting style and later tried, when I remembered, to put a new approach into place.

Perhaps here is the point for some thoughts on confidentiality of information, an area in which newer working methods have raised anxieties and practical problems. Confidentiality of information shared between doctor and patient has always been treated in the same way as the priests confessional and has been guarded carefully by doctors over the years.

The General Medical Council was always very strong in its attitudes to breaches of confidentiality. Over recent years with the changes in the nature of consultations often involving more than one member of a practice team and with records which are accessible to others the issue has become somewhat more difficult and blurred at the edges. In these circumstances it must be made very clear to all staff with access to records that inappropriate disclosure will be considered a serious disciplinary offence, possibly leading to dismissal

An interesting idea was that patients often thought that doctors told their spouses about patients` illnesses and often said when they met my wife "didn't your husband tell you". The answer was always No and this made things easier for her too. The only exception was to avoid embarrassment when someone mutually known had died, information which was anyway in the public domain.

A more open attitude to illness by patients and their families and discussion of it with others has contributed to the difficulties. It however must remain paramount that any information which the patient wishes to keep confidential must remain so, even if this means not making notes about it. If not trust may be lost for ever. This is particularly true for consultations by teenagers or even younger children who may wish to consult on contraception or pregnancy or on abuse by others without the knowledge of parents.

A very significant court ruling in 1982 concerning confidentiality in these circumstances was the Gillick case. Mrs Victoria Gillick had five daughters and was very anxious that they were not put on the contraceptive pill without her knowledge and consent and she took the Health Authority to court to try to achieve this. She lost and the result was the establishment of the legal principle of Gillick competence which is achieved "if a child achieves sufficient understanding and intelligence to enable him or her to understand fully what is proposed". This did make it very much easier and safer for us at the time to advise children without parental consent, although it was always accepted good practice to try and persuade the child to involve the parents.

Attempts are being made by some at the present time to prevent similar situations with regard to termination of unwanted pregnancies in young girls, often with the advice and support of social workers but without the knowledge of their parents, and sometimes their doctors.

Understanding of confidentiality by relatives is often different from that of the healing professions, for example if a person is ringing for the results of a spouses or partners tests. Obviously in most cases the patient does not object to the spouse knowing but there are times when the information is such that it should not be shared. Such situations cause problems for reception staff as they are perceived to be unhelpful and obstructive. Clear guidelines must be laid down and it is important that staff are supported if complaints are made.

Since the introduction of the Data Protection Act in 1984 many other organisations are now insisting on speaking with the named person and not with a spouse. This Act together with the Freedom of Information Act which itself has caused considerable problems at times for doctors and staff because the requirements and particularly the time limits were often not fully understood by either side.

The General Medical Council in its most recent guidance states that "Doctors hold information about patients which is private and sensitive. This information must not be given to others unless the patient consents or you can justify the disclosure. When you are satisfied that information should be released, you should act promptly to disclose all relevant information. This is often essential to the best interests of the patient, or to safeguard the well-being of others."

The nature and content of consultations has gradually changed over the years, from the completely undifferentiated, as they come, turn up and be seen and finish when the waiting room is empty pattern, to the more sorted, by appointment, at least partly selected list with some patients seen by the practice team, and with many attendances being known in advance as routine follow-up appointments and medication reviews. Patients used to accept coming to a waiting room and patiently waiting their turn, often collecting virus diseases at the same time. Now that they are given an appointment time they are more likely to complain if this is not adhered to. Constraints of appointment systems with continual clockwatching to keep to schedule does often result in truncated consultations and patients being told to come back again, whereas with an open system whatever had to be done tended to be dealt with at the time.

A new and very annoying, to doctors and patients alike, development is the telephone interruption of consultations, often on more than one occasion and leading to interruption in the flow of the consultation and often to things being missed or unsaid. Attempting to prevent this is another cause of friction between receptionist and patients.

Doctors and patients have come to a wish for increase consultation times and over the years various ploys have been adopted including changes in medical certification requirements, the issue of repeat prescriptions without seeing the patient each time, employing practice nurses and others. Some practices experimented with a system of multiple examination rooms with the doctor moving from one to another as happens in hospital clinics but the idea was not really appropriate or acceptable for general practice. Separate examination rooms are often available in new or converted premises so that patients requiring full examinations and time to dress and undress can be accommodated but even this can lead to a fragmented consultation. Many practices have not had premises which could be used in this way and in recent years most practices have been continually struggling for extra space.

In educational and psychological parlance the desk was seen as a potential barrier between doctor and patient. Most doctors looked upon the desktop as a convenient place to hold all the usual paraphernalia and a place to write on, but many did try to make consultations less threatening by having the patient sitting at the side of the desk rather than across it. Other doctors, including Dr Peter Elliott from Denbigh, tried to put patients at ease by doing away with the traditional desk and having patients and doctors sitting in easy chairs. The arrival of the computer meant that a desk was essential to hold it, and in itself did create new barriers. Poor I.T. and typing skills have meant that doctors appear to look more at the screen than at the patient.

Many practices now have an additional problem to surmount in the consultation, the increasing number of patients who speak a different language and who often need the help of interpreters to voice their symptoms. The significance and interpretation of symptoms, as well as personal sensitivity, can vary between different ethnic groups and needs to be borne in mind.

The major change in the clinical component of the consultation in recent years has been a change originally encouraged by College publications from dealing with the presenting symptom only and the switch to a preventative and proactive approach with enquiries about health style issues, smoking, alcohol, blood pressure, drugs, sexual issues and the like. More recently some of this has been target driven. The new 2004 Contract with increased emphasis on rewards for attaining targets and which has been well publicised in the media has unfortunately led some patients to question their doctor's motives in pursuing these genuine goals. One approach might be a preliminary consultation with a nurse (or even in some practices by the attached medical student) to discuss these areas but this might not always be acceptable to patients and would be time consuming.

Greater access to the internet and other sources means that patients are generally much more knowledgeable about their symptoms and about their diagnoses and are more likely to try to lead the process. Laudable but very irritating if they go about it the wrong way and especially if they are barking up a wrong tree. There is research evidence that an irritated doctor may be a less effective doctor. Of course the other thing which irritates doctors is the patient who turns up with a written and varied list of symptoms to be discussed. Unfortunately curtailing this list may result in the important complaint which the patient is embarrassed to voice and which is kept to the last may not be reached.

A significant indication of the way society now thinks and the changed status and perception of doctors is the need to consider the need for chaperones when examining patients. This was always considered a male doctor and female patient scenario but this is no longer the position. Female doctors examining males and also same sex examinations, male and female, now present a potential opportunity for abuse and the opportunity for unwarranted complaints either vexatious or because of a failure to understand the need for and the nature of examinations carried out in the course of routine investigation.

Even with routine medicals for insurance and other purposes it is necessary to carry out examinations which the person almost certainly has not expected to be subjected to and does not understand the reasons for and where explanation and informed consent needs to be obtained. The need may also extend to verbal communication between doctor and patient, or their families. The implications will have significant influence on the way consultations are carried out in the future.

It has always been a tradition within hospital settings for the doctor to be accompanied by a nurse, often a number of nurses and others in the retinue, but this has been the result of the way hospitals run, as well as the implied status of the specialist. Out in general practice the situation has been quite different with consultations and examinations usually taking place confidentially in a private one-to-one relationship within the consulting room or in the patient's home. Very often and especially in branch surgeries there has been no-one else on the premises at the time, and no-one expected anything different.

I have gone through a professional lifetime in such circumstances but it is unlikely today's young doctors will be able to do the same. On the odd occasion if one had a feeling of apprehension a doctor might call in a receptionist or a nurse if available to be present, although this could in itself send the wrong signals. With the usual staffing situation in practices this would inevitably mean delays and taking them staff away from the tasks they were already engaged in.

Home visits particularly out of hours were even more difficult. I well recall an occasion some years ago when I attended a call late at night to a patient of the other practice who was in an upstairs one-room flat and was complaining of severe abdominal pains. The door was opened by the youngish bottle-blonde patient dressed in, and only in, the short baby-doll nightdress fashionable at the time. The bed was a mattress on the floor and to make even a token attempt to examine her abdominal symptoms I had to be on my knees on the floor alongside the mattress. Luckily it was obvious that there was no serious problem and I gave her a couple of pills from my bag, advised her to attend the surgery next day for further examination, and departed hurriedly. A very worrying visit, although probably it was the only occasion when I can recall being really troubled.

On another occasion during my daytime round of visits I opened the front door as was my usual way, called out and went straight upstairs to find a young lady in bed. Unfortunately I was in the wrong house, she was not expecting the doctor and explanations had to be made. In today's climate this might have been interpreted differently.

Perhaps these sorts of situation provide further strong arguments in favour of all patients being seen in a surgery or out-of-hours centre since it would be quite impractical to be accompanied on all occasions by a nurse chaperone. In general terms the occasional use of an chaperone in itself draws attention to the potential problems and may in itself lead to the need for universal chaperoning. If there develops a perceived need to be chaperoned in the surgery and in the home, then this will require the employment and continual presence of a one-to-one assistant at considerable expense. It will also lead to a fundamental change in the nature of the consultation, removing the overriding confidentiality of the relationship between doctor and patient to its great detriment. Even if one tries to separate the initial presentation of symptoms from any chaperoned examination problems still remain. Very often it is only during or immediately after intimate examinations that patients finally admit to the true nature of their problem and their anxieties which they had previously been unable to reveal. How exactly the chaperone situation can be addressed and indeed whether patients wish this will take much debate to resolve. The GMC have issued revised guidelines but only time will tell whether these are practical. The trouble with guidelines is that there is always the danger of running into trouble if they are not carried out on every occasion.

The consultation will continue to evolve but will always remain as the cornerstone of general practice and that which sets it apart from other medical contacts. Non-medical researchers will continue to analyse it and make recommendations without fully appreciating the minutiae.

The Welsh language in medicine

Since NHS GP medical records are lifelong and pass from practice to practice when patients move home and in hospitals when they move from department to department, although not from hospital to hospital, they must be capable of being read by whoever is dealing with the patient at the time. While many consultations both in practice and in hospitals take place using the medium of Welsh it has always been accepted that in the interest of continuity of care that records be kept in English. This has been BMA policy for many years. It does not of course preclude informal telephone or other discussions between doctors or other staff and handwritten interim memos which are not intended to become part of the permanent record.

On a famous occasion in the seventies in Gwynedd a local GP sent in an X-Ray request written in Welsh to Ysbyty Gwynedd but was very surprised to receive in reply a report written in Punjabi. Obviously with the growth of a multicultural, multilingual and more mobile population in Britain the English-only principle is becoming more vital.

The Welsh Language Act in 1967 had given the language a status within the courts and judicial system amongst others but the passing of the second Welsh Language Act in 1993 which gave equal status to both languages has meant that documents need to be produced bilingually. All public bodies are now required to produce bilingual agenda documents and records and to allow speakers to use the language of their choice and they have to provide instantaneous translation facilities. The situation where the Welsh version of an official document often followed at some considerable time after the English version made mockery of the requirement. Problems arise when the need for translation results in delays in publication and this aggravates a situation where decisions and documents from England which also apply in Wales often have to be ratified by Welsh Office Government and the Assembly before distribution.

For smaller organisations within both the private and public sector problems arise from the availability of competent translators, and at times the quality of the translation from many bodies is not up to standard, sometimes the errors are very humorous. No doubt this will improve with time. There are also financial implications of bilingualism which are not insignificant. The Welsh Language Board has been willing to provide help to defray part of cost of bilingual signs in surgeries and similar places.

1981 saw the availability for the first time of bilingual death certificates, a significant advance welcomed by many families in the Welsh-speaking areas but blighted by the requirement to also fill in an English version, making the document very bulky and attempts were made to simplify it. An opinion from the BMA lawyers advised that there was nothing which stated that the completion of a death certificate had to be in a specific language but WGMSC were dubious about this advice and sought further clarification.

In many areas consultations have traditionally been held in Welsh even though records were kept in English, with a fair smattering of English words for diseases and diagnoses. The major advances in medicine and in technology at this time meant that new terms had continually to be devised and introduced, both in English and Welsh. Some claim that many of the Welsh terms were bastardised English ones with a different ending but in reality both derive from old Latin or Greek roots and so are likely to be somewhat similar.

In an attempt to encourage the use of Welsh as a living language in everyday medicine Y Gymdeithas Cymraeg, the Welsh Medical Society, was formed in 1975, holding its first meeting in the Conwy valley. It met twice a year for a weekend in residential hotel settings around Wales with all the lectures and discussion being in Welsh. Young and older doctors attended, many with their young families, and many longstanding friendships were developed. Some of the children have now grown up to themselves become prominent leaders of Y Gymdeithas. Lectures were of a high postgraduate standard and I was amazed at times how doctors living and working full-time in England and in English for many years could lecture in Welsh to such a high standard on esoteric subjects such as the DNA molecular structure or the biosynthesis of the insulin molecule, to recall a couple of subjects. This often necessitated the formulation for the first time of completely new words which by the end of the weekend had moved into everyone's vocabulary. I was persuaded to give a presentation once, on the work I had done on repeat prescribing in our practice, but I must admit it was quite an effort. Although our first language at home is Welsh I was brought up in Cornwall until I was eleven so I am not so fluent as I would wish to be.

To aid the development of the language a Dictionary of Welsh Terms had been published in 1973, and later several members of the Gymdeithas including Dr Ieuan Parri and Dr Tom Davies were involved with the University of Wales in developing a volume of Medical Terms published in 1986.Regular updating is obviously required.

The Welsh Assembly published a Study of Welsh Awareness in Healthcare Provision which recommended encouragement of awareness of the language by all workers but had little positive steps to offer. A volume of Terms for Health Promotion (Termau Hybu Iechyd) was published in 2001 by the North Wales Health Authority in association with the University in Bangor. Everything depends on the availability of Welsh speakers, both staff and patients, and encouraging them to use the language whenever appropriate. Many speakers however still find it easier to discuss medical symptoms in English and progress will remain slow but perhaps steady over the next few years.

Other ethnic groups have not figured prominently in North Wales and languages have not been a problem. However, recently a major influx of Polish workers and their families, some seventeen thousand in all, in the Wrexham area is causing some problems to local services.

Certification of illness and incapacity to work

If there has been one thing more than anything else which has caused aggravation and frustration to GPs over the years it has been the question of certifying sickness - or in many cases alleged sickness. The difficulties pre-dated the NHS and perhaps was more of a problems in areas with heavy industries, coal and iron and steel and in factories. Many symptoms of incapacity and illness such as diarrhoea and backache are not easily verifiable and the doctor has to depend on the word of the patient. Obviously working on a coal-face gives rise over the years to back problems which are recurrent and which cause difficulties at work. Similarly diarrhoea suffered a mile underground is not the ideal scenario but they both provided good opportunities for "plumbitis oscillans" or lead-swinging. Monday mornings were a favourite time for this, absenteeism on this day was much higher than on other days, often as a result of weekend over-indulgence. To try to curb the absenteeism the mines developed a policy of paying for six shifts if the normal five days including Monday were worked. Absences required a "susstificate", often (at times routinely in some areas) requested by the wife or mother rather than the patient himself in person. These were private certificates or "notes".

National Insurance certificates had strict rules attached, they stated that patients were to be "seen and examined" although proxy attendances were frequently tried and they could not be issued for more than one week, even if a patient had a broken leg which was likely to take months to heal. Patients attending casualty departments should have been issued with certificates there but very often were not. Many inappropriate visits were required just for certification purposes so it was no wonder that lax habits developed in some areas.

Final certificates could not be issued more than three days before returning to work so that if a patient was seen on a Thursday they had to be seen again on the Friday or Saturday to allow them to start on the following Monday. Problems about dating a Final Certificate arose when a patient would be fit to start on a Monday but his work shift rota was not due to start until the Wednesday or Thursday. If signed off on Monday the patient would receive neither pay or sickness benefit.

A most unfortunate event happened to one of my partners in the sixties. A patient with chronic chest problems had been visited and examined and was genuinely ill and unfit for work over a couple of weeks. He was not fit to attend surgery and his wife in the local tradition collected his later certificates weekly. He returned to work but unknown to him his wife continued to collect certificates and to claim benefit. The fraud was discovered after a few weeks and my partner had a very unpleasant court appearance. Again there but for the grace of God went many other doctors practicing in industrial areas at that time.

Blank National Insurance certificates could be a licence to print money and doctors had to be very careful not to leave them lying around on the desk if they left the room, although it was embarrassing to be seen to deliberately pick them up.

The GMC requires doctors to verify statements made in certificates and "any doctor who gives a misleading certificate renders himself liable to disciplinary procedures". In legalistic terms since N.I certificates are used to corroborate the patient's statement of incapacity strictly speaking no certificate based solely on the patient's statement in cases where there are no objective signs to verify the truth of this statement should be issued. If adhered to patients would be required to work when they were not fit enough but where there were no signs to back this up and administrative chaos would ensue. In addition the doctor/patient relationship would suffer. In practice doctors have always adopted a pragmatic approach and issued certificates when requested by patients unless there was some obvious reason not to. Doctors were not allowed to write "I don't know" on the certificate, the DHSS insisted on a diagnosis even when one was not possible at an early stage of illness. These problems really brought the system into disrepute with the doctor in the middle between the patient, the employers and the national insurance system and frequently acting illegally in the interests of their patient. The terms of service required the GP to issue to the patient certificates .... "reasonably required by them". .and so most doctors would only consider not issuing a certificate if there was definite evidence that the request was "unreasonable".

Many hours were spent in Annual Conferences angrily debating and demanding improved rules on certification but changes were achieved only very slowly and over many years. Gradually it became permissible to issue first and intermediate ones for longer periods and final certificates earlier. The first major improvements took place in 1966 allowing open certificates to be given for up to 28 days and a final certificate up to 7 days before the patient is fit to resume work which were a considerable advance.

Frustration increased until the Annual Conference of LMCs in 1969 passed a resolution "that this conference concludes that the issue of certificates by general practitioners for national insurance purposes is generally wasteful of medical time and is pointless, and may be harmful. It results in a wastage of medical manpower at a time when it is in very short supply, it has a harmful effect on the doctor/patient relationship, and it serves no useful purpose" followed by a rider "that National Insurance certification by general practitioners be abolished". The Annual Representative Meeting representing all branches of the profession adopted a resolution in similar terms the same year.

In 1970 at the request of the GMSC the Secretary of State agreed to set up a working group to "consider the operation of the present medical certification procedures and proposals for possible detailed changes to them". After the first meetings the group agreed to suspend its considerations until the Fisher committee on the Abuse of Social Security Benefits which had just been set up had reported'. When it did so in 1973, Fisher concluded that there was no acceptable substitute to certification by the family doctor and discussions were resumed on this basis.

Doctors were adamant that their primary concern was the prevention and treatment of illness whereas the administrative task certifying incapacity to work was becoming increasingly irritating. Under the National Insurance Acts independent authorities adjudicated on claims for benefit and whether the claimant had discharged the onus on him or her of proving incapacity for work. The National Insurance Commissioner had stated that "a doctor's certificate is not conclusive evidence of incapacity. It represents a particular doctor's opinion and has to be weighed with all the other relevant evidence in forming a judgment on the case......" The wording of the certificates was subsequently and significantly altered to " I examined you today/yesterday and "advised you" that ....

Further concessions were made as to the periods for which "open" and "closed (final)" certificates could be issued and life became somewhat easier although the ethical issues remained.

At a later date when resignation from the NHS was no longer a viable option or threat in negotiations the concept of refusing to issue NI certificates was proposed, a ploy which would certainly have caused an almost immediate effect and chaos. A consultation Green Paper on certification was issued in 1980 and at this time there was strong recommendation from us on the Welsh GMSC that to put increased pressure on government short term certificates should not be signed but GMSC in London felt this might prejudice on-going negotiations and it was not proceeded with.

An increasing problem in later years was the result of the early retirement on "health grounds" which were often tenuous of senior staff members who were no longer able to cope with changes in work patterns. While receiving their works pension they were also required to have National Insurance certificates or they would be required to continue to pay their insurance stamps themselves until they were 65 years old. Doctors often felt that that the incapacity seemed to disappear on leaving their job but certificates still needed to be signed. In other cases the patient might not be capable of carrying out his normal work but could certainly not be considered as incapable of any employment. There appeared to be no interest within the insurance system to actively tackle this issue.

There had always been an arrangement where if a doctor was uncertain about issuing certificates a referral to the Regional Medical Officer could be made and this would trigger an examination by him, provided that the patient did not ask to be signed off before then. This was at times very useful to the GP but many times the patient would sign off to start work but would very soon develop a recurrence of his complaint which would require him to go back on the "sick" or as often referred to "the Club"

By 1984 under statutory sick pay arrangements employers had been made responsible for the first weeks of sickness benefit with patients self-certifying and no NI Certificate was required for the first week, a great improvement, or it would have been if some employers including hospitals and other health service establishments had not started to insist on a private medical certificate after three days absence. Unemployment and job losses were becoming more significant at that time and this had the effect of discouraging some from staying off work.

Apart from National Insurance, doctors` certificates were required for a plethora of purposes, from claiming from social security to applications for re-housing, to applying to renew a gun licence and more recently to cancel foreign holidays. Certificates to cover school absences were very difficult as they were usually requested retrospectively. Very often the grounds were tenuous but a refusal offended. Housing certificates were a particular problem. If the doctor wrote a note and gave it to the patient it was taken to the desk of the housing department, opened by a receptionist who might already have told the client "there is a house coming up now, get a letter from your doctor and we will see what we can arrange" and comment that the doctor had not tried very hard or words to that effect. The Local Medical Committees decided that the medical certificates must be requested by the relevant department in writing and be addressed to the Medical Officer in charge, but problems continued as staff in the offices changed.

While problems do remain at times, particularly with private certificates and with a whole raft of other subjects which require to be certified, certification no longer appears regularly as an agenda item at LMC conferences.

The GP Contracts

At the start of the NHS GPs joined under an ill-defined contract which probably few of them read or actually signed and this sufficed for almost twenty years with many disputes and crises along the way.

In 1964 the profession faced another grave crisis of confidence. Family doctors again felt that they were working in a neglected and under financed branch of the NHS. They were very unhappy about the way they had to work and with the level at which they were paid. Morale was low and recruitment was again dangerously low. The Annual Conference of LMCs was held that year in Methodist Hall, Westminster, and was the first of many which I attended over the next thirty years. The GP leader and the chairman of the GMSC at the time was Dr A.B.Davies who came in for very severe censure about the lack of progress in negotiations with government and after a vote of censure was passed he resigned. At the next GMSC a young Scot, Dr Jim Cameron, was elected as Chairman. A new Charter was written in 1965 and negotiations with the government on a major review of the Contract and the Terms of Service were set in train.

The GMSC Charter for the Family Doctor Service set out as its view that

to give the best service to his patients the family doctor must

Have adequate time foe every patient

Be able to keep up-to-date

Have complete clinical freedom

Have adequate well-equipped premises.

Have at his disposal all the diagnostic aids, social services and ancillary help he needs

Be encouraged to acquire additional skills and experience in special fields

Be adequately paid by a method acceptable to him which encourages him to do his best for his patients

Have a working day which leaves him time for some leisure

It then went on to detail what would be necessary to ensure this.

Amongst the major aims was a reduction in list size to a maximum of 2000 (some urban doctors at the time had lists of up to 4500 patients) to allow adequate time for personal care, improved medical education oriented towards general practice and a payment structure related to workload, skills and responsibility rather than on list size with the choice of payment by capitation, item of service or by salary. A major change and significant improvement in the new contract was the introduction of the Ancillary Help Scheme whereby there was direct reimbursement of 70% of approved receptionist and practice nursing costs, the practice still being responsible for the remaining 30%, encouraging doctors to considerably increase staff to deal with new practice arrangements. Previously all these expenses were added to the Pool the following year and divided up pro rata between all doctors so that those investing heavily in their practices were disadvantaged compared with those who invested little.The question of what is a reasonable division between the direct doctor contribution and the indirectly reimbursed amounts has been debated frequently in subsequent years but remained at 70%.

The other major change was the development of the cost-rent scheme whereby practices were directly reimbursed for the investment in their premises, paving the way for greatly improved facilities for doctors, their staff and for patients. It led to additional space being made available to allow for the introduction of practice employed nurses working within the surgeries, to work alongside the District Nurses employed and administered by the Health Authorities. The interface and the relationships between these two nursing groups was an interesting one which has been considered earlier.

The subsequently negotiated 1966 Contract was welcomed by the profession, led to considerable improvements in patient care and Jim Cameron became a cult figure.It formed the basis of working arrangements until the imposed 1990 contract.

By 1977 GPs were again worried about the reduction in their living standards due to their relatively low remuneration and the Annual Conference asked for another new Charter, amongst other things to ensure that remuneration be comparable with medical remuneration in countries in the EEC (as it was then called). A GMSC New Charter working party published the following year concluded that "the substantial social and medical changes since the 1966 Charter merited a comprehensive review of all the major elements of general practice". It identified the ways in which practice was falling behind and suggested ways this could be improved. Progress subsequently was slow and piecemeal, with hard-won concessions wrung out of unsympathetic governments over the next decade.

One period when relationships with government were happier was when Mr Kenneth Robinson, himself the son of a GP and who understood some of the problems, was Minister for Health

The 1990 contract was a second major watershed in general practice representing major changes in requirements for GPs and their practice organisation. It was the first real effort by government to tell doctors in detail how to run their practices and to do their work.

GPs as independent contractors had, in legal jargon, a contract for service rather than a contract of services. The Terms of Service basically said that one should provide all such services as doctors as a group normally provided, and be responsible for care twenty-four hours a day and fifty-two weeks a year, but left doctors to run their practices and provide the service in a way they saw best fitted to their area and patients. The government`s draft new contract set out to change this.

Following the publication in 1988 of the White Paper "Promoting Better Health" detailed consultations with the profession's negotiators resulted, at least according to the government, in "agreement on all outstanding issues". The draft contract did introduce many of the developments which the profession had been asking for and moving towards for several years but much of the small print and the unnecessarily bureaucratic requirements were unacceptable. When put to the Conference of LMCs the draft contract was rejected.

Subsequently Kenneth Clarke, the then Secretary of State, in his usual rail-roading manner, unilaterally imposed the contract on April 1st 1990 which caused considerable angst and animosity and also engendered an attitude amongst doctors of wishing to co-operate fully only in those parts considered relevant to good patient care. He particularly offended doctors by accusing them in their response of "reaching for their wallets".

The stated aims of the contract were to give patients greater choice by providing them with more information and increased competition, to make the terms of service more specific to reflect clearly the requirements of good general practice that better practices already met in serving their patients e.g. health promotion advice, full preventative cover, ready availability to patients and services geared to their needs and to make the remuneration system more performance related, allowing GPs who provide high quality services to be better paid; strengthening the contractual relationship with Family Practitioner Committees to encourage the provision of good quality services; and ensuring that there is better value for money - a sine qua non for all governments in recent years (and one that is perhaps rarely achieved).

A major unacceptable plank was the transfer of more practice income back to headcount capitation fees, and which many feared would result in a return to the "bad old days" of the Pool before the 1966 Contract with competition for bigger list sizes and consequently less time for individual patients.

Amongst the major changes originally proposed, and which were subsequently conceded by government at least in part during negotiations, were the abolition of seniority payments to older GPs and the payments introduced in the 1966 contract which had encouraged doctors to form group practices of three or more for more effective working, major changes to the rural practice payments which would have made many practices unviable, single level target payments for childhood immunisations and for screening for cancer of the cervix both of which might result in undue and unethical pressure on patients to conform.

New features which were proposed and welcomed were capitation payments for newly registered patients who often required considerable time spent on getting to know and review their history and medication, higher fees for patients over 75 years who it was generally acknowledged required more consultations and care, payment for providing child surveillance which had previously been done by health clinics, payment for carrying out minor surgery and for running health promotion clinics within the practice, and for the time spent in teaching medical students in the practice which it was anticipated would become much more extensive in the following years.

While these introductions were welcomed it was the detail of how they were to be carried out that caused problems at the time and later. Extra payments were to be made to patients of GPs practising in areas of deprivation, mainly but not exclusively in inner city areas, to encourage more to work there. These when introduced gave rise to many anomalies and to gross distortion of incomes and this aspect will be explored in more detail later. Many of these doctors found that there income rose so significantly that there was no real incentive for them to carry out the new work which was being encouraged. The Law of Unintended Consequences had reared its head again.

One proposal which did not go down well with many city doctors was a lower night visit fee for doctors using commercial deputising services, and there were many of these doctors in the larger conurbations, rather than providing the service themselves. The first deputising service in the UK was set up by Dr Pollock in 1960 covering south London below the Thames and the concept spread later to most of the conurbations, Air Call being the predominant provider, with doctors switching over to them each evening and at weekends. The BMA were actively involved over the years in overseeing the working of the Air-Call service. There were only deputising services in Cardiff, Swansea and Newport. The rest of Wales did their own on-call or sometimes worked in strictly limited rotas with adjoining practices.

Doctors claimed a fee for each night call between midnight and seven a.m on a form which required the patient's signature, a requirement which was not always easy to obtain if the patient was ill and distressed, and was much resented by doctors. To allegedly counter fraud a sample of claims were checked by the FHSA writing to the patient later to confirm visit had been made, objectionable because some patients formed the impression their doctor and the practice was being investigated. Better drafting of the letters would have been helpful. Elderly slightly confused patients often could not remember whether or when a call was made. Since the fee was only in the region of £15 there was no real incentive to fiddle anyway although the occasional doctor did.

The 1990 contract reiterated that doctors had to be responsible for their patients on a twenty four hours a day basis, but then went on to impose "availability" criteria which specified at least twenty-six hours in face-to-face consultation a week spread over five days "at times convenient to patients". In recognition of the work which some GPs do elsewhere on health-related activities in the public service this five day commitment could with the agreement of the FHSA be reduced to four days. For most doctors the 26 hours a week certainly was not a problem but for those of us with extensive involvement both with health authorities and with professional bodies even the four days was a problem in some weeks. Since these requirements were for forty-six weeks a year, allowing for holidays, any weeks where a query was raised were considered part of the six holiday weeks.

Patients were now to be allowed to change their doctor immediately even if they had not changed their address. Previously unless they had moved they had to notify the FPC and wait a week before the new doctor could treat them, a hangover from the old panel days when patients sometimes moved en-masse.

Practice leaflets were to be produced which detailed doctors full names, gender, date of birth or year of first qualification, surgery hours, information on how to make appointments and arrangements for home and out of hours visits, and the arrangements for off duty cover, access for the disabled, as well as what special clinics and other services the practice provided, all information which was already easily obtained from the surgery office. Commercial firms stepped in and offered to produce the practice leaflets or brochures, which were often quite elaborate, funded by advertisements. This was a major change as in my early days advertising or any publishing of one's skills or clinical interests was seriously frowned upon and might lead to a referral to the General Medical Council. A single plate outside the surgery premises giving the doctor's name and registered qualifications were all that would be acceptable. Nor was it acceptable to have signposts on lampposts or corners pointing towards the surgery, although gradually by the eighties much bigger signs advertising SURGERY were appearing, particularly in poorer urban areas and some were even illuminated.

Even more rigid was the forbidding of referral to or association with unqualified practitioners such as homeopaths, osteopaths and manipulators, many of whom one knew could provide more effective treatment at the time than the doctor could. It was forbidden to direct patients to named professionals such as private physiotherapists and to pharmacies and particularly to be associated with these and share premises with them. This did make things difficult at times when patients or relatives specifically asked for guidance. Often guidance would be given in the form "if it was my family I might be thinking of Mr X ". It was even more difficult if one of a medical couple was a doctor and the other a pharmacist or physiotherapist. Now it is becoming not unusual for commercial pharmacies to be located in the same buildings as the non-dispensing surgery. Obviously in all referrals any possible interest has to be declared.

Strangely enough no such requirement to provide information has been required of doctors within the NHS secondary care services or in private practice. According to established practice and GMC guidance these should only see patients after referral by a GP and the assumption was that the GP would be aware of the skills and interests of the specialists to whom referral was proposed. This was probably true in the early days when referrals were virtually all to the local hospital and where there might be only one or two consultants in each specialty. More recently the number of specialists has often quadrupled and many have never met local GPs. Patients are requesting referrals to other parts of the country, perhaps for the convenience of relatives, to specialists NHS or private, and to hospitals unknown to the referring GP, and a new situation exists, one which has not yet been satisfactorily addressed.

On top of this was a requirement in the 1990 Contract to prepare a detailed practice annual report. to the FHSA, with again the contents specified in detail. All these requirements would take time and cost to produce, but no extra staff or finance was available. This was a new field for doctors but as no guidelines were set down to enable these to be in a standard format which would allow the information to be statistically correlated. and practices compared much of the value was lost.

Whereas previously doctors attended courses which they considered relevant to their own needs the new contract specified that in order to qualify for a new Postgraduate Education Allowance postgraduate or continuing education would be required to fit into a programme which required attendance at a minimum of two courses in each of three areas, health promotion and the prevention of illness, disease management, and service management over a five year period. From a strictly educational position there was some logic in this in that it was well known that doctors and others tend to go on courses on subjects which interest them rather than perhaps those of less interest but where their knowledge may be deficient. A complex central mechanism for the accreditation and classification of courses and for certifying attendance had to be set in train. The arrangements failed to recognise that keeping up to date could increasingly be done in a variety of other ways which did not involve "bums on seats" in lecture halls.

The contract introduced the concept of Health Promotion clinics which required at least five patients to be seen in a session before it was recognised for payment. It failed to appreciate that it was generally accepted that GPs were the most effective providers of health education and advice and that this was best accepted when provided as part of routine consultations.

Over 75's visits were one of the most irritating of the new requirements particularly in our practice which had some 20% of the list in this age group, arguably the highest in Wales by some degree, and many of whom were active as golfers or in other social activities. The requirement was to offer them all in writing a home visit at least annually to see the home environment and to find out whether carers or relatives were available and to do social assessments of their lifestyle and relationships as well as their physical condition. It did cause a lot of administrative work to ensure that the offer was made and some patients did want to take it up even though one had to negotiate a suitable time to fit in with their social calendar. In the end we decided to employ one of the partner's wives who was a nurse to do this work for us, although we could have found more useful and productive work for her. Perhaps the requirement may have been perceived to be sensible in some of the deprived or ethnic areas in the cities but it certainly was not in North Wales. It may arguably be more useful now when home visiting has decreased to a very large extent and the home conditions are not often seen. Home visits did provide a lot of useful feedback in the past and one occasionally came across unexpected and eye-opening situations.

The new contract also introduced the new Complaints Procedures discussed elsewhere.

Perhaps this summary indicates the causes of the dissatisfaction with the 1990 Contract, the better parts were readily accepted and are now part of standard good practice but also why ever- resourceful doctors attempted to find was to circumvent some of the onerous requirements. Local discussions with our cooperative and understanding health authorities over the following months and years helped ease the burden and smooth the unnecessarily jagged edges, ensuring that the spirit rather than the letter of the contract was followed.

Changes and modifications occurred over the years until discussions started on the next major review, the 2004 Contract, which was introduced after I had retired and so was not personally involved. The requirements for recording and paperwork have increased considerably. It has also importantly allowed the LHBs with the doctors locally to agree on new work to be undertaken in practices and for work transferred from hospitals to be paid for. The full impact and effect has not yet been fully assessed.

Out of Hours Care

Patients in rural areas have had a massive shock at new arrangements for out of hours care in the last few years and especially since the introduction of the 2004 Contract. Those in the conurbations have experienced deputising care for many years.

In my early years in practice there were often several small practices in each area, often single handed and competing for patients and not wishing to let their patients come into contact with other local doctors lest they be enticed way. This meant there were large numbers of doctors, and their wives, tied to telephones 24 hours a day and 7 days a week. Tied meant being housebound as phone transfer arrangements phones which could be carried into the garden were not available, and mobile phone networks had not been invented. Answering machines were starting to come in during the early sixties. Frequently one had to rush in from the garden, kicking off Wellingtons en route, to answer the phone before it stopped (no 1471or 1571 recall of numbers was available then), sometimes carrying mud on to carpets and causing displeasure. Outside bells were necessary and neighbours were not pleased if one forgot to switch them off at night. Many patients did not have telephones and a knock on the door was not unusual..

Doctors began to practice in groups to share the on-call and as competition and headhunting for patients became less neighbouring practices began to cooperate out-of-hours. Even then most doctors were in a rota of five or less.

In the larger centres extended rotas of local GPs began to be formed, working on a knock for knock basis, while in the biggest conurbations commercial deputising services were set up with the doctors who opted to work for them being paid on a sessional rate. Call handling was centralised and drivers were provided when necessary. These deputising services were visits only, there were no arrangements for seeing patients at a centre or giving telephone advice. Patients in these urban areas often used the hospital casualty (later A&E) departments as their out-of-hours centre.Many doctors in these areas did no evening or weekend work Wales only had commercial deputising services in Cardiff, Newport and Swansea. In the Swansea area doctors split about fifty-fifty as to whether they used the commercial service or the alternative doctors' cooperative and this sometimes caused problems when partners within the same practice used the different systems. The commercial service also acted as a call-centre for the Neath and Port Talbot area doctors.

Over the past ten or fifteen years extended rotas covering larger rural and semi urban areas have been developed on a knock for knock basis between local doctors.

Locally the Morfa-Doc consortium was started as an informal cooperative covering a large part of Glan Clwyd catchment area. Morfa-Doc became a limited company in 2001 but still dealt directly with the GPs. Another co-op, Dee-doc, was based on the Deeside Community Hospital and extended to the English border. They and the Chester co-op provided reciprocal cover for patients who crossed the border. A further co-op Menai-doc was developed based on Bangor and later still Aberdoc based at Llandudno Hospital and covering the Conwy valley was started. Our practice at Penrhyn Bay did not join as it was of no practical advantage since it was necessary to cover the police work every night. All these co-ops provided considerable relief to the practices but all who participated had to do sessions in their turn.

Some practices because of their geographical situation and distance from the centre could not be covered by these arrangements. South Meirionydd had a particularly large area to be covered by a rota which covered Barmouth, Dolgellau and Tywyn and this led to some difficulties, both in winter and in summertime when the population at risk increased markedly with the influx of temporary residents. Cover for another very large area, but one with considerably less patients, in the latter years was provided by a rota of the Cerrig-y-drudion, Bala, and Corwen practices.

On Anglesey before the A55 across the island was completed Holyhead was considered too far to be covered by Menai-doc at Bangor and the local practices had to form their own rota, while Amlwch at the other corner of the island was isolated with no-one willing to cover them. In the east the only major problem was with Llangollen with the Wrexham co-op, which later amalgamated with Shrop-doc covering the English borders, unwilling to extend its area to Llangollen and the Dee valley. Inability to form extended rotas made it increasingly difficult for practices to attract new partners.

The major breakthrough came in the 2004 contract with the negotiation of the right of GPs to opt out of out-of hours work completely while at the same time giving up a proportion of their practice income. Responsibility for providing out-of-hours cover became that of the Local Health Boards who then sub-contracted to new commercial providers based largely on the existing co-ops. Aberdoc merged into Morfa-doc. The LHBs had also to assume responsibility for the geographically difficult areas of south Meirionydd. The new providers employed any local GPs and qualified non-principals who so wished on a sessional basis and many have opted to do some sessions, some more than others. Morfa-doc operates from purpose built premises in the grounds of Glan Clwyd hospital which allows patients to be transferred across easily if necessary. Patients have their symptoms checked by a triage nurse who has access to protocols and who assesses whether a visit is necessary or whether the patient should attend the Centre. Occasionally if the symptoms suggest this is the appropriate action patients may be referred direct to the Accident unit. The idea of a nurse being allowed to assess symptoms and make decisions would certainly not have been acceptable to patients or to doctors a few years ago. Two or three doctors supported by receptionists and nursing staff are on duty at all times, one available to go on visits when necessary, with a driver who knows the area and with global positioning systems and radio communication.

Patients in community hospitals had been looked after by local G.Ps so it was necessary at the same time for the LHBs Trusts to negotiate cover with the new providers.

Home visits even during office hours have not been a feature of health care in other countries, attendance at surgeries or admission direct to hospitals and nursing homes being the norm. It has taken some time for patients and their relatives to accept that they should come into the centre but most are now realising that facilities for examination, investigation and treatment are better there and also that they are seen much sooner than when they used to wait at home for a visit. Many falsely and incorrectly still believe that home visits are no longer done.

Doctors and their families are now feeling liberated. A large number still work on a sessional basis for the new providers but at times of their own choosing. However political and public pressure is building up to restore longer opening hours and weekend surgeries and this may well become the next major battle to be fought.

NHS Direct

NHS Direct was set up in 1999 as part of government attempts to improve patient access to the services of the NHS through a single telephone number. It was to function in two ways, by providing general advice on a 24 hour-a-day basis about services available nationally and in a local area, and in specific instances to assess patients' symptoms, give simple advice, and to suggest where and when was the appropriate place to seek further advice and treatment. Call centres were set up with specially trained nurses working to computerised protocols.

In some ways the concept has been successful and has been well used by the public Some of the GP out-of-hours organisations have used NHS Direct as their triage centre, others have preferred to use their own in-house triage by receptionists again working to protocols. Some have suggested that the NHS nurses add some of their professional experience and views to colour the set protocols and that this leads to inappropriate referrals being made. Certainly the view of many GPs is that the advice is not always appropriate and often excessively defensive. Costs have proved to be higher than estimated and changes may be necessary.

The ambulance service has seen an escalation of out-of-hours calls since the new arrangements were introduced. In informal discussions with ambulance-men they have complained to doctors of an avalanche of silly calls which "in the past you would have dealt with yourselves on the telephone"

Police work

In Penrhyn Bay in addition to our practice work we took responsibility as police surgeons for the Llandudno Division and did so in rather tragic circumstances.

The South Parade surgery had undertaken this for some years and Dr Emyr James in particular was very keen on this work Unfortunately Emyr died suddenly at an early age, a considerable loss to his colleagues and the community as a whole. The remaining partners were not so keen on the work and commitment and resigned and we were appointed in their place. One of my partners Rod Gilmore developed a considerable interest in the subject and later sat and passed the Diploma in Medical Jurisprudence. Rod was the official police surgeon and we were listed as deputies but in fact all did an equal share of the rota duties, which we combined with our practice on-call, and which at times caused a conflict of priorities. This was perhaps more of a problem during daytime when a call to the police station was requested at the start of a long surgery. Payment was by a retainer plus call-out fees.

Many of the call-outs were very routine and were to see prisoners taken into custody and they initially increased following the introduction of PACE, the Police and Criminal Evidence Act, which laid down strict guidelines on the care and examination of those in custody. Many regular offenders taken into custody knew their "rights". Some complained of alleged injuries sustained during arrest, often very minor and some obviously much older than claimed. A number had bleeding injuries and it was necessary to be particularly vigilant to avoid the risk of hepatitis and HIV from contamination and from needle-stick injuries in these higher risk groups. Others wanted narcotic drugs and would claim that they were attending drug withdrawal clinics in Manchester or Liverpool and needed to continue their medication, although none had any documentation to support this and it was often impossible to check on this. In many cases they were given a small dose, to keep them happy overnight. Others alleged they suffered from agoraphobia and could not be kept in a cell. On occasion the requests were quite facetious, once I was rung at 2-0.a.m by the custody sergeant who said that a prisoner was complaining of being unable to sleep in the cell, the reply being " neither can I now you have woken me". The number of calls certainly depended on the attitude and toughness of the custody sergeant on duty at the time.

An interesting aspect was that prisoners in custody are not eligible for NHS treatment and any prescriptions we wrote had to be taken to and dispensed privately by a local chemist. They are of course still entitled to full medical confidentiality and this could on occasion create some difficulties as the custody sergeant needed for the prisoner's good to be aware of some issues. There was the ever present worry of a prisoner being found dead in a cell, particularly so with drunks and with head injuries. Records were of course kept by us personally rather than at the station and reports might be requested by solicitors months later. Occasionally a summons would be received to attend Crown Court, often at Caernarfon, and usually on an inconvenient day. It was not unknown to be present for two days waiting to be called as witness and then to be told one was no longer required. If an appearance was cancelled the day before no fee was payable even though one had spent much time preparing and perhaps employing a locum.

Another task was taking blood from motorists who had failed or refused a breathalyser test. This was a very straightforward procedure with no opinion required, other than if the driver was suffering from any other significant illness or disability, a far cry from older days when drivers were tested by being required to stand on one leg, walk along a straight line and repeat tongue- twisters such as "The Leith polith deceiveth us. ." On one unfortunate occasion somewhere in North Wales, certainly not on our patch, the duty doctor arrived to find his partner already there. On enquiring why he was there as he was not on duty the reply was that unfortunately he was the person to be examined.

One of the anxieties of police work is of missing or of disturbing forensic evidence at a scene of crime, particularly when it was not immediately obvious that a crime may have been committed. The ability to use DNA testing was not available at that time. Calls to cases of sudden death were not uncommon, often to confirm the fact of death and allow further action to proceed. If possible the patient`s GP was called but often this information was not available. There has always been a difficult circumstance where either an ambulance or the police had been called and found an obviously dead person. Regulations required that they were unable to confirm this and unable to leave the scene until a doctor had confirmed death. Nor were ambulances allowed to convey an obviously dead patient to a hospital. In these circumstances it was not unusual to have to leave a waiting room full of patients to confirm a death and allow them to leave, to the unnecessary inconvenience of those waiting. Common sense has at last prevailed and under defined protocols police and paramedics can confirm the death and immediate attendance by a doctor is not necessary. Some years ago I sat on an NHS complaints panel hearing an appeal against a finding of breach of contract against a lady doctor from London who refused to visit a patient who had collapsed and died at home. Her defence at the hearing was that she had no prior knowledge of the patient and therefore could not certify death. Obviously legally incorrect and the finding was that she was required to attend to confirm death even if unable to certify the cause of death.

Deaths in certain circumstances have statutorily to be reported to the coroner and the body cannot be moved before he gives permission. This can give rise to problems at times.Where obvious trauma or injury is present this does not present a problem. The requirement also includes patients suffering from certain prescribed illnesses, for example asbestosis, to be reported but at times the attending doctor may not be aware of this aspect of the past history. Another required situation is when a patient dies within a month of an operation, and this particular requirement did give us a problem in our practice on one occasion. A very elderly patient in a Residential Home died during the night, a not unusual occurrence bearing in mind the huge number of nursing and residential home beds in the area. The carer on duty rang my partner to report the death, was asked whether the death was expected and told this was so and that another partner had seen her the previous day, and he gave permission for her to be moved as was the local custom to a chapel of rest. Residential and nursing homes always liked to move bodies out under cover of darkness. Significantly what he was not told was that the patient had fallen a month before, sustained a fracture, had been admitted to hospital and a plate inserted into her femur and she was then returned to the Home. The Coroner was not at all pleased when this became apparent and both this partner, and another partner whose only fault was that the patient was registered on his personal list, were both required to attend the inquest and severely reprimanded. Headlines in the local press are always embarrassing and never welcomed. Luckily I think this was the only time during my time in practice.

In most of the major crimes a forensic pathologist is called in direct and there is no local involvement. In our time this was usually Dr Don Wayte from Bangor, who I knew well from contact in other areas within the service, and who became a very respected witness. During our time as police surgeons I managed to get Dr., later Professor, Bernard Knight who was at the time one of the most senior and respected forensic pathologists in the country up to talk to one of our College meetings.

A more frequent involvement in serious crime was in alleged rape or sexual abuse cases, either to examine the victim or the alleged assailant, but never both because of the potential risk of cross-contamination being used as a defence. In these circumstances another partner had to be called. The nature of these examinations and the intimate specimens which had to be taken made this an unpleasant task for both doctor and examinee. In latter years there has been a demand from the women's lobby to have a female doctor carry out the examination of rape victims and where possible this was arranged. While this can more easily be done in larger conurbations which are so busy that the doctor may be present and busy continually all night in North Wales the number of female doctors willing to be called out was very small and uncertain. Improved facilities were initially provided by carrying out female examinations at our surgery rather than at the police station, and more recently a special and quite luxurious rape examination suite was set up by the Police Authority.

We did both the practice and the police on-call at the same time, but the development of the local on-call doctors co-operative based initially at Llandudno and later at Bodelwyddan Hospital caused a dilemma. The NHS on-call commitment was much reduced but the practice had to be continually available for police calls, which had in any case reduced in frequency. By this time I had retired and new doctors had joined, resulting in a difference of opinion as to whether to carry on. A further change was the building of a new police station at St Asaph with the intention to carry out all the custodial work for a large area there. Rod Gilmore has continued to do the work individually, along with Dr. Hugh Jones of Prestatyn, one of my ex-trainees.

The Ambulance Service

This is a service which has seen major expansion over the years. In the early years there were a few ambulances operated by the District Councils under the Medical Officer of Health and based locally, together with many local voluntary ambulances staffed by part-timers and by the St John organisation. Hospital out-patient attendances were few and patients usually attended by public transport. The majority of emergency calls in rural areas went direct to the local GP and most were dealt with on the spot and not admitted. Only the most serious injuries went direct to hospital. Perhaps the situation was different in the conurbations where many patients used the casualty department for all injuries and many other complaints as well. GPs and the local ambulance-men knew and trusted each other. Strictly speaking ambulances were only allowed to take patients to hospitals, not to surgeries even if miles closer.

Hospital out-patient letters routinely included "if you need transport tell your GP" (not ask!) which put the doctors and receptionists in a difficult position when they thought an ambulance was not necessary. At times ambulances did not collect on time and this led to an irate call to the surgery which then had to check with the ambulance centre. The ambulance service have now taken direct responsibility for all ambulance bookings and arrangements directly between themselves and the patient, to the great relief of many receptionists.

The inexorable rise in outpatient attendances together with the loss of public transport services has meant an ever-increasing demand on the ambulance service. A two-tier service had to be organised, the true emergency service and a sitting service to outpatients which at times was provided by the contracting of local taxi services. Two types of ambulance vehicle were required, one being more highly equipped to cope with more serious cases, some of which needed to be transferred much longer distances and at great speed with. more experienced and better trained crew and this led to more centralisation of services.

Highly trained paramedics began to appear and provided excellent on the spot resuscitation and care together with better supervision during the journey to hospital. They carried equipment such as ECG machines and defibrillators together with intravenous fluids and a variety of drugs, facilities which were not available to local GPs at the time. Most GPs would acknowledge that ambulance crews were better able to provide on the spot treatment than they themselves could provide. A few GPs did take a special interest in this area. I recall Dr Peter Gratton Parry from Portmadoc who early on experimented with flashing lights and radio communication and who appeared at meetings all kitted out. Another was Dr Chas. Parry-Jones from Benllech who was an enthusiastic member of the organisation BASICS. One practical problem did arise in extending the paramedic service to all the peripheral stations. Many of the crew were locals who had been there for years and understandably not all wished to retrain and upgrade.

GPs ordering an ambulance for admission and which ws not a "blue-lights" emergency situation were asked to give an acceptable "in-hospital" time, say within the hour or within two hours. This put a degree of medico-legal pressure on the GP if the condition of the patient worsened in the meantime. Ambulance response times have achieved much greater political prominence in recent years with target times being reduced and this has led to the situation where crews sit and wait in their vehicles in strategically placed locations rather than at their home base. Comments in the press are not uncommon when emergency amulances fail to attend within the target times.

The rural nature of much of Wales and the mountains where many people get into difficulties together with the occasional childbirth in snowbound farmhouse has led to the services of the RAF helicopter services being called in from Valley on Ynys Mon or from RAF Brawdy in the south to evacuate patients to hospital. Many have been very grateful for this assistance. More recently Air Ambulances have been developed by public fundraising.

Over the years the service has moved from a local to a county and then to a North Wales service. In 1988 an All-Wales Ambulance Trust was formed and for once the administrative centre was based in the north, at the H.M. Stanley Hospital at St Asaph. Costs have exceeded budgets and this year has seen a major crisis with three Chief Executives in one year and a wish-list for major financing for new vehicles. A system whereby all 999 calls to the police, ambulance, or fire services go to a central control is being introduced since very often more than one need to be involved at the same incident. The Trust may consider involvement in the GP call centres and is taking responsibility for running NHS Direct in 2007.

The service over the years has provided an excellent service much appreciated by doctors and by the public, a service which has usually been provided with a smile and a cheery word for the users.

Vocational Training for general practice

In pre-NHS times doctors qualified and usually went directly into general practice, even single-handed, without any further experience or training. Many would become assistants in one or more practices before becoming a partner in the practice or setting up their own practice, learning the ropes by "standing next to Nellie " as the saying in the factories went. They might wait up to ten years or more before being offered a partnership, or at least an offer to buy into the practice. Even then it was usually a junior partnership doing most of the calls and most of the night work, and taking only a small share of the practice profits. How different from today when supply and demand often dictates that new partners expect parity of workload and of income from day one. Older readers will no doubt remember the very popular series Dr Finley's casebook on television - Dr Finlay being the young doctor with new ideas working as an assistant with the old-fashioned Dr Cameron. A generation later my personal experience was not too dissimilar.

No further formal training after qualification was required for the whole of the GP`s professional life. Hospital doctors were required by their Royal Colleges to undergo specified training before being appointed to specialist posts and this difference in training often resulted in them looking upon the GP as a second class doctor.

The 1940's during the latter stages of the World War and at a time when great plans for the future were being conceived, amongst them the concept of a comprehensive National Health Service available to all and free at the point of delivery, saw major proposals for medical training. Two reports by Sir Henry Cohen, later Lord Cohen of Birkenhead, identified the need for GP education and proposed specific training for general practitioners, although it took a couple of decades before this was available. Lord Moran,. physician to King George and to Winston Churchill in evidence to the Spens committee in 1946 famously described GP`s as "doctors who had fallen off the specialist ladder", a comment which rankled for many years. The Report was mainly concerned with remuneration but did recommend that after the completion of the required pre-registration house appointments doctors wishing to enter practice should spend a period of one year and preferably two as an assistant, and even suggested that doctors who intended to become specialists would benefit from a year as an assistant in general practice.

The Platt Report in 1961 on Medical Staffing in the Hospital Service pinpointed the benefit of additional experience by undertaking a minimum of two years after registration and recommended that for doctors intending to go into general practice these posts should include specialties such as obstetrics and paediatrics but it also stressed that this additional training was for educational development rather than for the service needs of hospitals.

In 1963 the Annis Gillie Report from the Standing Medical Advisory Committee on The Field of Work of the Family Doctor covered the whole topic but made important recommendations in its chapter on "Education and the Family Doctor".

The parlous state of affairs emphasised by the Collings Report in the BMJ in 1951 and the generally poor morale within general practice following the introduction of the NHS led, as already described, to the founding in 1952 of the College of General Practitioners with the aim to raise standards and to boost morale,

The Fifties, following The Medical Act 1950, saw the first formalised requirement for any postgraduate study and resulted in the setting up of Postgraduate Education Committees in all regions to cover both hospital doctors and general practitioners. The requirement was for all new doctors qualifying from 1953 onwards - two years before I qualified - to undergo twelve months pre-registration experience in surgical and medical hospital posts (six months in each) before full registration was granted and the doctor could practise independently, electing either go into general practice or continue another career path. There was still no requirement for any exposure during undergraduate training to medical life outside hospitals although by this time some medical schools were encouraging and facilitating students to spend a few days in a GP practice. The first independent University Department of General Practice was created in Edinburgh in 1957 but other Universities were very slow to follow suit although encouraged by the recommendation in the Todd Report. By 1986 the Mackenzie Report which studied the position was able to identify that all Universities would have some sort of department of general practice by the end of 1987.

The Spens committee in 1946 had recommended that after completing house appointments a doctor who wished to enter general practice should spend a year (or preferably two as an Assistant in General Practice at a fixed salary and that the principal to which the assistant was attached should also receive a supervision fee plus a contribution towards the additional necessary expenses. The first Trainee Assistant scheme was introduced in1948, administered by the Executive Councils on the advice of their LMC who appointed Selection Committees for the appointment of trainers who were then allowed to appoint their own trainees. The only influence the University had was the right of the Postgraduate committee to appoint a representative to the selection committees. It was all very informal and unstructured and not taken up by all Executive Councils or by many trainee assistants. As explained elsewhere I believe I was one of the few to do so in North Wales in 1958-59. The Denbighshire and Flintshire LMC later approved Drs Wharton, Dr Anderson,and Dr REH "Bob" Jones, as GP trainers.

The Trainee General Practitioner Scheme which had been in existence for fifteen years was reviewed by the GMSC in 1963. It identified a number of criticisms of the scheme as currently run and pinpointed the lack of overall supervision and the abuse of the facility by some practices but it supported the principle of the Scheme and made recommendations about the selection procedures and the educational content during the trainee year.

The Royal Commission on Medical Education (the Todd Commission) in 1968 recommended a total period of five years vocational training for general practice. In 1971 a working party of the Advisory Committee on General Practice of the Council for Postgraduate Medical Education in England and Wales formulated proposals for a programme of vocational training. It was an aim to set up the full five year period of training which had been recommended by Todd but GMSC at that time were strongly opposed to any more than a three year programme. It was accepted that the only realistic and practical step which could be taken because of the manpower situation and the need to develop the necessary facilities for training was that a three year programme be set up The subsequent development of vocational training in the UK was overseen by the establishment of General Practice sub-committees in each of the Regional Postgraduate Committees in 1971

An early call for training for general practitioners had been made at the Welsh Postgraduate Committee by Mr McInroy, a general surgeon at Llandudno Hospital, but his ideas entailed all the training being in hospital posts. This was fairly typical of the attitudes of many consultants at that time. While welcoming his interest the Postgraduate Committee rejected his suggestion. A contribution of inestimable value towards the setting up of training for GPs in Wales and based on a sensible wide vision was that of Professor C.R.Lowe, Professor of Public Health and Industrial Medicine in Cardiff, who chaired the Welsh Postgraduate Committee of the Senate of the Medical School for some years. The committee was reformulated as The Committee for Postgraduate Education in Wales. Many of the postgraduate issues were dealt with at the main committee level while responsibility for Vocational Training for general practice in Wales was delegated to a new Sub-committee in General Practice of the Welsh Postgraduate Committee which held its first meeting on 26th April 1972 called by Mr Arnold Aldis, the Director and Dean of Postgraduate Studies and which elected Dr. Robert Harvard Davis to the chair. I was not present at the inaugural meeting but arrived to represent WGMSC at the third meeting and was there for over twenty years. Gwyn Thomas was there representing the College from North Wales

Meetings were always held in South Wales and it was one of the many committees Gwyn Thomas and myself spent many hours and days travelling to. Since most of the other members worked within an hour or so of Cardiff they were very accommodating to us in arranging meeting times, either at about 4.0pm or about 11am. - either time made for a long day and drive but at least we could do it in a day and we normally travelled together. Over the period of some twenty years the roads to Cardiff improved considerably with the building of the M4 and a number of by-passes but it remains poor in many places to this day. Most find it easier to go down through Shrewsbury and Hereford rather than round the longer M5-M6 route. On a couple of occasions we tried the embryonic air-service from Hawarden to Rhoose, Cardiff, but the timings were more geared to those travelling from South to North rather than the way we wanted to go. Nevertheless an interesting experience and a great aerial view of Wales. The new commercial air service recently commenced from Anglesey to Cardiff still suffers from the same poor timetabling as far as users from the north are concerned.

Train journeys to all meetings in Cardiff were long and rarely used as the service was so bad with no meals available. On occasions people from North Wales drove to Shrewsbury and picked up the train there, not very convenient and later it was found to be easier to drive a little further to Craven Arms where station access and parking was much easier. All in all we found it easier to drive all the way giving flexibility to timings and allowing stops for refreshment when required.

Robert Havard Davis was the first chairman of the sub-committee, later followed by my namesake Dr R. C.(Cen) Humphreys from Crickhowell, by Dr John Owen from Porthcawl, by Dr William Roberts from Aberystwyth and then Dr Geoff Morgan from Cardiff. In the early days the main focus was on vocational training, later when this was well established the Sub-committee turned its attention more to the new continuing medical education (CME) developments as discussed later.

The Sub-committee was responsible for setting standards required within training practices and for appointing and training the trainers. Meetings were interesting with occasional battles between academia and practicality, but always friendly. I was there together with Denzil Davies from Barry as a WGMSC representative with our remit being to allow things to develop at a reasonable pace without causing too much distress to some of the educational die-hards on GMSC in London. This at times brought me into conflict with the chairmen, in particular Dr William Roberts who was parachuted in from the main committee as chairman. The results in the MRCGP examination from Wales were never good and William had set up a very effective MRCGP course which improved results considerably. His great desire was to introduce a criterion that trainers should be required before appointment to hold the MRCGP by examination (at a time when many of the trainers were older and pre-dated the examination) and that all trainees should be required to pass the examination on completion and this led to frequent but friendly conflict. Since Wales is a medical village and we all knew each other well from other committees there was always a good rapport within the group. When he vacated the chair I was nominated along with Geoff Morgan from Cardiff and the College - unsurprisingly he won.

The central figure around which the organisation of vocational training revolved was the Postgraduate Adviser, for many years Dr Derek Llewelyn of Bridgend. He was appointed in 1971 as the first Postgraduate Adviser in General Practice in Wales (in England his colleagues were known as Regional Advisers but Wales was considered a Principality not a Region).We insisted at the outset that the Adviser should spend at least half-time in clinical practice so as to be in touch with practicalities and developments at the coalface but the demands of the post steadily increased. On a UK basis vocational training was supervised by the Joint Committee for Postgraduate Training in General Practice, the JCPTGP, about which much more later. On his retirement in 1990 he was succeeded by Dr Terry Reilly from the same Bridgend practice and one of the first trainees in Wales. The other vital component of the training programmes was the Course Organiser in each local scheme. They were all very enthusiastic and hard-working but were initially unpaid until we managed in 1974 to amend the Regulations so that they could receive the same grant as the trainers received.

Textbooks on general practice and on training started to be written, one of the earliest in 1971 being the Principles of Family Medicine edited by the Bridgend practice. The following year The Future General Practitioner from the RCGP set out in five areas the curriculum to be covered during training.

Trainer selection was by Standing Area Selection Committees with a membership consisting of the Postgraduate Adviser, another member of the Sub-committee, an LMC member, a local Postgraduate Organiser and a local Course Organiser. Appointments had subsequently to be approved by the Sub-committee. An appeal mechanism was available for rejected candidates but after informal discussions and helpful advice was virtually never used.

Trainers were initially voluntary and it was important not to be too demanding of them but in later years payment was built into the pay structure. Criteria for trainers and training practices were introduced and these were strengthened as training developed High standards came to be expected both of the training provided and the practice premises and organisational standards. Attendance at trainers courses was encouraged and later made mandatory. The first course was run by Robert Harvard Davis at the teaching unit at Cardiff and courses were later set up in Swansea and in Bangor.

One of the earlier standards set for training practices in Wales was the improvement in medical records with letters filed in date order and also the setting up of an age-sex register, very easy now but quite difficult to do on cards and to keep up to date before the introduction of computers. Even the FPC registration systems were manual at that time. As interest and the requirement to undergo formal vocational training developed the number of training practices increased, some taking trainees from within the scheme and some finding their own trainees usually from amongst those who had already completed some of the necessary modules and were constructing their own programmes.

Following the retirement of Terry Reilly as postgraduate organiser the post passed to Dr Simon Smail, senior lecturer in the Department of General Practice at Cardiff Medical School. The increasing workload had also led to the appointment of Dr David Wood as associate adviser for North Wales. All have contributed immensely to general practice education in Wales.

The first V.T. scheme in Wales was set up in 1971 as a pilot by David Coulter and Derek Llewelyn in the Bridgend practice, followed a year later by one based on Rhyl in North Clwyd. The initial meeting of our scheme in Rhyl was attended by consultants Dr David Meredith, Dr Charles Hilton Jones, Mr David Aiken and by Gwyn Thomas and myself as representatives of the Denbighshire and Flintshire Local Medical Committee as it then was. Later Dr Ellen Emslie who replaced Charles Hilton Jones as Postgraduate Organiser and Mr Pal the A&E consultant joined.

Gwyn Thomas had been shadowing the Bridgend development for the previous year and was elected chairman and Course Organiser, a position he held for twenty-three years. In so doing he held the record for the longest serving course organiser in the UK by far. Subsequently the course organisers have been Dr. Peter Elliott for four years, followed by Dr Alison Park from Betws-y -coed, and then Dr Tim Peskett and my partner Rod Gilmore shared the role.

In 1973 when my family were visiting an old friend Professor Philip Worthington (formerly Consultant Oro-maxillary surgeon at St. Asaph) at the University of Washington in Seattle I was able to briefly visit John Guyler, Professor of Medicine at the University to see how training for general practice (known there as Family Practice Residencies) was being developed in the United States and was able to bring back useful ideas.

The UK approved course consisted of three years, two in hospital posts usually medicine, paediatrics, obstetrics and casualty and two six-month periods in two approved training practices. Initially locally the trainers were Dr Denis Wharton in the Rysseldene practice in Colwyn Bay and Dr P.M. Anderson in the Russell Road surgery in Rhyl, his partner Brian Bracewell joining him two years later. The first trainees started in August 1972. Dr Leask who was later in practice in Conway was in the second year and one of my partners Patrick Edwards was in the third wave. Drs JG Jones and Hardway in Kinmel Bay also acted as trainers but outside the scheme and advertising directly for their trainees. As the intake expanded from two trainees per year to four Pendre surgery in Holywell and the Beech House practice in Denbigh joined the scheme Trainers and trainees were the terms officially used but educational purists later emphasised that the aim should be to educate broadly and that "training was something done to circus animals". With the rapidly changing role of the GP over the years a wider education became essential, with increasing emphasis on management and leadership and on ethical issues. Those hospital consultants who agreed to participate in the new scheme deserve thanks for their vision and help, but as a consequential perk they probably had a consistently higher standard of SHO in their departments than they would sometimes have obtained by advertising in the open market. The development of a good training scheme also meant a supply of well-trained new partners into practices in North Wales.

There was always a considerable conflict between the service needs of the hospital department and the need of the trainees to participate in the GP training requirements, particularly in the Half-day Release scheme. This was one of the success features of the scheme, allowing trainees once a week to meet up together and with the other GP trainers and to remind themselves and others that although they were at the time in hospital posts they were actually training for general practice. It was not always popular with consultants who had to release their SHOs from their hospital duties. At the outset trainees had to travel all the way to Liverpool to attend a day-release at Dr York's practice in Maghull but this was not really practicable. Later while the numbers of trainees was still small a combined day-release with the scheme at the Wrexham Maelor Hospital which started the following year with Dr Matt Sampson of Overton as Course Organiser but the travel time factor and difficulty getting away in time again made this unsatisfactory and the joint programme ceased after some three years. The day release module was one of the more popular aspects of the scheme and provided an opportunity for subjects relevant to general practice which would not otherwise be encountered to be laid on such as a visit to the Point of Ayr colliery, meeting the undertaker and the Macmillan nurse. Later as the number of doctors wishing to train increased other practices including my own became approved as training practices. Ysbyty Gwynedd in Bangor started a scheme in August 1973. Since undertaking Vocational Training was voluntary an additional Allowance was built into the pay structure on entering practice for those who had undertaken it.

Most of the doctors going through the Scheme entered practice in North Wales at the end of their training. An advantage to both sides was that during the training period trainees got to know the training practices and other doctors and practices in the area so that the formal and often unhelpful references received previously were no longer required. Of the many trainees going through our practice only some five did not enter local practices so one felt one had some responsibility for the raising of standards through the area. My particular interest in the medico-political field meant that our trainees received perhaps more insight into this field than they might otherwise have had and I am pleased that several have since continued this interest and are now making they own very significant contributions in this field.

A very successful feature of training in Wales was the Welsh General Practice Vocational Training Day held each June in Llandrindod Wells and attended by both trainers and trainees. The morning session was split allowing the Welsh Association of Trainees to meet by themselves to discuss problems and develop constructive criticisms to present to the afternoon plenary session while the trainers and organisers held a seminar on a topic related to training. During the afternoon the whole conference under the guidance of the Postgraduate Adviser would discuss feedback he had received from trainees questionnaires and comments arising from the trainees morning session. Constructive full and frank discussions took place and the report of the Conference was relayed back to the Sub-committee in General Practice for further discussion and action.

A few years ago when entry into general practice became a less attractive option the number of trainees applying diminished and some practices found they had periods without a trainee in the practice. This had arguments for and against, some arguing that the practice should not become dependent on trainees for the service component of their training. On the other side the increasingly monitored requirements for becoming and remaining a training practice including the requirement for set-aside teaching time with perhaps the need to drop other commitments outside the practice to allow for this, together with the need to provide additional accommodation and library facilities make gaps inconvenient. With the increased number of doctors leaving medical schools and a proportion of these training for practice the need for training places has increased again recently. Since a large number of these are women special arrangements to allow for part-time training have been introduced. Somewhere along the line at their instigation there was a name change from trainees to Registrars to reflect more accurately comparability with hospital training grades and also to improve their perceived status by patients.

Alongside the need to accommodate the registrars there has been a considerable need for practices to provide much more experience for medical students and also for nurses and social workers in training. Accommodation within the premises has become an increasing problem and some practices have expanded them more than once in recent years. Others have been less fortunate in not being able to do so adequately because of their sites. Trainer manpower problems are arising. One area in England has reported a practice which normally accommodates one or two registrars being told to prepare for up to six simultaneous registrar placements, in addition to medical students. Obviously in such circumstances considerable changes in the format of teaching will need to be introduced.

There has for many years a fairly strong lobby suggesting that all hospital doctors in training should spend a period in general practice so that they become more aware of patients' lives outside hospital. A worry by some GPs was that a disenchanted and disgruntled specialist registrar forced to spend a period in practice would not be easy to handle. Now all doctors will in future receive experience in practices during their two postgraduate Foundation Years training.

Since I left the sub-committee in 1994 at the time I also left the GMSC the attention of the Sub-committee has been largely directed at the development of a system of accreditation which will tie in with the GMC proposals for re-validation of doctors when details of this are finally agreed, while at the same time continuing development of vocational training and of the Summative Assessment requirements which we imposed on them from the JCPTGP, of which more later. The appraisal scheme for established principals which is being developed in Wales under the guidance of Professor Malcolm Lewis is receiving considerable acclaim nationally and by the GMC.

The development of vocational training has been a long but fascinating and largely successful process which I have been fortunate to be able to contribute to on a local as well as on a Wales and UK basis. All in all a very enjoyable part of my experience.

The JCPTGP - the Joint Committee

The Medical Practices Committee reported that of forty doctors filling single-handed practice vacancies during the year to September 1975 only twenty-four had any previous experience of general practice. The Joint Committee for Postgraduate Training for General Practice (hereafter called the JCPTGP or the Joint Committee) was set up in 1974 with equal representation from the then "divided tribes" (Dr Brian Keighley`s description) of the GMSC and the College of General Practitioners a year after the first preliminary committee meeting.

Its functions were to advise professional and educational bodies on the standards required for postgraduate training for general practice, to monitor regional training arrangements and to recognise programmes which furnished educational experience of the required standard. It was also the prescribed body to carry out functions related to certification as specified in the Vocational Training Regulations. Until then arrangements for training GPs had been completely voluntary and were being developed in a piecemeal fashion across regions in the UK.

The JCPTGP had wide representation from the Conference of Postgraduate Advisers in General Practice and of Postgraduate Medical Deans, from the Joint Consultants Committee, the Association of University Teachers of General Practice, the Armed Services GP Approval Board, from the Association of Course Organisers, and also from the Ministry of Health so all interested bodies were represented. Trainees themselves were represented by one from each of the RCGP and the GMSC.

There were Joint Secretaries, both practising GPs and one from each group, and the Chairmanship rotated on a three yearly cycle between the two. There has been some mutual suspicion between the two main groups over the years with the young and expanding College always striving for higher standards and looking for a five year training period, in line with hospital specialist training and as recommended by the Todd Royal Commission, while the GMSC were keen to move at a speed which was practical, affordable, and acceptable to the profession as a whole and looking at a three year training. Three years was accepted as an initial programme but the five year programme has throughout remained a firm aim of the Royal College.

The National Health Service (Vocational Training) Regulations were passed in 1979 and required all practitioners entering practice after February 1981 to have completed a three year programme, defined as two years in recognised and varied hospital posts and twelve months in recognised training practices. This was defined as Prescribed Experience. To allow for doctors already having considerable experience, sometimes abroad, and perhaps wishing to make a career change an Equivalent Experience mechanism was introduced which allowed doctors to set out their past experience and for them then to be told how much of this was acceptable and what other training they were required to undertake. Some doctors wished to count experience in EEC countries. None of these countries had the equivalent of the UK Royal Colleges who inspected posts for standards and gave educational approval and it was often difficult to obtain satisfactory confirmation of the quality of the training which had been received in posts in these countries. The hospital experience was in service posts, already existing and therefore already funded, whereas the general practice training posts were not previously in existence and so considerable additional service funding was necessary and often extremely difficult to obtain.

At the end of the required period of training the JCPTGP issued a Certificate of Satisfactory Completion of Prescribed or of Equivalent Experience, although in practical terms there was no difference between the two. JCPTGP Certificates of Satisfactory Completion of Training were issued purely on the confirmation of completion of the required programme with each trainer signing that the period had been satisfactorily completed.

Supervision of Training schemes and standards had been delegated to Regional Postgraduate Committees with the JCPTGP from time to time publishing its Recommendations for the Establishment of Criteria for the approval and re-approval of trainers. It set out its expectations for Trainers as doctors and as teachers and for the organisation and management of the practice. Doctors training within the Armed Forces were supervised by the Armed Services General Practice Approval Board with which Dr. Mike Jeffries from North Wales was actively involved for many years. Mike also served as Medical Adviser to the Joint Committee in 1989 but this post was later discontinued.

Organisation of the training was delegated to Regional Postgraduate Education Committees who in turn delegated to their Sub-committees in General Practice. The Principality of Wales was considered as one Region and within it there were local Training Schemes, usually based on a District General Hospital, with ours at Glan Clwyd being the first to be up and running after a pilot at Bridgend.

Each Regional Committee was inspected regularly by the JCPTGP using a team of peers, usually Regional Advisors from other regions, who would look at arrangements in the region as a whole and also visit and inspect in detail one of the local training schemes. Very detailed reports were submitted and debated at meetings of the JCPTGP who would confirm any remedial action which might be deemed necessary and usually give approval to the Region for a further period of three years. On only one occasion was re-approval not given to a Region. It was soon after I had been asked to become a GMSC representative on the JCPTGP in 1987 and this was the start of a very interesting period.

Dr Dorothy Ward from Glasgow and the GMSC was the chairman at the time. In 1988 after receiving evidence from inspecting teams over several years that standards in training practices in the region were repeatedly unsatisfactory a momentous decision was taken by the JCPTGP to withdraw recognition of the North-East Thames Region from 1st February 1989.The Royal College Council as a consequence withdrew its recognition of the Region and the eligibility of trainees from the Region to take the MRCGP examination. It subsequently "reiterated that College recognition of vocational training and entry to the College examination have now reverted to the College itself". and set out its views clearly in an editorial in its Journal in June 1988.

This decision because of its potential consequences involving about 175 trainers and a similar number of trainees reverberated for several years. One immediate need was to safeguard trainees already part-way through a programme. Those on self-constructed schemes were protected until 31st January 1990 and those on three year schemes until 1st May 1991.This was the only occasion when withdrawal of approval from a region was necessary although as a result of visits some schemes were required to be reorganised and some hospital posts had their recognition for general practice training withdrawn.

The words "satisfactory completion" of training were not defined in the early days but later gave rise to considerable debate as to whether any examination or other testing at the completion of training was required. The question of the meaning of "satisfactory completion " came to a head in the late 80`s and arose because there was anecdotal evidence of doctors who had completed vocational training but whose knowledge and practice was subsequently found to be grossly deficient. Deficiencies in training appeared to be almost exclusively within the hospital components of the programme. Estimates suggested that about two per cent could come into this category and obviously there was criticism of the GP trainers who had not spotted this and who should have refused to sign them up. There was a practical problem however in that there was within the Regulations no mechanism for a trainee not signed up to undertake a further period of approved GP training and this gave the trainer who had doubts no room for manoeuvre as the trainee would be left in limbo and unable to enter practice.

There had been an examination requirement for entry to membership of the College since1965 and they wished to use this as a compulsory end-point assessment for vocational training. The examination did however have a fairly constant failure rate of between 20% and 30%. Obviously the GMSC could not accept that this number of doctors would not be given what was now a mandatory Vocational Training Certificate and who therefore would not be allowed to enter practice, that is to work in their chosen field, particularly as there was no possibility of them undertaking a further period in a training practice. Arguments raged about whether the College standard was too high an entry standard and that there should be a lower standard which was acceptable to enter practice, but allowing the College to maintain its examination at a higher level for membership of the College.

There was an additional difficulty in that doctors could not sit the MRCGP examination which was held twice a year until after they had completed training whereas doctors often wished to start in practice as soon as they finished training and the JCPTGP certificate was issued. In fact the certificates were in practice issued a few days before completion to allow this.

The RCGP published a Policy Statement on Quality in General Practice in 1985 which was discussed by JCPTGP in 1986. At the same time UEMO, the European body representing general practice across Europe, were working towards training in the other countries which could be recognised across frontiers. An EEC Directive in 1986 required countries to set up regulatory authorities so that certificates could be issued by 1990, although the minimum prescribed training period was two years, which could be exceeded if wished. There is no doubt that the training for general practice, if it existed at all, was in none of these countries up to the level of the UK and in some it was still very rudimentary. Complexity was introduced in 1993 with the introduction of the Directive on Free Movement of Labour within the E.U.(the EEC as it was then) allowing doctors who had completed training in other EU states to practice in this country without further questions.

Having accepted that some assessment method at the end of training was necessary the question arose as to how. Various papers on assessment methods were produced and published including The Assessment of Vocational Training in General Medical Practice by the University of York in 1988.

In 1988 Dorothy Ward passed the chair on to Dr. Donald Irvine from the College. Donald was a powerful figure with very high aims and expectations on the attainment of quality and who was very keen to press the College view. He later went on to become President of the General Medical Council and to set out upon its reorganisation.

Representatives to the LMC Annual Conference in 1988 were still very suspicious about the changes being introduced into medical education and "invited the GMSC to prepare a report on the legal position and powers of the various bodies involved in training such as the Regional general practice subcommittee, the JCPTGP and the course organisers, as concern has been expressed that they may be assuming powers to which they re not entitled". One particular issue was that some regional sub-committees were attempting to insert a requirement that trainers should hold the MRCGP before appointment. The resulting report from the BMA lawyers cleared the air, clarified the situation, and indicated that in most instances powers were being correctly exercised.

Discussions on "satisfactory completion" continued to rumble and as in all such situations where there is a marked difference of opinion or emphasis the holding mechanism of setting up a working party "to consider methods for ensuring a doctor's competence to become a principal in the NHS" was adopted, although it was obvious that a report that both sides could agree to and on which action could be taken was essential. In September1989 the JCPTGP under the chairmanship of Donald Irvine received the final report of its Working Party on Assessment and Vocational Training for General Practice.

The issue of "satisfactory completion" was finally laid to rest by the publishing in 1990 of a joint letter signed by Donald Irvine as Chairman of the JCPTGP, Denis Pereira Gray as Chairman of College Council and Ian Bogle as Chairman of GMSC stating that " certificates… (of the JCPTGP)…do indeed indicate that doctors have achieved a satisfactory standard of competence and performance" The next phase was to attempt to produce some acceptable way whereby a trainee's competence at the end of training was satisfactory could be made. All agreed that this was necessary, the disagreement was as to how.

At the end of Donald's three years in 1991 the chairmanship rotated back to the GMSC and unexpectedly Ian Bogle, the GMSC chairman who had himself previously been a Joint Secretary and knew its problems well, asked me to take the hot potato of the chair of the JCPTGP. Considerable persuasion was necessary before I agreed.

To carry the implementation of satisfactory completion forward a further working party was set up under my chairmanship in 1992 to produce a blueprint for end-point assessment. I was very lucky in the committee's selection of the other members. Drs. John Toby, Robin Fraser, Brian Keighley and myself together with the two Joint Secretaries Malcolm Freeth and Bill Styles, who while having considerably different viewpoints, were willing to discuss and compromise and over a period of months we agreed a report which after considerable debate at the main committee and at the parent committees was finally accepted without significant amendment in 1994.

We had managed to agree that Satisfactory Completion would require more than just completion of the programme and would require competence to have been demonstrated in four ways, a process which came to be called Summative Assessment The four areas were to include an assessment by the trainer, a test of factual knowledge, analysis of consulting skills by use of video-recordings, and the completion of a project which could be an extended case study or an audit. The whole concept of Summative assessment with the possibility of failing to achieve a certificate and thus being unable to enter general practice was obviously not a popular one amongst trainees and also amongst many of their trainers.

Following its adoption by the JCPTGP the introduction of Summative assessment in itself gave rise to further debate about the mechanisms and the standards required, about the relative place and educational significance of Formative Assessment and Summative Assessment. It was agreed that formative assessment should be seen as educational, should take place regularly throughout each period of training and should be the opportunity for progress to be discussed between trainer and trainee and further needs assessed. It was seen as a mechanism whereby deficiencies in knowledge or its application could be spotted early and corrective measures introduced so that no-one arrived at the Summative stage unprepared. Summative Assessment was seen as a pass or fail assessment at the completion of training, and it was argued as to whether the results of formative assessment could have any place to play within the Summative process. Since then considerable fine tuning of assessments methods has continued.

Both my predecessor Donald Irvine and my successor in the chair, Professor Denis Pereira Gray, were subsequently given knighthoods in the Honours Lists which makes me feel I went wrong somewhere!! In truth they were knighted in recognition of other and wider achievements over a number of years, but at least I felt I had been in good company.

During my period of office I was very lucky to be supported by three excellent Joint Secretaries, Dr. Bill Styles and then Dr. Justin Allen from the College and Dr. Malcolm Freeth from the GMSC, as well as being able to lean on the invaluable advice and counsel of Mrs Hilla Gittins who had been administrative secretary of the JCPTGP for many years and of Brian Keighley of GMSC who followed on in the chair after Denis Pereira Gray.

Trainees, or registrars as they are now called, have themselves changed considerably over the years as have their expectations. Improved working conditions within the hospital posts has led to different expectations within general practice. A high proportion of them are female and expect to work part-time both during training and afterwards. It is not just the female doctors whose ideas have changed. Many of them come into the so-called 'Dinkys' category- double income, no kids - and want a lifestyle to suit. I was shocked when attending a National Trainee Conference as part of my chairmanship to discover one of the male trainees talking about only wishing to work in practice on four days and wishing to spend the fifth day doing forestry.

The Joint Committee continued to work very successfully, continually striving to improve standards and receiving plaudits for its functioning. However in 2002 the Chief Medical Officer in England in a Report identified that large numbers of SHOs or doctors in training were being taught to widely varying standards. The Modernising Medical Careers (MMC) programme was set up with its objective of helping to establish national standards for doctors in training. As part of this it was decreed that the JCPTGP should be abolished, together with the Specialist Training Agency (the S.T.A.) responsible for hospital specialist standards where the influence of the various specialist Royal Colleges had been perceived to have possibly compromised best regulation, and sub served into a new body, the PMETB (Postgraduate Medical Education and Training Board) which was given responsibility for postgraduate medical education and training for all specialties. First proposed as the Medical Education Standards Board in the NHS Plan of 2000 after a rocky ride and resignations it finally went live in September 2005. It set explicit standards for both the training curriculum and the assessment of the completion of training in all specialties including general practice and it will issue the certificate of completion of training (the CCT). Dr John Toby took the Joint Committee chair over the last few difficult years and has tried to make sure that the interests of general practice have been safeguarded in the new organisation.

Following the MMC recommendations all graduates will follow a two-year Foundation Programme rotating through more specialties than was possible with the previous system and will then choose which specialty they wish to enter. This will ensure that all doctors have experience of general practice and life outside hospital walls, something general practitioner representatives have been advocating for years. Immediately after this doctors will need to start to train in their chosen specialty and are likely to have increasing difficulties if they subsequently wish to change career course. Unfortunately the introduction of the new arrangements has resulted in a chaotic system for application for posts and has created a crisis within the junior doctors ranks.

The PMETB highlighted failings in all the specialties' assessment methods at present and has also said that it is no longer acceptable to have two standards of assessment and that Summative Assessment must be phased out with all new GPs being assessed in a new programme leading to the MRCGP. The Royal College has finally achieved its goal and the five-year training recommended by the Todd Royal Commission in 1967 will have been achieved. To date the new body has had major problems with long delays in the processing of the applications and is now imposing very large charges for certificates which were previously issued free.

Dr Liam Donaldson, the Cheif Medical Officer, in his recent consultation paper on revalidation and the GMC suggested that the PMETB should take over responsibility for medical education from the GMC. Whether this and his other suggestions will be implemented remains to be seen

My anxiety is that under this general umbrella organisation the vast practical expertise which the JCPTGP has developed over the years in developing the practical, economical, and very detailed day to day oversight of training standards and training practices across the UK will be lost.

Lifelong learning- postgraduate education

In the early days doctors went on "refresher courses", later came "postgraduate education", but currently doctors, like everyone else, are expected to take part in "life-long learning". "Refresher courses" was obviously a wrong term as much of the time one was learning about new developments, many of which would have been considered to be in the realm of fantasy at the time when I qualified. The methods by which doctors learn have also changed markedly.

Certainly in the early years all lectures and courses were run by consultants, no GP would consider putting themselves forward to talk to their peers, and this changed only gradually. Perhaps this was a carry-over from undergraduate days when all teaching was hospital oriented and based. When the change did occur the content became much more relevant to everyday practice, although the need for updating in the rapidly changing specialist fields was recognised.

Sir James McKenzie, a northern GP who developed an interest in heart disease in his practice, moved to London and went on to become one of the founders of modern cardiology wrote in 1919 "the teacher of practical matters must be one who experiences what he teaches. We all recognise that the best teacher for one who wishes to be a shoemaker is the man who is in the habit of making shoes. Unfortunately this common sense idea is rarely applied to medical education".

The Spens Committee chaired by Sir Henry (later Lord) Cohen included a paragraph which read "the committee does not, therefore, accept in its full implications the often re-iterated view that the aim of the curriculum should be to produce a competent GP. General practice is a special form of practice which must be treated on basic principles and appropriate postgraduate study".

In the late fifties it was common for doctors entering into practice to sit one or two diplomas, either the DCH (diploma of child health) or the DRCOG (obstetrics), or occasionally the DPH (public health). It was unusual to sit any other higher qualifications such as membership of the Royal Colleges unless one was thinking of pursuing a hospital career. I sat and passed the DRCOG in 1960 soon after starting in Ruabon. It was at a time when domiciliary midwifery was encouraged and homebirths reasonably common. It had after-effects in that every year or so a completely unfounded rumour would start that I was leaving practice to be a hospital obstetrician. Strangely enough, similar rumours spread several times again while in the Penrhyn Bay practice. On one occasion at Ruabon I was approached by a mother who thanked me very profusely for my skill and attention to her daughter who had just had a baby. I must say I did not recognise her and could not bring to mind who her daughter was, but I accepted the plaudits graciously. It was the following week that I discovered that there was a newly appointed consultant at Wrexham Hospital whose name was also Humphreys, first name Arnold. For some reason even to this day hospital managements seem very loathe to inform local GPs that a new consultant has been appointed, possibly because they are afraid patients will be referred to him or her. As it happened he also drove a car similar to mine, a sporty Kharmann Ghia conversion of the Volkswagen Beetle, of which I was very proud.

One invaluable monthly Journal which supplemented the BMJ and The Lancet and was more geared to GP level with articles on a specific topic each month was The Practitioner which had been published for many decades but which closed down in the sixties or seventies. New free journals paid for by advertising such as Update and Update plus took its place and were equally valuable.

One very valuable learning aid for doctors in the periphery was that developed by husband and wife members of the College, Drs John and Valerie Graves, who developed and ran from their home an audio-visual postal library lending system based on tapes and photographic transparency slides which were coming into use at that time. They ran it for some years until it became too big and was taken over by the College.

Postgraduate Education in Wales has been under the control of the Dean of Postgraduate Medical and Dental Education who controls the training of doctors after leaving medical school. Dr Donald Makinson was Postgraduate Dean at first but for most of the time I was involved the Dean was Dr Tom Hayes who has contributed immensely to an excellent set up in Wales. He was supported by a representative (invariably a Consultant) in each hospital or district known as the Postgraduate Education Organiser responsible for supervising all training locally.

An important feature was the development in 1963 of Postgraduate Centres with pilot centres for Wales in Swansea and Wrexham. These provided facilities and administrative support to organise meetings of various kinds, some on specialist subjects and some specifically for general practice. Later the GP Vocational Course Organisers were also based there. It was interesting that while GPs attended the specialist lectures consultants were rarely seen at GP events unless they were contributing. I was at Ruabon when the Wrexham centre opened and it was a very major asset with a library named after Mr John Spalding who was surgeon at the Maelor. The Postgraduate Centre in Rhyl, the first purpose built centre in Wales, opened in a prefabricated building at the Royal Alexandra (later moving to Bodelwyddan) and one at Bangor developed later. The Postgraduate Organisers played an important role in developing high quality education locally and the ones I recall in North Clwyd were in turn

Drs.D.E.Meredith, Charles Hilton Jones, Ellen Emslie, F.K.Wright, B.K.Bhowmick, and D.Q.Borsey.

We were very lucky at Bodelwyddan to have for many years a very helpful and cooperative postgraduate centre secretary Mrs Gwyneth Stringfellow who went out of her way to help the newly developing GP led events. The RCGP appointed volunteer College Tutors at each centre until in 1992 we were able to persuade the Department of Health to fund paid GP Continuing Medical Education (CME) Tutors at each one.

GPs being independent contractors were required to fund their continuing education themselves whereas hospital salaried doctors were entitled to study leave. The GP position was recognised under Section 63 of the Health Services and Public Health Act 1968 which provided for expenses to be refunded for attendance at courses run by Universities for the independent contractor professions, the GPs, the dentists, pharmacists, opticians and for ancillary staff employed by GPs. This was an important consideration in encouraging doctors from the periphery to go on courses involving travel and overnight stays, often to study topics which could not be covered locally and which at the same time led to cross-fertilization of ideas. This facility was particularly important for doctors in North Wales who often had to travel some considerable distance to attend approved courses. I was frequently amazed that doctors would travel fifty or sixty miles each way after completing an evening surgery to hear an hours lecture at the postgraduate centres. On talking recently to the postgraduate secretary at Ysbyty Glan Clwyd I was told that very little GP CME takes place there now as it is arranged on a LHB level and in GP surgeries, beneficial in some ways but resulting in less interchange between doctors from different localities. Meetings involving both GPs and consultants are very infrequent.

In 1983 a budget overspend resulted in the reduction by the Department of Health of the allocation for that year to the Postgraduate Deans who had responsibility for organising Section 63 as it was universally referred to although in Wales it was strictly speaking Section 2. The Sub-committee in General Practice had an important role in advising on the educational approval of courses, many of which were by this time being organised by bodies other than Universities, and on individual claims if queried. In particular there was a suggestion put forward that only courses in Wales could be attended and this had to be resisted vigorously. Gradually over the years GPs became more certain of their role in teaching each other and the quality of courses and meetings improved considerably. A Postgraduate Training Allowance was introduced into the G.P. remuneration structure in the 1966 contract to encourage doctors to attend.

Continuing medical education was not confined to attending courses, doctors often met together in small study groups and a number of Welsh GPs undertook higher Masters degrees. Weekly publications such as Pulse and General Practitioner as well as providing news produced good educational supplements and a number of other free circulation publications such as Geriatric Medicine appeared. Initially audiocassettes were produced so that doctors could listen to them in their cars and later these became videocassettes. It was not always possible to convince those in authority that these were often a better way of learning rather than the bums on seats at lectures approach.

On a personal level I have already described my first residential post-graduate course in Manchester. Over the years I had had an interest in forensic and medico-legal topics and even as a boy used to read Sherlock Holmes and other crime stories. I read with interest accounts of the famous trials involving forensic experts such as Bernard Spilsbury and the barrister Sir Patrick Hastings. The post-mortem room at the medical school was always of interest and a highlight was the visit of Professor Keith Simpson, the doyen of forensic pathologists at that time. One Cardiff pathologist was always worth watching at his work and I well recall one occasion when he had completed a post-mortem without finding an obvious cause of death and in his inimitable cockney style said "well, I guess I must have killed him myself". It is interesting to note in view of the recent Alder Hey body parts scandal that retaining diseased organs for preservation in pots and subsequent use for teaching purposes was quite normal and there was no question of consent being sought. Learning pathology would have been much more difficult without the many pots of normal and abnormal specimens which had been kept aside over many years. Professor Bernard Knight who has gone on to become a very eminent forensic pathologist was a contemporary at medical school. He showed his talent for writing by editing the Medical School magazine and has since made use of this talent and his experiences from his forensic work in writing murder novels under a pseudonym.

In 1986 when our practice were acting as police surgeons for the Llandudno area and when much of the medico-political discussions within the committee structures revolved around proposed or existing legislation and regulations there was an opportunity advertised for anyone with an existing health-related degree to study for a Masters degree in Law (LL.M) at the University of Wales Cardiff over a 12 month period, largely by course work and a few weekends in Cardiff. I discussed this with my son Gareth who had fairly recently qualified as a solicitor with LL.B. after three years in Cardiff and a year at Christleton law college and who was not impressed that I would get a higher qualification than him with only one years' part-time study. The issue was resolved when something else intervened and I did not pursue the idea.

A further interesting continuing education diversion occurred in the seventies when I attended a weekend hypnotherapy course at Abergele Hospital. We were very fortunate to have living in retirement in the area in

Deganwy Dr John Hartland, a retired consultant psychiatrist and President of the British Society of Medical and Dental Hypnosis and who was the author of a seminal but easily readable work, Medical and Dental Hypnosis and its Clinical Applications. Dr Jock Morison, medical superintendent of Abergele Hospital at the time, was also a keen user of hypnotherapy particularly in the management of asthma, while a third local expert was Dr Fred Peach, the Medical Officer of Health for Colwyn Bay. Some dozen of us turned up over a weekend to be introduced to a completely new concept which we had previously only seen on the stage as entertainment and which was rather frowned upon by the medical establishment because of the degrading exhibitions which hypnotised members of the audience were then subjected to.

Split into pairs I teamed up with Deri Thomas, a dentist in practice in Wrexham and brother of Dr Gwyn Thomas, and somehow we managed in turn to hypnotise each other, at least to the first level. Jock Morrison demonstrated some severe asthma patients with very dramatic improvement in their condition and marked reduction in re-admission rates, particularly in those patients who learnt to self-hypnotise during the onset of an attack. A branch of the Hypnosis Society was formed locally to continue the interest. I did subsequently attempt a little in the practice, with some success, but the sessions tended to be time-consuming and as I was single-handed at the time I could not devote enough protected time to it. One of the peculiar features of NHS general medical practice has been that one is forbidden to charge a patient on one's list for any treatment, even if that is quite outside the range of "treatments which the general practitioner normally provides", although one could charge a patient not on the practice's list for the same service. Deri however pursued the interest in his dental practice in Wrexham for many years and became very skilled at it. One of the skills learnt was the ability to self-hypnotise and I have found this very helpful, a short session when tired and exhausted making one immediately feel better. Hypnotherapy has been tarred with the same doubts as other alternative therapies over the years and has been neglected within the NHS as a proven means of therapy. Major operations are carried out under hypnosis and without anaesthetic in China and some years ago major surgery was successfully carried out in the Newcastle-on-Tyne region. Perhaps with the recent wider acceptance of alternative therapies it will become more regularly used. At least it does not give rise to the side-effects that many modern medicines do. One aspect which does need to be considered is the need for chaperoning during sessions, patients being by definition in a very suggestible condition, to avoid possible misunderstandings and complaints later.

Medicine and the need for continuing education or lifelong learning as it has been renamed remains vital but the methods by which this is achieved are continually evolving. The internet now provides a huge resource for learning with modules on most subjects available for doctors to study and importantly with the arrival of re-certification and re-accreditation a record to confirm the study and results.

Medical Audit

Mention audit to many people and their concept is very much a numerical exercise, a sort of bean counting activity equating what is actually present with what should be present, and with overtones of some sort of investigation by management and possible penalty if the audit does not add up. Medical audits while to some extent doing this should be much more about the quality of work done and the standards achieved compared with that of ones peers.

Although many individual doctors and departments within hospitals had long been sporadically reviewing their work audit as a centrally required activity was first beginning to be discussed in the late seventies. The concept was greeted with considerable alarm by many, particular those who had knowledge of the audit activity required by doctors within the American HMO`s (Health Management Organisations), initially with checks on surgeons on the number of cases of "negative pathology " found in operation specimens and later spreading to other specialties, and who were aware of the sanctions which could follow which included the withdrawal of admitting rights to the hospitals. Their Department of State issued an ultimatum to doctors that unless they set up an acceptable system of peer review by 1972 then the state would institute its own system. A Professional Standards Review Organisation (PRSO) was set up and started in 1974. Dr DEP Shapland, a GP from Brecon, was granted extended study leave to visit the USA in 1975 to study PRSOs and later reported back to the Sub-committee in General Practice.

Knowledge of audit amongst Gps generally was often scanty and hearsay, enough to create anxiety and resistance to the introduction of medical audit in Britain, but within medico-political circles the view was expressed that we must do it before it was imposed on us. A major educational exercise was required to counter the view of doctors but also to persuade politicians and health service management of the different viewpoint and of what form of audit should be pursued and which would be acceptable to the profession.

A WGMSC working group chaired by David Williams and which had included representatives of the hospital consultants had produced a report in 1975 on Medical Audit by Peer Review, emphasising that audit should be carried out by and with one's peers rather than by administrators and should focus on quality and identify errors rather than be simple numerical counts. In Dr Williams words " if Quality Assurance, Peer review or Medical Standards Control, call it what you will, is to be widely accepted then personal threats needed to be removed and it should be a review of the practice of medicine rather than of an individual practitioner; a review by equals not superiors; of how we do our work not how they do theirs. It must not be allowed to be a criticism of the generalist by the specialist or vice versa nor should it pretend to judge those who bear the heat and burden of the day by unrealistic, theoretical or academic standards". Progress has been achieved because these basic principles have been followed.

In 1977 the BMA ARM "instructed Council to investigate methods of audit within the profession and to report back" and again in 1979 "required Council to review alternative systems of medical audit and to make practical recommendations".

The anxiety amongst the rank and file of the profession was such that the word audit was deliberately sidelined and the concept of "clinical review" was adopted.

Audit has been an area where the Royal College and the GMSC have worked closely together and a major joint conference on Audit in General practice was held in 1980. In Dr David Williams` words at that conference " if audit or peer review were to be accepted, the personal threats had to be removed". He also presented a major paper on Quality assurance in Medicine at the BMA Congress in San Diego in 1981.

Trainers' workshops in Wales had been actively discussing and promoting audit and other local groups of principals and trainees had also been active in developing the subject. The Postgraduate Adviser, Derek Llewelyn, proposed that the clinical review / audit groups should be formalised across Wales and that an annual Symposium should be held in mid-Wales. This idea was accepted by all the relevant bodies taking Wales considerably ahead of the field in other parts of the UK.

The College at this time was very active in extending the literature and in developing expertise in audit skills while the GMSC were anxious to ensure that there was no undue pressure on practices to conform until the necessary resources were made available. These included adequate computer systems to facilitate the work. In 1989 Derek Llewelyn devoted his Harvard Davis lecture to the issues of audit taking as his title "The iron fist in the velvet glove" There is no doubt that the development of audit in general practice was streets ahead of that taking place within the hospital service.

In the new 1990 contract there was a requirement on all Health Authorities to encourage audit and FHSAs were required to set up Medical Audit Advisory Groups (MAAGs) in their areas with the intention of introducing the concept to practices and to facilitate their early efforts. As I had been involved with audit issues centrally I was asked to chair the Gwynedd MAAG although I must admit that the amount of my own practical audit experience at the time was fairly limited. We were very fortunate to have Dr. Medwyn Williams from Bodedern, now medical director of Ynys Môn LHB, as the secretary of the Gwynedd MAAG and his practical experience and computer know-how was invaluable.

A MAAG was set up at the same time in Clwyd with Dr Huw Lloyd as chairman but on reorganisation in 1996 both were initially amalgamated into a liaison group (NWMALG) and then into the multidisciplinary North Wales MAAG with Huw Lloyd continuing in the chair and with Mrs Chris Bladon as administrator.

Initially MAAGs were doctor-only groups but it soon became obvious that clinical review was not entirely a doctor or nurse activity but involved the activities of the whole practice team. While it was for the professionals to make sure that the relevant information was collected and recorded diligently and completely and in a standard format so that valid comparisons could be made, there was no reason why the ancillary office staff could not do the searching and collating of records part of the exercise and present the results back to the doctors for discussion and appropriate action. The way forward was to encourage and develop the skills of the practice team, the practice managers and the receptionists together with the practice nurses in those practices which employed them at that time. They were the ones responsible for ensuring the completeness of data entry and for doing the necessary but boring data extraction later. Doctors on the whole are not good at seeing things through and tend to get side-tracked into other issues. There is a very true saying which goes - "Ask a doctor to do something and he or she will do it for a week, ask the receptionists and they will do it for a month, ask a nurse and she will continue to do it until someone says stop" - something to do with the way they are trained I think. In 1994 Dennis Williams of Pwllheli took over as chairman and continued until the amalgamation with Clwyd MAAG. The administrative support for the MAAG was admirably supplied by Sue Hughes, by Chris Williams (now Turner) now working for Ysbyty Gwynedd Trust and by Grace Lewis Parry, now Chief Executive of Gwynedd LHB

One of the first lessons to be learnt and promulgated to doctors as an encouragement to undertaking audit was that the emphasis which one was seeking and striving for was improved quality of care across the profession and encouraging "good practice" and that one was not looking for the "bad apples" with a view to punishing them. The suspicion that this was the hidden agenda was very difficult to eradicate but the MAAG tried to emphasise it was voluntary, formative and that the results could be very interesting. It emphasised as a carrot that by identifying work not currently being done, or often being done but not recorded, in the practice there was a potential increase in profits for the practice.

Given the important new role of the office staff considerable time had to be spent in training them in the data recording and retrieval techniques. While a few practices at this time were using computers to record all consultations and results, in many practices retrieval would still require considerable time and manual effort. Of course this did presuppose that there was spare capacity amongst the staff to undertake this. Additional office staff was required but very often this could not for financial budgetary reasons be sanctioned by the FPC. The message was that in order to make medical audit easier a different format of medical recording, manual or computerised, was necessary and unfortunately there was never sufficient central input, guidance or support for this.

Another form of audit which was not numerical but could be very effective and which involved the team members on a more personal basis was known as Significant Event Analysis and involved looking critically at the management of things which had gone wrong or which could have been handled better with a view to learning from mistakes. It could be used to highlight good practice which could then be passed on to others. Audit exercises were often uncomfortable events but if done well and auditing the right areas it could be of enormous benefit to the team and to patients in the future.

Wales had been in the forefront of developing the concept of clinical review and as mentioned earlier the first Annual Clinical Review Day for practices from across Wales, run jointly between WGMSC and RCGP, was held in 1981 at Llandrindod Wells, a town which. has over the years developed into a venue for all-Wales meetings for many different organisations because it has been the only place in mid-Wales which has had adequate facilities for large conferences. It has been labelled "equally inconvenient to all " but at least it was possible to make it there and back in a day from all areas. The format was for expert contributions on aspects of audit, followed in the afternoon by two to four individuals presenting audits carried out in their practices. Over the years the Conference was indebted to drug companies including Pfizer who sponsored prizes awarded to a practice who submitted an idea and who were then required to present their audit at the Clinical Review Day the following year. In 1984 the topic was repeat prescribing and I was lucky or unlucky enough to be awarded one of these to carry out a study of prescribing in our practice, very time consuming in a pre-computer age and with the information which the Prescription Pricing Authority could supply at that time. The conducting of the audit was as nothing compared with its presentation to some hundred and fifty of one's colleagues at the Review Day. There was no complex audio-visual technology, computerised slide shows or power-point available in those days. The following year I presented the results in Welsh to Y Gymdeithas Feddygol (the Welsh Medical Society), an even bigger challenge. The Annual Clinical Review Day continues more than twenty -five years later but as to be expected its format has changed over the years and it now runs over two days.

For many years hospitals had used the international classification of diseases (IUCD) codes to record illnesses and to aid comparisons but this coding system was relatively useless to record many of the minor illnesses and the undiagnosed symptoms seen in general practice. Dr. James Read, a general practitioner, started to develop an alternative and more appropriate coding system which general practitioners started to use and which was gradually expanded to cover a wider disease base including minor illnesses and symptomatology. After some years the government bought the system from him which provided more resources for its continuing development in which he continued to be involved. Without such a universally applicable system meaningful audit on any scale would not be possible. The European Union (the EU) has now adopted an alternative system, the ICD10, which means further change may be necessary at some stage. Hitting the wrong keys in entering a Read code has produced many an unusual diagnosis in the patient's medical record. The old computer adage "garbage in, garbage out " still holds true however.

The need for trainee practitioners to be taught audit skills meant that the training practices were expected to be ahead of the field in auditing their activities. An annual audit prize of several hundred pounds was offered by Syntex to each vocational training scheme It was competed for regularly by trainees on the Clwyd North scheme and presented at an annual informal gathering of trainers and trainees and their spouses and by Sue Jones, the local Syntex rep, and which helped considerably to develop good relationships within the area and continued longer than in any other part of Wales.

The 1990 Contract discussed elsewhere required accurate recording of activity and much time-consuming quantity number-crunching auditing of workload and to some extent held back the wider introduction of audits of the actual quality of care. As payment within the contract has increasingly been linked to performance and recorded data the need for verification and access to records by the Authorities has increased. There has been considerable anxiety amongst many doctors and their representatives about patient confidentiality arising from lay professionals searching clinical records and from data-sharing. Strangely, the anxieties about patient confidentiality have troubled doctors far more than they appear to have troubled patient representative organisations.

The new 2004 Contract with its financial emphasis and carrot of the Quality and Outcome Framework (QOF) points requires considerably more auditing of performance but much of this becomes easier with the newer computer software packages, provided that the data is entered accurately While the Read Code continues to be developed it is never up to speed in producing the more detailed coding required for statistical and fiscal purposes.

In all this number crunching it must not be forgotten that the real purpose of audit is to ensure improved care for patients and not just to improve target figures for both practices and the government. There is already a suspicion held by some patients that screening and other services being offered, even pushed, by doctors and practice nurses is more for the financial benefit of doctors rather than themselves.

One of the results of accurate and detailed recording of every consultation, diagnosis and medication is that for the first time accurate information and figures are becoming available to government and to planners about the incidence and prevalence of diseases in the community. There remains a substantial difference between the actual incidence as recorded in general practice and the hospital figures on which planning of services have been based.

The MAAG as its name implied covered only general medical practices. When the arrangements for LHGs were made in 1996 in other parts of Wales the Audit and Clinical Effectiveness groups continued but the North Wales Health Authority decided to abolish the MAAG and split the money between the six LHGs to support the concept of clinical governance. The six soon formed the North Wales clinical governance forum consisting of their medical directors and the clinical governance (CG) facilitators and it was made clearer that its remit was to cover all the contractor professions and practices. An attempt was made to involve the CG leads within the Trusts but this was unsuccessful. It has in my experience unfortunately never been easy in any field to arrange cooperative arrangements between primary and secondary care providers.

In all auditing and checking within any organisation it is very important to get the right balance between checking and trusting. One of the major anxieties for clinicians in recent years has been the perceived lack of trust in their integrity and doubts about their motives and this does not lead to a comfortable and happy workplace.

Clinical Governance

Back in the eighties quality as a wider issue was being actively pursued and encouraged by the RCGP with its publications such as What Sort of Doctor, Quality in General Practice and those on audit. Closely related to but wider ranging than audit was the concept of Clinical Governance introduced in the nineties. This followed on from the acceptance of the concept of TQM (Total Quality Management) as a vision to aim for. This concept, developed within Japanese manufacturing and other industries, emphasised that a focus on quality within every part of the process was essential for the efficient working of the whole and aimed to make individuals conscious of and responsible for their personal task. This led on to their reputation for reliability at a time when so-called Friday afternoon cars and other shoddy products were coming out of British factories. It involved talking to see what customers really wanted and then working out how to supply it cost-effectively. It should however be remembered that customers` wants are not necessarily customers` needs. Henry Ford once said "if I'd listened to my customers I'd have just ended up designing a faster horse".

At around this time as a result of a number of alleged scandals in British public life there was general concern in many quarters about probity in parliament and in the public services and this carried through into the health services. A government commissioned report produced a series of seven Nolan Principles which it was felt should be considered and adhered to at all times. The principles included selflessness, integrity, objectivity, accountability, openness, honesty, and leadership.

In 1997 there was increasing anxiety about the use and the confidentiality of patient data, an area to which GP leaders had been drawing attention for a number of years without much response. Doctors had always insisted that any data from practices should be anonymised and aggregated to such a number that individual patient data could not be identified. The Caldicott Committee reviewed this issue in 1997 and expressed increasing concern about the way patient information was being used within the NHS and the need to be wary that confidentiality was not undermined and it drew up confidentiality guidelines.One of the new requirements was that each practice was required to appoint a Caldicott Guardian, usually a senior partner or practice manager, to be responsible for adherence to the guidelines

The use and sharing of personal and clinical information about individuals was one which had worried GPs and their leaders for some years. Many doctors had been loathe to share information because of uncertainty as to how far it would subsequently be spread. As an example one particular area of concern was when there was an early suspicion of child abuse within the home but GPs would be reticent in involving the health visitor because she had a duty laid down to report any suspicions to her superiors. Another annoyance to GPs had been the failure by social services to report back action taken, or not taken, after a referral had been made to them. The profession considered it very important to ensure that when performance data were being published that it was aggregated to the extent that individual patients and doctors could not be identified. The climate has now changed considerably and practice aggregated data are frequently circulated. Perhaps what has been surprising is that doctors over the years have come under much more scrutiny than the other healing professions such as dentists, opticians and nurses, certainly their actions have been publicised more.

Clinical governance follows the aims of TQM of developing a quality service but across a wider spectrum of organisations working towards improved care. As a concept it was first announced in 1998 in the document "Putting Patients First" and it took some time for its remit and its extent to be appreciated. The breadth of what was included within clinical governance was vast and it was important to recognise that it was not just "a doctor thing" but involved all care workers.

It was defined by Welsh Office in 1999 (in Quality and Clinical Excellence) as "a framework through which NHS organisations are accountable for continuously improving the quality of their services and safeguarding high standards of care, by creating an environment in which excellence in clinical care will flourish". Emphasis was to be put on creating the right environment.

Quality was to be achieved through National Service Frameworks (NSFs) and by the National Institute for Clinical Excellence (N.I.C.E), discussed in another chapter, setting out clear standards of service and by patient and public involvement into clinical governance, underpinned by modernised professional self-regulation and extended lifelong learning leading to a dependable local delivery. The achievement of standards would then be monitored through the National Performance Framework, the Commission for Health Improvement (CHIMP), and a National Patient Survey. The importance attached by government and the profession to quality is demonstrated by the new remuneration structure in the 2004 contract which is heavily based on Quality of Outcome Framework (QOF) points.

In developing clinical governance of the Quality of Care the professional committees reiterated that there was a balance to be struck between, on the one hand, the legitimate desire to drive up "standards", to monitor and to regulate and, on the other hand, the need to give them the support they need when, inevitably at times, things go wrong, and freedom from excessive stress.

There was another balance to be struck between, on the one hand, the time professional people have to spend dealing with complaints, monitoring their colleagues and worrying about management targets and on the other hand, the consequent loss of clinical time for patient care. This has been a recurrent issue over recent years.

Dr. David Williams was again a leading figure in this debate and he had the ability to put potent and sometimes very innovative arguments across directly to the political party leaders as well as through the committee structures. Re-reading some of his documents and papers on a wide range of issues has shown how influential he was at both Welsh and UK levels.

Identification of poor standards may at times involve whistle-blowing, a relatively new concept in medicine as in other fields of public and private life. In earlier years it would certainly not have been thought acceptable, except perhaps in the gravest situations, to report colleagues to employers or to the GMC, but it has now become the required norm so that failure to report in itself has become an offence. Patient questionnaires are seen increasingly as a means of obtaining feedback. Another avenue is the use by the Community Health Council of Mystery Patients attending for treatment in selected departments and who are supplied with a pack of questionnaires to be filled in at each attendance. Since they volunteer themselves for the task then perhaps they may not be a true representative sample. Suggestion boxes sited in surgeries rarely seem to come up with ideas which have not already been considered or which are feasible.

Already discussed are the ways in which general practitioners have become involved in improving care through the efforts of the RCGP Quality Initiatives and its publications and through GMSC. Locally clinical governance committees were set up in the Local Health Boards working alongside their Audit Committees and their early role was to clarify and inform providers of their expectations as regards quality standards. They brought together all local activity for improving and assessing clinical quality into a single programme which everyone could be a part of and work towards. Frustration and disillusionment is then likely to set in when the necessary resources cannot be made available.

The areas to be covered included consultation and patient involvement and partnerships, risk management, clinical audit, clinical effectiveness and research, staff management, education and training and personal development and the use and sharing of information. In some areas such as audit and personal development the profession had perhaps been ahead of the field but other areas such as risk management had not really been a part of everyday thought except on a purely personal level, at least consciously. The story of the little girl who suddenly learnt to her surprise in an English lesson that she had been speaking prose all her life and did not know it comes to mind.

For individual doctors and practices the increasing burden of administrative work in drawing up protocols, training staff and ensuring adherence to them meant that practice managers were required to adopt a much wider role.When practices first started to appreciate the need for a practice manager the role was still envisaged as a relatively simple role and often a senior receptionist was appointed without any specific training. Later, and this probably started in many practices with the 1990 contract and the introduction of fund-holding at about the same time, the need for a different level of management was appreciated. Many practices unfortunately found themselves with an existing manager who could not be removed or moved sideways as in other organisations. Some of the managers set out to acquire additional qualifications. Unfortunately practice staffing, paid for 30% by the practices and 70% by the FHSA came out of a budget which was capped making it difficult to get agreement for more and upgraded staff. Practice management has certainly moved on considerably and as a result of changes in the 2004 Contract which is with a practice rather than with individual doctors some managers are becoming profit-sharing partners. The success of clinical governance within practices will to a large extent be dependent on them.

On the wider view the Government's health service reforms may soon see the trickle of patients from the NHS to the independent sector turn into a flood, with barriers disappearing and traditional models of care changing. Whatever happens quality control issues will remain important. Common methods of measuring quality, overseen by the Healthcare Commission, need to be in place across both the NHS and private sectors. "Intelligent information" needs to be developed which can be used as a basis for decision making but there is a risk that information which can be compared across sectors may mean information which is potentially misleading for patients. Yet another watchdog is the National Patient Safety Agency which has highlighted significant variation in error rates across areas in England and Wales although emphasising that the error rate is low considering the number of patient episodes, with about one million consultations a day within primary care.

An important area of clinical care continues to evolve, becoming more complex as care becomes more multidisciplinary and multi-agency.

The investigation of complaints

Understandably there are occasions where patients or their relatives are unhappy with the management or the outcome of illness and wish to complain about this, and there have always been complaints mechanisms in place to allow them to do so. There are also occasions when the doctor is unhappy with the behaviour of patient or relatives and would like to tackle this but no formal mechanism for doing this within the NHS was available for many years. It was not always thus. In pre-NHS days patients treated under Friendly Society arrangements had a medical card showing their entitlement to treatment but also listing a number of obligations on the patient, which if not adhered to could lead to loss of privileges.

The history of the formal NHS complaints procedures was never a happy one, with patients and relatives as complainants and the doctor as respondent both very unhappy with the system and it is pertinent to look at why this has been so. The major reason was that the process was always adversarial rather than constructive and conciliatory and was very drawn out.

Patients were registered with the doctor whose name appeared on their Medical Card and any complaint had to involve this doctor even though the doctor was not personally involved and may even have been on holiday at the time. Sometimes it was another doctor in the practice who was being complained about, but on occasions a complaint against the actions of a locum who could not later be contacted had to be answered.

The contract with the health authority requires a doctor to "render to his partients all necessary and appropriate personal medical services of the type usually provided by general medical practitioners", a loose definition which could be all-embracing but which was certainly open to interpretation, and of course the services usually provided have varied over the years, and in practice very much from area to area.

There was a need to judge on the circumstances of practice. In inner city areas practices were often single handed with lists of 3500 or even 4500 patients, all within an area defined by arterial roads. If patients crossed the road to live they would be considered out of area and be transferred out. All homes were within walking distance, home visits if necessary could be done on foot and the doctor did not need a car. Out of surgery hours calls were transferred to a deputising service. One practice in Birmingham. was run by a doctor who commuted daily on the train from London. These practices had to be compared with an area like North Wales where there was often only one or two practices and where all night work was carried out by the practices themselves. Standards were generally higher but so was the expectation and the trigger level for complaints.

A complaint had to be made by the aggrieved party (the patient) except if it related to the death of the patient. Often the patient was satisfied with the care received from the practice over the years and did not want to complain about a particular episode but was pressurised by relatives, some of whom were rarely seen in the vicinity. The complaint had to relate to a breach of the doctors "terms of service", a concept that complainants have never understood. In particular attitudes such as rudeness were never a valid reason for a complaint although patients wished to do so, and complainants would often get round this by adding some vague clinical component to their complaint. There was also a time limit for a complaint to be registered, a reasonable requirement given that the details as opposed to the main points of any consultation and conversation were not routinely recorded. Telephone calls at home were a particular problem as patient records were not available to make notes and the exact timing of any call was not regularly recorded by most doctors. Sometimes exact timing was of great significance if a complaint involved alleged delay in visiting. Patients or relatives who felt they had cause for complaint would be aware of this immediately and make notes whereas the doctor might not become aware that a problem was looming for many weeks.

Successive authorities, the Executive Councils, Family Practitioner Committees and Family Health Services Authorities were required to have broadly similar complaints structures known as Medical Service Committees. The arrangements were cumbersome and long drawn out but in particular it was an adversarial system and as such contributed nothing to rectifying the initial problem. Doctors dreaded receiving notice that there had been a complaint and that this was to be formally investigated. No attempt could be made at this stage to discuss the problem with the complainant and perhaps in a few minutes resolve the dispute to everyone's satisfaction. Continuing to care for the complainant while investigation was ongoing was difficult and as a result patients and their families either voted with their feet to another practice, not always easy in rural areas, or were sometimes taken off the practice's list by the doctor. Complaints which might not otherwise have been pursued often result from previous indiscretions and problems between doctor and patient.

Service committees had a lay chairman, often a solicitor, and equal numbers, usually three, of lay members of the Authority and GP peers chosen from panels of six nominated by the LMC. Caernarfonshire and later Gwynedd were very fortunate to have Mr Guyse Barker, a Llandudno solicitor, as chairman for many years. His hearings were always conducted with courtesy and fairness and both sides felt they had had a fair say. He was succeeded in July 1995 by a school friend of mine, Gwyn Morris Jones who again always ensured a fair hearing to both sides.

Dentists and opticians had their own service committees if the practitioner was providing services under the NHS but many of the services they provided were in the private sector. Problems in investigation could occur when part of the treatment was provided under the NHS and part as a private service. They sometimes arose when the financial nature of the treatment had not been fully explained or was misunderstood.

Problems also arose when practitioners from two different disciplines were involved and a joint service committee had to be set up. Difficulties arose when a GP and a district nurse were involved in the same complaint and where the Trust would not allow the nurse to be part of a service committee but wished to investigate the complaint under their own disciplinary machinery.

Provided that the initial complaint was in order it resulted in a letter to the GP asking for comments and an explanation which was then made available to the complainant who could comment further. Since very often it was the first time the doctor had been in such a situation one of the things we tried to instill into doctors was that they should seek advice from the LMC and usually from their Defence Society before penning the first reply to the letter of complaint. Many a doctor has prejudiced their chances by a hurried and careless reply. Sometimes with overseas doctors there was a language or interpretation problem.

The chairman would then decide if a formal investigation was necessary. GPs often formed the impression that formal hearings were sometimes decided upon even when there appeared little basis for the complaint purely to satisfy the complainant and family. There then was a wait of some weeks while a convenient date was set. No formal rules of evidence were used and no paid advocate was permitted although both sides could be accompanied by a friend, the doctor often being accompanied by a member of the LMC. However for some reason only the defendant or the friend, but not both, could present the defence.

For both sides the experience was daunting and on occasions complainants without explanation did not attend in which case the complaint was dealt with in their absence and formally dropped. GPs were obliged to attend. Following both parties giving evidence and cross examination, together with questioning by the panel both parties left. Witnesses could be called on matters of fact but not as expert witnesses to give an opinion. A decision as to whether there was a Breach of the Terms of Service, or No Breach, was made and the decision formally communicated to both parties in due course, not that day. The six-member panels were fifty-fifty medical and lay but very often it was the doctors who were the more ready to condemn if appropriate. On a finding of a breach the doctor could be fined and would be directed to adhere to his terms of service more closely in future. There was no constructive advice attached. Whichever party lost usually felt dissatisfied or aggrieved, often about the actual rules of procedure which they did not understand. Complainants often said that they did not wish to penalise the doctor but rather they wished to ensure that lessons were learnt to avoid the same thing happening to others. There was never any publicity about the case or the issues so there was no educational benefit and whether this hearing procedure was the best way to do this is very doubtful.

An appeal within three months to the Secretary of State for Wales who was responsible for the conduct of the Health Service was an option to the aggrieved party. The appeal process was either determined within the Welsh Office or in some cases as an oral re-hearing heard by a nominated GP and a Welsh Office doctor with a lay chairman which could take many months to be arranged and held and many further months before a decision to uphold or quash the findings was made by Welsh Office. No wonder that neither the GP`s committee or patients groups were satisfied with the system and changes were finally introduced in 1994 following the 1990 Charter.

Luckily complaints were not usually of such a serious nature that other patients were immediately at risk. The Health Authorities while they could refer a doctor to a Service Committee had no power to suspend a GP, unlike the hospital trusts who could suspend their consultants, which they sometimes did for years at a time, pending a decision.

GPs have always felt themselves under multiple jeopardy from complaints, from the above procedure, from legal action for negligence in the courts and from referral to the GMC (to be discussed later) and have often worried that a health service complaint was being used as a dry run for a formal legal procedure at a later date.

On average a GP might expect a formal complaint every 10 years or so, some areas having more than others. Personally I was involved as defendant in only one hearing during my time in practice and on that occasion the complainant failed to attend. It concerned an alleged failure by me to refer her immediately at her request to a gynaecologist for a hysterectomy. She then saw a consultant privately and unethically without a referral and was admitted to a private hospital for operation the following week From the consultant's correspondence one felt that the operation may not have been strictly necessary and certainly was not that urgent. An NHS referral would have resulted in some weeks delay for a consultation and more weeks or months on a waiting list, if in fact an operation was considered necessary. It demonstrated one of the ways private medicine could create problems for GPs. Since I had been a GP member of hearings in the past I was knowledgeable about the procedures but it still gave rise to weeks of anxiety as well as many hours of preparation. For GPs with no previous experience and facing more complex complaints the anxiety must have been intense. Many doctors shot themselves in a foot by their initial reply to the official notification of a complaint. Others had never really considered what exactly the vague words terms of service implied and needed guidance from experienced doctors from the Local Medical Committee

I was pleased from time to time to have the opportunity to act as a colleague's friend and adviser both before and if necessary at the hearing, and also to participate in the Welsh Office appeals procedures. The doctor's friend par excellence was Dr David Williams who loved to get his teeth into anything to do with the NHS Regulations. He was for some years the chairman of the GMSC Statutes and Regulations committee looking very carefully at all the legal issues arising from the numerous NHS regulations and schedules, from the Red Book, and other matters. He was particularly in his element defending at appeals. Very often when John Lynch, David and myself were travelling back from London on the train he would try out his intended defence on us looking for possible flaws. Those train journeys, on which we were often joined by Mr John Chawner, the Bangor obstetrician and gynaecologist who was chairman of the CCSC, the central consultants committee, and sometimes by Dr Mollie McBryde from Chester who was the Secretary of the RCGP at the time, provided great debate and much enjoyment as well as indoctrination into the arts of negotiation for me as the junior member of the group.

A few examples may help to illustrate the type of complaints and also the inflexibility and perhaps the absurdities of the service committee complaints system as it was operated. Some complaints result from deficiencies in knowledge of procedures by inexperienced doctors. The majority concerned perceptions by the patient or a relative that insufficient care had been provided or delays had occurred before the correct action was taken. One involved a complaint about doctor who refused to visit a patient who had collapsed and died at home, her defence at the hearing was that she had no prior knowledge of the patient and therefore could not certify death. The finding was that she was required to attend to confirm the fact of death even if unable to certify the cause of death and she had breached her terms of service.

Occasionally the complaint had a management basis. A practice in Clwyd ran a small branch surgery in the local church hall. Like many branch surgeries the facilities were far from satisfactory but served their purpose up to a point. As tenants they were unable to deal with the broken window and other defects. David's graphic description of the "consulting area" was that it was in the anteroom to the gent's toilet. An FPC inspection decided that the facilities were unsatisfactory for purpose and that it should be closed immediately. The practice were unable to find alternative and satisfactory accommodation in the village, applied to discontinue the surgery and no surgeries were held. Permission to close was refused. The FHSA then formally charged the practice with a breach of their terms by not providing a surgery and imposed a hefty fine each week while no surgery was held. The practice appealed to the Secretary of State and the issue went on for months during which time the quite substantial weekly fines continued to be levied.

Caernarfonshire and Llandudno unfortunately had over a period of many years one recurring and persistent complainer, who usually had a number of other complaints on the go at any one time, against the police, the Local Authorities, various consultants and hospitals and GPs. Each body felt it had to investigate each complaint and much time and expense were expended in dealing with usually unfounded or unsubstantiated complaints. On one occasion he had notice to attend a hearing at Caernarfon and had the temerity to ask his GP, the doctor he had complained about, for a lift to the hearing. The request was refused!. For some years and because no-one would put up with his attitude and intolerable behaviour he was moved around the local practices in Llandudno by a formal allocation by the FPC every three months. On the third time round our practice, and partly to protect another GP`s family who lived very close to him, made a pact with him that we would keep him provided his behaviour improved. It did not really improve but we did keep him for some years until he moved out of the area and started to intimidate other practices in Clwyd. He never actually dared put in a complaint about our practice but we all, partners, wives and reception staff did put up with frequent and foul language abuse on the telephone, demands for immediate visits at unsocial hours, face to face abuse and threats that conversations in his home were being recorded. For some years I kept very securely a tape-recording of a telephone call from him to my home which I felt could be of assistance at some time in the future. However it could only have been listened to after the nine-o-clock watershed. I made an attempt to make a pre-emptive complaint against him at Welsh Office as a vexatious complainer but they would not take any action. I suspect they would listen more attentively now. Luckily he was a one-off, in our area anyway.

On another occasion a single-handed GP was the subject of a complaint by the FPC because of frequent absences from his practice area without providing cover. On the day of his hearing a telephone call to his practice resulted in a recorded message saying he could not answer as he was in a meeting in Caernarfon many miles away. Some people never learn.

While most complaints were run of the mill another interesting one arose many years ago, again in Clwyd. Doctors could claim an annual mileage payment for patients living more than two miles from the main surgery. The Family Practitioner Committee queried the mileage payments to one practice and formally lodged an investigation. The practice had initially been started in one village and later a branch surgery was opened in a neighbouring town.

Over the years the second surgery outgrew the original one but the practice continued to claim from the first main surgery whereas the FPC took the view that the second surgery was now the main one and that overpayments had been claimed. Other issues relating to the practice prescribing were also investigated. The situation was difficult in that the doctor involved was at the time Chairman of the Authority which was investigating him and he refused to stand down. After many months of very detailed investigation no evidence of any malpractice was found.

In addition to participating in the formal complaints procedure the LMCs always had the so-called Three Wise Men arrangement. These were senior members who were available to deal on a semi-formal intra-professional way with doctors about whom doubts may have been raised by colleagues or by the administrators about the way they were practising, about their health or about abuse of drugs or more often alcohol. Sometimes a visit by the Wise Men would persuade the doctor to seek professional help before it was too late. I recall being involved in the Wise men procedure on two occasions, one where there were persistent but unconfirmed rumours about the social behaviour of a doctor within his practice area. The other was where the doctor's standard of practice had been sub-standard for some years with a number of complaints on which successive administrations had failed to act decisively and where we were able to persuade him to retire voluntarily before punitive action by the GMC or in the courts was taken.

It was finally agreed that the existing complaints procedures were in no-ones interests and there was a major change in 1994. The new complaints procedure was to be a practice-based conciliatory one with early resolution if at all possible. Each practice was required to appoint a complaints manager and to write and publicise its complaints procedure arrangements with a timetable set down for dealing with them and resolving problems to satisfaction. If local resolution was not possible there was also a procedure for an Independent Review by the Health Authority.

A further review of the Procedures was held and changes came into effect in 2003, mainly to the Independent Review mechanism which now became independent of the NHS. Where a complainant asked for an Independent Review the complaint would be considered by two independent lay people appointed by the Assembly, and where necessary supported by a clinical adviser, who would consider what else might be done under local Resolution or what advice might be given to the health authorities. They might decide to set up an Independent Panel of different lay persons and clinical assessor to consider and investigate further. A final appeal to the Ombudsman was to be available. Hopefully these new mechanisms will satisfy complainants better than the old Service Committees and also lead to better practice.

The immediate reaction of some GPs to a complaint being made against him or her by a patient and where no attempt is made by them to resolve this informally is that because of the very special relationship which exists them and which has broken down is to feel that he or she cannot continue to care for them and removes them from their list. Sometimes it is the attitude of relatives which aggravates the situation. With larger practices it is often possible to transfer care to a partner and both the GMC and GMSC have produced strong guidance and encouragement as to how to manage the situation.

Over and above the NHS complaints procedures doctors may be taken to court for negligence, the breach of a legal duty of care which results in damage caused by the defendant to the plaintiff. This is in itself a complex area

When a GP agrees to attend a patient whether under the NHS, privately or as a good Samaritan a contract is established whereby the practitioner has a duty to exercise reasonable skill and care. Negligence may be defined as "an omission to do something which a reasonable man guided by ordinary considerations would do. Or doing something which a reasonable man would not do". However the GP is not necessarily to be judged by the standard of the consultant. The judge in the Bolam case in 1957 set out the standard expected and within this said "that it is sufficient if he exercises the ordinary skill of an ordinary competent man exercising that particular art "The judgment also stated that "there may be one or more perfectly proper standards ... if he conforms to one of these standards then he is not negligent if he has acted in accordance with the practice accepted as proper by a responsible body of medical men skilled in that particular art". Medicine in many ways remains an art and not an exact science.

The Medical Defence Bodies

All doctors belong to one of three Defence Bodies, the oldest of which, the Medical Defence Union (the MDU) was formed in 1885 to assist doctors in trouble and last year celebrated 120 years of uninterrupted service to the profession. Interestingly it was not started by doctors but by seven laypersons, "five gentlemen and two solicitors" following on poorly conducted defence of doctors who had been wrongly found guilty and imprisoned. One case involved an allegation of abuse when evidence of the patients hallucinatory episodes was not presented to the court. The Union has remained a mutual organisation, with a large reserve fund derived from members guarantee of £1 by each member. The initial subscription was ten shillings(5p)a year, later raised to £1 and still available in 1945 for the same amount. The subscriptions have escalated since but remain a very essential part of a doctors armamentarium.

In addition to defence issues the Defence Bodies provide invaluable and immediately accessible advice and guidance to individuals on practical and ethical issues and produce regular Journals which are essential reading, drawing attention to new legislation,to GMC interpretations, and documenting cases where one at times feels "there but for the grace of God...."

The GMC has also been much more active in recent years in producing guidelines on Good Practice and interpretation of legislation.

The Defence Bodies emphasise that complaints and claims are not good indicators of poorly performing doctors. Neither investigates professional competence and variable factors unrelated to patient safety can influence outcomes. Complaints vary widely both in specialty and in geographical areas. One of the Defence Bodies has recently stated that a cosmetic surgeon might face a claim every two years while a radiologist would have to practice for 75 years before he or she would have to defend a claim.

Complaints, like death, are likely to be unavoidable in the long-term and doctors at these times need good friends to guide and support them.

The hospital service has had its own disciplinary procedures which are outside the remit of this work but at times seems to work extremely slowly and with consultants on "gardening leave" on full pay for long periods.

An interesting hospital case in which the Local Medical Committee became involved happened in 1976 and which went to the highest level with the Health Service Commissioner (the Ombudsman) being involved. It was specifically reported in his Annual Report of 1977-78 and raised several interesting clinical issues. A complaint against the Clwyd Health Authority (which at that time had responsibility for the hospital services) was made to him by the son of an elderly patient who had died and who had been unhappy about the Health Authority's response. The Ombudsman duly investigated the complaint and criticised both the hospital doctor and the Health Authority. The Authority discussed the issues with the Secretary of State for Wales and subsequently set up its own inquiry. The Medical Committee of the Authority and the LMC strongly criticised the Ombudsman's report, deplored his criticism of the hospital doctor who he had criticised as "inhuman" and expressed no confidence in the Ombudsman system generally. There had been no criticism of the actions of the GP but the LMC felt that a doctor's "clinical judgment" had been unfairly called into question. They called on the Ombudsman to resign, all very strong stuff.

The complaint, which was well publicised at the time and is common knowledge, concerned an elderly 103 year-old patient who had a fall in the nursing home where she lived and after being seen by a GP was taken to the accident unit at Rhyl with a suspected fractured femur. She was seen by the SHO who arranged x-rays and as these were normal and as her general condition was very good for her age said she could be taken back to the nursing home by ambulance, even though it was in the early hours of a very cold night. There were differing recollections about her repeated requests to be sent back, and about whether there were beds available in the hospital at the time. Regrettably the patient died soon after returning to the home. Whether the decision was the right one or not the decision had been made after full examination and investigation and after full consideration of the circumstances. It has often been said that elderly patients run less risk of infection if not admitted to hospital.

The issue was such that the Select Committee of the House of Commons as part of its review of the Ombudsman's Annual Report looked into the circumstances and held a hearing at which the Health Authority and the LMC were represented, the latter by Drs Chowdhury, John Lynch, Eddie Davies and David Williams. It reported in favour of the Ombudsman's handling of the complaint, but it was an interesting episode and showed the LMC`s support for hospital colleagues making difficult decisions.

The General Medical Council and regulation of the profession

The General Medical Council, the GMC, is probably the one body apart from the BMA which the general public has heard about, although most have little knowledge of its complex function. In their eyes it is the body which punishes doctors, the regulator of the medical profession. It does this but it also has had a continuing role in setting standards and by publishing its Register allows the public to know that a doctor is bono fide and considered fit to practice. Its statutory purpose is "to protect, promote and maintain the health and safety of the public by ensuring proper standards in the practice of medicine."

The General Medical Council has over the years been a kind of bogeyman to practising doctors and was really the only way (short of being sent to prison) in which they could be deprived of a living by being struck off the Register. A complaint to the GMC was the start of a sometimes drawn out and very worrying process for the doctor, the practice and the family with the ultimate penalty, erasure from the list a catastrophe. It could also be traumatic for the complainant.

While the public in general hears only of the GMC in its judicial role with at times lurid press stories the Council over the last few years has been regularly producing and often updating guidance notes on the duties of a doctor and on the management of a wide range of moral and ethical issues, on confidentiality, research, withholding of fluids from terminally ill patients and similar difficult issues which arise for practising doctors.

Judicial decisions have traditionally been reached on the basis of what a reasonable doctor would have done in the circumstances, akin to the concept the "opinion of the man on the Clapham omnibus " recognising that individual circumstances might influence decisions. Debate still continues as to whether doctors should be named in the media with lurid publicity while a case is on-going and before a decision has been made. Referral to the GMC could be by official bodies but could also be done by individuals with a grievance and who would make threats of referral to the GMC to frighten doctors.

The GMC was first established under the Medical Act of 1858 and was initially a purely professional Council whose function in addition to dealing with erring doctors was to keep a list of doctors registered as fit to practise. It had an entirely medical representation, dominated bynominees of the Royal Colleges and the medical schools and had gradually become very large and cumbersome. Registration with the GMC was free for doctors for many years but in 1970 doctors were asked by the GMC for the first time to pay an annual registration fee of £5, a sum which has progressively escalated enormously to £290 a year at present. A BMA Special Representative Meeting agreed to a n annual fee, subject to the majority of the members being elected by the profession. Alec Merrison, a university vice-chancellor, chaired a government inquiry into the regulation of the profession and following this the Medical Act of 1978 provided for a new composition and framework. and gave the GMC new powers to coordinate all stages of medical education.

It was always the view that because of the severity of sanctions available and the frequently complex nature of the cases that the profession should be self-regulating and that the Council membership should be composed (largely) of doctors The many GMC members there as nominees of medical schools were often thought of by rank and file doctors as not subject to the pressures of day to day clinical practice. It is true to say however that doctors at any level sitting in judgement on their peers and not wanting to be seen as condoning bad practice are likely to be more *severe* than perhaps a lay person would be.

In recent years as a result of consumer pressure lay representatives were gradually added and as a result of professional pressure the number of elected members rather than representatives of the medical Schools has increased. The composition now is 19 elected doctors, 14 lay members and two doctors appointed by educational bodies.

In my early days advertising or any publishing of one's skills or clinical interests was seriously frowned upon and might lead to a referral to the General Medical Council. A single plate outside the surgery premises giving the doctor s name and registered qualifications were all that would be acceptable. Nor was it acceptable to have signposts on corners pointing towards the surgery.

Gradually by the eighties much bigger signs advertising SURGERY were appearing, particularly in urban areas and some were even illuminated.

The 1990 contract saw a major change in the situation with doctors being contractually required to produce practice leaflets which specified the full name, qualifications and gender of the doctor, date of birth or date of qualification, together with surgery times and allowing any further relevant information.

At the same time it was forbidden to direct patients to named professionals such as private physiotherapists and pharmacists and particularly to be associated with these and share premises with them. This did make things difficult at times when patients or relatives specifically asked for guidance. Often guidance would be given in the form "if it was my family I might be thinking of Mr X ". It was even more difficult if one of a couple was a doctor and the other a pharmacist or physiotherapist. Obviously in all referrals any possible interest has to be declared association with and directing patients to a named pharmacy was strictly frowned upon over the years but it is now becoming common for pharmacies to be developed alongside a non-dispensing surgery.

Even more rigid was the referral to or association with unqualified practitioners such as homeopaths, osteopaths and manipulators, many of whom one knew could provide more effective treatment than the doctor could at the time. Many of these are now becoming members of their registered Societies and it is now acceptable to refer to these, but not to practitioners who are not so accredited.

Strangely enough no such requirement to provide information has been required of doctors within the secondary care services or in private practice. These should according to established practice and GMC guidance should only see patients after referral by a GP and the assumption was that the GP would be aware of the skills and interests of the specialists to whom referral was proposed. This was probably true in the early days when referrals were virtually all to the local hospital and where there might be only one or two consultants in each specialty. More recently the number of specialists has often quadrupled and many have never met local GPs. Also patients are requesting referrals to other parts of the country, perhaps for the convenience of relatives, to specialists NHS or private and to hospitals unknown to the referring GP, and a new situation exists, one which has not yet been satisfactorily addressed.

Doctors accused of negligence or improper behaviour have always felt that they were in a position of double or multiple jeopardy with formal local NHS complaints procedures initially, and then if the case was referred to the GMC complainants and their legal teams had the opportunity to wait for the result of a hearing before deciding whether to pursue a complaint through the courts. Things have become worse recently with the GMC now sometimes taking the step of referring its own decisions to the Council for Healthcare Regulatory Excellence (the HRE) asking them to consider referring the decision of its professional committee to the High Court for review because it may have been "too lenient ". Since its establishment in April 2003 the HRE has referred twenty-three health care workers of which ten were doctors to the High Court.

Complaints to the GMC have escalated and it now receives complaints concerning around five thousand doctors a year although many of these relate to hospitals rather than to doctors. It takes forward about 1200-1500 to investigate further but only takes action against 250 doctors each year. The current chairman of the GMC, Sir Graeme Catto, who is overseeing the on-going changes has expressed concern that the GMC is needlessly investigating and worrying around 1000 doctors per year.

Dr Shipman who murdered so many of this patients with injections of controlled drugs has changed the landscape significantly. The review by the High Court Judge Dame Janet Smith of the issues arising from the case of Dr Shipman was wide-ranging and looked particularly at the performance of bodies responsible for monitoring primary medical care and in particular the GMC.

There have been two views strongly held, one that Dr Shipman was a murderer who happened to be a GP and had access to the means and that the profession should not be considered accountable for him, and on the other hand that adequate systems were not in place to have identified his actions much sooner. These systems did not only apply to GPs, the arrangements for certifying and registering deaths were inadequate. The review has raised anxieties and made numerous recommendations which if accepted will have very major implications for medical practice and also for other administrations. Although changes within the GMC were already on the move they were not considered sufficient to satisfy her that perceived fundamental defects in the system were being sufficiently addressed. Several years later she believed that the case had broken the pillar of trust between the public and the profession, that blind faith should be replaced by transparent standards, and that doctors who fail against such measures "should be removed from practice."

In particular she believed that when there has been a conflict between protecting the public and being fair to doctors the Council has taken the side of doctors, whereas if the GMC was to retain the confidence of the public and of parliament then it should put the public issues first. She also identified that the GMC has been both prosecutor and judge, a situation which conflicts with the Human Rights Act 1998, and that the proposed ways round this were not sufficiently robust.

However long before Shipman there was a general acceptance within the profession and elsewhere that a system which allowed a doctor to qualify and then continue practising for perhaps the next fifty years without any formal checking of his or her continuing competence could not be condoned. There was already universal agreement in the profession that some sort of regular revalidation was necessary and that passing final examinations on qualifying was not an adequate assessment of a doctor's competence years later. The question was how.

Ideas started to crystallise on two layers, regular appraisal which would take place annually between the doctor and his appointed appraiser and within the practice in a formative manner identifying good and not-so-good aspects of his or her care and setting out any necessary programme of continuing education and improvements. This would be organised and carried out on a regional level. The second level would be a formal revalidation by the GMC probably every five years.

Appraisal started off slowly, the whole concept was very new and the first ones were merely paper exercises of no real value but after three years appraisals are now infinitely more substantial and meaningful than the first ones - it is a developmental strategy. As appraisal becomes more robust then revalidation itself becomes more robust. Neither should however take up too much clinical time which should be better spent caring for patients.

On the new proposals for the revalidation of doctors and guaranteeing fitness to practise which were due to come into effect within months in April 2005 Dame Janet believed that the proposals would not achieve the required effect and concluded that "a doctor will fail to be revalidated only if his or her performance is "remarkably" poor". As a result all the preparations for the introduction of revalidation were put on hold at the last minute. The law defines revalidation as "an evaluation of a medical practitioner's fitness to practise". In all the discussions which have taken place on the introduction of revalidation there has always been the conflict between a system which was taxing but not excessively so and considered practical within the daily working schedule and resources and a system one which would require an excessive amount of time and resources for both the doctor and the assessors. The GMC now feels that this delay has been beneficial in that it has allowed the ideas and the methodology to be refined and more effective.

There is evidence however that the public has not lost trust and faith in their GP and see Harold Shipman as a one-off. There is also general acceptance that no system of revalidation would have identified Shipman as a serial killer, but his name will long to remembered as the catalyst for major changes in the way doctors are regulated.It appears that, apart from his propensity to murder a number of his patients over the years, Dr Shipman was not a bad clinical doctor and he ran a good practice and was well thought of locally by his patients and colleagues Whether these changes will be effective in preventing future major scandals only time will tell. Dr Bodkin Adams, a GP and convicted serial murderer of old ladies in nursing homes on the South Coast in my early days of practice in the nineteen sixties, had much less impact on the future.

Doctors had been discussing changes in this field with government for some years, covering both educational and administrative arrangements.. There has long been a recognition that certification of death and cremation arrangements needed to be reviewed. The BMA and other bodies has recognised for years that the system was flawed and needed review. New death certificates had been introduced but the situation needed to be tightened up together with the whole coroner system and the requirements for referral of deaths to coroners. One anomaly of referral was the generally held view amongst the public that a post-mortem would have to be held if a patient had not been seen by the doctor within two weeks of death. Certainly in the seventies and eighties when cremation was much less common than it is now some Medical Referees of crematoria would require a post-mortem in these circumstances, the difference being that if the coroner requested one he paid for it from his budget whereas if it was the Medical Referee who required it the cost fell on the family. Some patients are known to have visited their doctor regularly just to ensure that this would not be necessary. The government decided not to proceed on suggested changes but support for reform and an exhortation to revise their policy has come from a recent Commons Committee Report.

One of Dame Janet Smith's criticisms of the GMC was that there has not been adequate accountability of doctors for their actions. On the other hand Onora O'Neill in her Reith lectures argued that attempts to replace trust with accountability may have gone too far saying "the efforts to prevent the abuse are gigantic, relentless and expensive: their results are always less than perfect". There is strong evidence that excessive accountability is already distorting management within the Health Service and in other organisations. The BMA Council chairman has warned that delays in introducing revalidation following from root and branch changes could set the process back years.

The GMC were now talking about a four-layer model of regulation- personal regulation, team-based regulation, work-place regulation and professional regulation. The end result would certainly make for better care and better protection of patients. However it is not in the interests of patients for doctors to be oppressed by the regulator. Its proposals did not find favour with Dame Janet Smith or with others who wished for a much more radical change in the GMC. The Government requested the Chief Medical Officer for England, Dr Liam Donaldson, to review the problem and come up with ideas. After very considerable delays his proposals have just been published. The initial reactions are that they are not generally acceptable and an interesting debate is sure to follow. One of the more contentious issues is a change in the burden of proof as currently in use within court cases in the UK from "beyond reasonable doubt" to "on the balance of probabilities". This is not acceptable when a doctors livelihood could be in question.

Welsh members who have provided distinguished service on the GMC over the years have been Dr David Parry from Portcawl, Dr Jane Wood from Clwyd and now Dr Malcolm Lewis from Swansea who is also Sub-dean and Director of Postgraduate GP Education in Wales and who has been responsible for organising the Welsh Appraisal Scheme which has been very well received nationally and by the GMC.

The future of the GMC is very uncertain at present as very fundamental proposals are currently being consulted upon, both as to the composition of its membership and its role in the oversight of medical education. Dr. John Reid while Health Secretary said that he wanted to "put to an end to the idea that the GMC is a representative body for doctors. It is not. Its primary role must be to protect patients". Many doctors are starting to say that if this is to be so should the profession continue paying for it.

A salaried service

The NHS has since the outset of the Health Service always functioned on the basis of general practitioners acting as independent contractors. They have valued highly and fought to retain this independent contractor service contract and the right to run their practices as it suited their neighbourhood and themselves within a loose general framework set down by the service. They provided and financed the premises and their staff. Much of medical politics over the last decades has been centred around retaining this independent contractor status which involved having a contract for services with the local health authority, rather than as an employee having a contract of services. The exact legal distinction is not entirely clear cut but has been seen in the following way in a court ruling which stated *"An employer was considered to have the right to "control" the manner of executing the work, the right to say both what shall be done and how it should be done. More recently the test of integration has been used and asks "Does the worker carry out tasks which are fully integrated within the organisation of the employer?. If the answer is "yes" he is probably an employee."* The distinction is of practical importance in regard to the fiscal advantages of being taxed as a self-employed person and what class of national insurance payments should be made. Of greater importance is that employees have certain rights arising from various Acts of Parliament which are not conferred on the self-employed independent contractor. Much has changed in the last few years and the advantages are not so obvious. The number of single-handed practices has dropped markedly across the whole country. Practices are much larger and as a result individuality has been lost and they tend to conform to the norm in the area. Much tighter control, budgetary and otherwise, from the LHBs and their control of new surgery provision and developments limits the actions of the practice.

The option of a salaried service for general practitioners had been considered at the inception of the NHS in 1948. It was rejected because of opposition from the profession who were prepared to accept the onerous 24hour a day / 365 days a year contract in return for the freedom to organise their professional lives themselves. The salaried option had been considered in 1920 by Lord Dawson of Penn in his Report to Parliament on the Future Provision of Medical and Allied Services. He wrote *" The alternative of a whole-time salaried service for all doctors has received our careful consideration and we are of the opinion that by its adoption the public would be serious losers. No doubt laboratory workers, and medical administrators who do not come in personal contact with the sick can, with advantage, be paid entirely by salary.*

The clinical worker however requires knowledge not only of disease but of the patient; his work is more individual, and if he is to win the confidence so vital to the treatment of illness, there must be a basis not only of sound knowledge but of personal harmony. The voluntary character of the association between doctor and patient stimulates in the former the desire to excel both in skill and helpfulness. It is a true instinct which demands "free choice of doctor "and there should be every effort, wherever possible, to make this choice a reality. In no calling is there such a gap between perfunctory routine and the best behaviour, and the latter in our opinion would not be obtained under a whole-time State salaried service, which would tend, by its machinery, to discourage initiative, to diminish the sense of responsibility. and to encourage mediocrity". Consultants and GPs remained independent contractors but in 1948 the consultants opted to become salaried within the new service.

Penn's clear statement, in spite of many reorganisations in the way health care has been delivered over the last eighty years and of major advances in treatment and care, fundamentally sets out the position which many general practitioners still hold dearly. From time to time there have been individuals and organisations who would prefer to have a salaried service. On the whole these have in the past arisen from those with views towards the left of centre and who have felt that the practice's profit or take home pay may be influenced by the way it works and that if doctors had a fixed salary this would not happen. The Medical Practitioners Union put forward proposals for a salaried service in their Blue Book in the early sixties soon after I had entered practice.

The great variation in the size, the location and the demographic structure of geographical areas and of practices would make this very difficult to organise where there were fewer doctors and especially in the shires and rural areas while at the same time it would limit patient choice. Provision of out-of-hours care except in major conurbations would have been difficult in the thinking of those times, although the advent of cooperatives and extended rotas together with wider availability of patient transport and more recently the new 2004 GP contract has changed the whole concept, although perhaps not yet the perception of patients. The vast majority of general practitioners as demonstrated through many resolutions to the Annual Conference of GPs over the years (1979, 1985, 1986, 1990) would fight very hard to retain their independent contractor contract.

In 1989 after the then Secretary of State Kenneth Clarke announced his intention to impose the "1990" contract on general practitioners despite the rejection of acceptance of this by a large majority, the GMSC as part of a wide consideration of alternative strategies for coping with the new contract formed a Working group under Dr. Ronald Gibson" to investigate a salaried service option and possible action." Although the vast majority of the submissions to it were in favour of the retention of the status quo, the Working group did conclude that the implications of the new 1990 contract severely undermined the traditional arguments in favour of the independent contractor status and that it would be perfectly possible to organize a system of care based on salaried GPs and to separate the normal hours from the out-of-hours elements of care. The report also concluded that the cost to the exchequer would be much higher although they did not quantify it. Dr David Williams in his inimical way later produced a paper for WGMSC which suggested that it would require two and a half times as many doctors to run a system based on sessional work. The Working Group did not feel that overall patient care would be adversely affected by a salaried service, but this view was not widely accepted. The loss of continuity of care was seen as major disadvantage.

The Medical Practitioners Union produced another document "A salaried service for General Practitioners " in 1991, one of the co-authors being Dr. Brian Gibbons, now the Minister for Health in the Assembly Government. This emphasised that many of the traditional arguments for the independent contractor status had been considerably eroded as a result of the requirements of the 1990 contract, with clinical direction and economic coercion and the increased administration going with it. It also argued that a salaried status would be more acceptable to the increasing percentage of new graduates who were women

In 1997 Dr Julian Tudor Hart wrote a discussion paper on behalf of the Socialist Health Association entitled "Going for Gold - a new approach to primary medical care in the South Wales valleys". The valleys had a long history of chronic unemployment and deprivation and high medical demands which were largely catered for by a number of small medical practices working independently. Many of these doctors had originally come from Ireland or from the Indian sub-continent, were nearing retirement age and recruitment to practices was likely to become a major problem. He argued that this was an ideal area for a pilot of a salary based medical service with greater teamwork and liaison with other services.

The contract of 1997 which introduced the concept of Personal Medical Services (PMS) practices where doctors in designated practices worked on a salaried or sessional basis was taken up in some areas in England but was not introduced in Wales.

Since the 2004 contract for the first time agreed what were the "core (or essential) services" that general practices should provide it left other "enhanced" services which the practice could contract with the LHBs to provide. These include Directed Enhanced Services covering areas such as access to general medical services, provision of anticoagulant services within the practice, and minor surgery. There were also National Enhanced Services which practices could bid for covering areas such as care for the homeless, intrapartum care and minor injury services. All these had detailed specifications to be adhered to.

The concept of Alternative Private Medical services providers has been introduced allowing Local Health Boards to contract with individuals or with private companies as well as with doctors already on their performers list to provide a defined service not covered by the usual contract. These may well be services which are currently within the hospital trust field. There is a danger that private or commercuial organsations will cherry-pick the easy services and leave others to provide the rest.

By 1999 both Dr Tony Calland, (a chairman of WGPC, a national negotiator and now chairman of BMA Welsh Council), and Dr Andrew Dearden (now chairman of WGPC and a central negotiator had both produced documents on "A Future Model for General Practice 2000-2010 "(Calland) and " Plurality: The Way Forward for General Practice in Wales"- A Discussion Document on a salaried service (Dearden). All discussion documents emphasise that a salaried service and an independent contractor service need not be mutually exclusive and there can be a two-way movement between them.

Perhaps times have moved on and with larger practices, out of hours cover being the responsibility of LHB`s, and the development of practice nurses and nurse practitioners together with out-reach services in the community by hospital services the concept of individual care has already been diluted, if not lost. There is no doubt that with the very high proportion of women graduates, many of whom favour flexible part-time working without financial commitments in the structure of the practice, and with many of the younger male doctors having similar views, salaried doctors will continue to increase in number. This change has been recognised in the new 2004 Contract where the contract is between the Local Health Board and the practice rather than with each individual doctor as in the past. Significantly the practice partners can now include practice managers and nurses so long as the practice contains at least one doctor.

Surprisingly in all these discussions about a salaried service over the years the views of the patients have not been actively canvassed or recorded.

Sessional doctors,
formerly known as non- principals

The term non-principals, of recent coinage, covered a numerically increasing and practically important group of doctors within general practice. It encompasses assistants, salaried partners, retainees and locums and the changes in recent years in registration and re-accreditation mean that their special needs have to be recognised and catered for.

While many of them are members of the BMA there was until very recently no formal representation within the central or local committee structure. Indeed it would have been difficult to achieve this as there was no recognised list or an "electorate " or any local structure through which they could be accountable. LMCs did what they could to assist them locally on an individual basis and co-opted a willing doctor if they could. From time to time a "permanent locum" has been elected to GMSC from the Annual Conference. For some years now Dr Ian Banks from Northern Ireland has been in this position and has been a very able advocate on their behalf. The Medical Practitioners Union recognised this hiatus and have been active in attempting to recruit within this group of doctors.

The name was later changed to sessional GPs and The National Association of Sessional GPs (NASGP) was formed in 2001 to look after their interests and to provide support and guidance to ensure an equal playing field with traditional principals within the NHS.

Assistants were a regular feature of general practice in the earlier years of the NHS, and before that, but the additional allowances available within the NHS fee structure did not encourage their employment. The rules laid down in Regulations about the amount of work and their work pattern were not always appropriate to the needs of the practice. It was generally much better to take on an additional partner if the approval of the Medical Practices Committee could be obtained. .

"Assistantships with a view" were frequently advertised in the early years but later, and particularly after the introduction of vocational training, the market place dictated that new entrants to a practice came in as partners immediately. The old system of coming in on a smaller share and gradually working up to parity (often over many years) largely disappeared and new partners expected to come in on parity or close to it.

The downside of this was that the usual period of six or twelve months mutual assessment disappeared and incompatibilities between the doctors (and at times between their marital partners over practice shares or perceived workload) within a practice became more frequent leading to partnership splits, sometimes with fairly dire consequences. Since all the partners were on the FPC or FHSA list they could set up a new practice in opposition just down the road. One had the impression that this situation was common in the Valleys. In the early years the partnership contained a restrictive covenant forbidding practicing within a designated number of miles but this concept became more easily challengeable. On occasion a partner would split off but refuse to move out of the premises and I recall several instances where a second entrance and second reception area had to be provided. Many practices did not have a written agreement anyway, in spite of frequent exhortations to do so by the LMC and the BMA.

Another group of non-principals were those on the Doctors Retainer Scheme. The need for women doctors who were taking time-out for family or other reasons to have the opportunity to continue to keep up their skills during this period was recognised with the hope that they would rejoin the workforce at a later stage. The Retainer Scheme was set up and allowed them to work in a practice for one session a week, the salary and costs to the employing practice being subsidised by the NHS. It was intended to cover a relatively short period of up to five years but we found that some doctors had been in the Retainer Scheme in the same practice for many years to their mutual benefit. When the organisation of the scheme in Wales was taken over and supervised by Dr Simon Smail, the sub-dean and Director of Postgraduate Education for General Practice, it was identified that as the total budget was cash-limited new doctors could not be accommodated and it was necessary for the Sub-committee in general practice to address this issue. At a later date it was recognised that occasionally some male doctors would need to make use of the opportunities and they were included in the scheme.

The Scheme was improved in 1998 when retainees could work for up to four sessions a week including their educational sessions and could become part of the NHS pension arrangements.

Locums make up the bulk of non-principals. They have always played an important role in general practice both to cover short-term absences and by providing regular cover over a longer period, sometimes years in a single practice in circumstances where being employment as an assistant was not appropriate for either the practice or the locum.

Locums themselves can be divided up into broad groups, those seeking permanent posts or in between posts, and those who have been principals and are now retired. More recently these include those who have taken early retirement to escape the stresses of general practice but who are happy to continue to work and to enjoy it without the commitments of being a principal. Women doctors who have family commitments are another important group of potential locums.In my earlier years, before the complexities of practice and the requirements of mandatory vocational training made it impossible, it was not infrequent for hospital consultants to undertake general practice locums during their leave periods, often in small rural practices where the demand was low and the fishing good. Many of these consultants had been in general practice before being appointed as consultants in the early years of the NHS.

There have always been a number of doctors in the large conurbations who have worked almost exclusively for the commercial Deputising Services, preferring to work out of hours during nights and weekends rather than during normal working hours.

Doctors seem to divide into two groups in their interest in working as a locum. Some seem to love working without the administrative and other ties related to being a principal and continue for years, others have no real interest in working in this way after retiring. I fell firmly into the second group. I had undertaken a few locums over several months in late1959 while looking for a permanent position, and this did allow me to experience different types of practices and to try to assess which sort of practice I would be happy in. Since retiring in 1996 I did no more than a handful of half-days in my old practice in Penrhyn Bay and a single fortnight in a small rural practice at Llanfairtalhaearn which I must admit was like a rest cure. Llanfair T.H. as it is familiarly known was run for many years by a highly respected part-time doctor, part-time farmer Dr O.L. Jones who had organised the practice and the patients well, and his successor kept this going. With the changes in practice, both clinical and administrative, since my retirement I think it would be impossible to go back now.

The 1990 contract introduced a requirement of compulsory retirement as a principal at age seventy but with no age restriction on being an assistant or a locum and a number of doctors continued to work in this way. It is highly unlikely that many doctors would wish to do this now.

For many years there was no requirement for locums to attend post-graduate courses and to be able to demonstrate this, although many did. Unlike principals and assistants locums were not eligible for reimbursement of course fees and expenses under the Section 63 arrangements and of course while they were studying they were missing out on potential earnings.

The employment of locums had potential hazards on both sides. Arrangements were usually made by telephone and often in time of crisis, sometimes by a doctor's wife whose husband had died suddenly and who had never had to arrange one before. A locum arriving at a new practice had no idea of what to expect or the working arrangements and hours, the principal had no knowledge of the personality, the clinical competence or the social habits of a locum employed through an advertisement. Nor indeed whether they would turn up as there was no form of contract. There was often no opportunity to check their GMC or defence society status beforehand There was also the worrying requirement within the Terms of Service that the principal would be clinically responsible for the acts and omissions of a locum and could possibly be brought before a Medical Service Committee hearing even though he or she might have been out of the country at the time.

The introduction in 1994 of mandatory vocational training requirements required all doctors working in general practice to have a VT Certificate from the JCPTGP, or else to be exempt under a grandfather clause because of previous experience before that date. This requirement included locums and Health Authorities were required to keep an up-to-date list of locums who were eligible to work within their jurisdiction. With the introduction of re-accreditation for general practice locums will also be required to comply and some may face difficulty in providing the necessary paperwork on which re-accreditation will be based. With these requirements together with the contract being with the practice rather than with an individual doctor the risks are diminished although still present.

There has never been an adequate availability of locums in general practice to cover planned and unplanned absences and the need now for partners to be absent from the practice much more frequently to attend various representative committees has worsened the situation. It is not unusual for two or three partners in a larger practice to be absent at the same time attending various committees and working groups.

Welsh Office as well as many statutory committees and other organisations over the years have failed to recognise that attendance usually means that a locum has to be employed or someone has to cover the work and have been loathe to compensate for this. Official "loss of earnings" payments which could be claimed for some NHS bodies were set at a fraction of the true cost and additionally only covered the time attending the committee, with no allowance for travelling time. For us from North Wales the meeting might last an hour or two but the total time including travelling might amount to twelve hours or more. Welsh Office had a peculiar wording saying that it was " work in the public interest" and for many years they did not accept that a partner covering in one's absence was acting as a locum and that this should be recognised financially. Thankfully this has now been corrected.

Until recently locums were a disparate group of individuals with no central coordination or formal negotiating rights. The BMA and GMSC have however kept an eye on their interests over the years and did for years publish a suggested list of fees for locums but this, together with other suggested fees for other activities, but this was considered to constitute price-fixing and in breach of the Competition Act 1998 and had to be discontinued on the advice of the Office of Fair Trading.

The interests of this diverse group of doctors are now looked after nationally by the Non-principals committee, now renamed the Sessional Doctors Committee, of the GPC.

Their individual needs, including their educational needs, have also been recognised and in North Wales have been catered for under the umbrella of Meddwl, run very effectively from the North Wales Medical Trust office in Llandudno by Dr Bridget Osborne, a former partner of mine at Penrhyn Bay. It provides a central reference point for advice on a number of issues ranging from personal health problems to clinical governance and developing educational issues, and also ensures that necessary educational opportunities are available.

Underprivileged and deprived areas

It has long been acknowledged that socially poor areas have a significantly higher incidence of diseases and of medical problems. In the late seventies various publications and reports including the Royal Commission on the National Health Service and Inequalities in Health (the Black report) drew attention to the problems in specific areas of the UK. Black used the words socio-economic deprivation rather than poverty to emphasise that the disadvantage suffered by those who through no fault of their own found themselves at the lower end of the social scale was multifaceted. It was not merely financial, they were often condemned to live in squalor with unhealthy lifestyles and with no easy access to educational and cultural opportunities. The Black Report was so damning that following its submission to the Secretary of State in April 1980 it was not printed and published as was usual by the DHSS or HMSO but 200 duplicated copies were made available in the week of the August Bank Holiday with major organisations within the NHS including Health Authorities not receiving copies, in modern parlance "a good week to bury bad news". The move backfired and press publicity including in the BMJ and the Lancet resulted in wide dissemination of the findings.

The particular problems in Inner London were highlighted in the Acheson report, Primary Health Care in Inner London, in Medical Problems in Inner London, and in the Survey of Primary Care in London by Dr. Brian Jarman. The problems were not however confined to the inner cities, they existed also in the industrial South Wales valleys and, perhaps surprisingly to many, areas of under-privilege and social deprivation were to be found in apparently attractive rural areas of Wales. Within underprivileged communities the elderly and the mentally ill fare even worse than the general population. At the same time as the Black Report in 1980 a working group of WGMSC members working in South Wales practices and chaired by Dr W.B Davies from the Rhondda valley looked at the "Workload, manpower and net remuneration of GPs in South Wales" and reiterated the problems there. The South Wales valleys, and indeed Wales as a whole, have for many years had documented higher consultation rates, higher incidence of chronic disease and higher benefit and prescribing rates than the UK. As will be discussed later the highest prescribing rates in the UK were consistently in Caernarfonshire in the north and Merthyr Tydfil in the south. The statistical evidence was very clear.

One of the facets particular to the South Wales coalfield valleys was the lung condition pneumoconiosis which caused severe breathing problems and cough. Pneumoconiosis was a notifiable disease and sufferers were entitled to compensation. Diagnosis of its degree was based on X-ray films but often these did not correlate well with post-mortem findings. Professor Jethro Gough, my professor of pathology at the medical school, had pioneered a technique of taking very thin slices of lungs at post-mortem and sticking these on to paper for use for comparison. This did not help the patient when alive but it did mean that compensation to the many widows became much fairer.

Within the Valleys there were long-established attitudes to entitlements and rights, dating back to the pre-NHS and pre-Lloyd George days of working-men's clubs employing a doctor to give medical care and who was in fact their "servant" and subject to discipline by the lay committee of the Club if thought not to be sufficiently attentive to the needs of members. I mention elsewhere that a similar situation had previously existed in my old practice in Ruabon which was part of the North Wales coal-mining area.

As the chapels and churches, the previous focal point of the community, became less well-attended the clergy became less revered and were no longer seen as leaders of the community. Following the introduction of the comprehensive education system many of the teachers, once so respected in South Wales, no longer lived within their community and were not held in such high esteem.

Over-attendance at surgery has long been a feature of South Wales practice and the report stated that all the evidence suggested that the people of South Wales as a result of the chronic stress in their lives had a low "giving-in" threshold, and that as a consequence any general practitioner working in these circumstances in turn was bound to "give in" to the demands of the community, otherwise life for him would become intolerable.

Dr Julian Tudor Hart working in a very deprived valley in Glyncorrwg in west Wales had postulated his Inverse Care Law in an paper in The Lancet in 1971.which stated that patients with the greatest need normally received the poorest care services and this is frequently quoted. He regrets that the second clause which postulated that the malign effect was the consequence of market forces has been conveniently ignored.

Many of the Valleys practices had been originally staffed by the influx of doctors from Ireland and later from the Indian sub-continent following an appeal from Mr Enoch Powell, the Health Minister in the late sixties, for doctors from abroad to come to help with the increasing workload within the NHS. Many of the latter took on partners from the same culture but reputedly treated them badly in terms of workload and remuneration which led to partnership splits and a number of small practices on bad terms competing with each other for patients.

Following the report WGMSC recommended that a similar committee should be set up by the GMSC in London to look at the problem and to identify criteria of deprivation set by the profession (as opposed to those set by politicians) and which could be incorporated into the fiscal structure.

Evidence to the Acheson committee in London suggested that social characteristics were thought to be more relevant to pressure on primary care services than perhaps intrinsically medical problems. In 1980 a group led by Brian Jarman, a London GP who later became Professor of General Practice at St Mary's, Paddington, looked at the problems in London and wrote to 4000 London GPs, the replies confirming their workload problems. In trying to get to grips with this problem it was thought necessary to differentiate between the problems of the population served, however assessed, and those of the services provided. The former were the responsibility of central and local government, the latter involved GPs amongst other healthcare workers and the conditions under which they operated.

In his attempt to identify those areas where the difficulties were greatest (later referred to as under-privileged areas or UPAs) and the factors which most influenced their workload or pressure on their services a questionnaire was sent to a representative sample of GPs throughout the United Kingdom asking them to score social and service factors according to the degree of impact on them and local services. These scores were averaged and used as weightings for a number of variables from the 1981 census figures and together formed a basis for identifying "underprivileged areas".

Factors which affected a GPs workload or pressure on his services included consultation rates and times, visiting rates, prescribing rates, morbidity and mortality rates, and practice working conditions. Very relevant was the amount of support available from others such as ancillary staff, community nurses, social services and the local hospitals but it would be difficult to obtain precise measures of individual workload based on all these factors.

In analysing the evidence submitted to various groups it became clear that there was a clear consensus that certain social characteristics of the population such as the proportion of elderly persons living alone, recent change of address, poor housing, social isolation and unemployment rates were thought to be associated with increased pressure on primary care services. Medical conditions with the exception of psychiatric problems were mentioned less often, and deficiencies in local provision of services were thought less important than social conditions. Following further questionnaires to clarify and expand some of the initial impressions it was decided to use social factors alone to measure workload associated with deprivation. Using up to ten weighted criteria it was thought to be possible to map out areas of deprivation or underprivileged.

The GMSC sub-committee which had been set up following Brian Davies' WGMSC report and of which I was a member looked into possible solutions in close co-operation with Professor Jarman. An early Jarman formula when applied to Scotland resulted in about 37% of the country being identified as underprivileged which obviously was not politically acceptable and their formula had to be modified. While the nature of the topography between inner cities and the Welsh industrial valleys was diverse the social factor criteria were generally considered equally relevant. In due course a considerable sum of money was set aside for distribution to GPs under a formula using the agreed criteria, modified slightly by us in Wales to reflect our views and those of Welsh Office. This happened during the time I was chairman of WGMSC. A small group including myself and Bryn John, my vice-chairman, and Welsh Office officials sat down with maps and played around with various modifications of the criteria and their relative weightings. One model suprisingly threw up Aberdaron amongst other communities as a deprived area.

My initial shocked reaction was that I would have difficulty in selling the idea that Aberdaron, an idyllic village on the beautiful Llyn peninsula was an area of deprivation. At that time no-one had really considered the concept or the extent of rural deprivation and poor access to care. Subsequent work has shown that mortality rates for road accidents, asthma and cancer are worse in rural areas with the last being diagnosed at a later stage. Active intervention for coronary heart disease is less common and patients are admitted to hospital less frequently. Secondary and tertiary care are less accessible involving travel and inconvenience which disproportionately affects the most vulnerable. Patients in remote communities are less likely to be able to exercise choice, something which governments now rate highly in their reforms. The inverse square law operates as much with rurality as with other indicators of deprivation. In the end Aberdaron did not show up in the finally agreed criteria but other small pockets were identified across North Wales and came into the scheme.

In due course deprived area payments were added to the GP remuneration structure, both to encourage doctors to move to work there and to improve the remuneration of those already there because many were having difficulty achieving target payments in areas such as smears and immunisation. They also recognised that in the absence of other services problems are brought to the easily accessible GP and added to their workload. Unfortunately in themselves the payments gave rise to anomalies. Statistically it was impossible at that time to identify small enough enumeration or post-code areas and in some districts quite affluent properties were included within the designated areas. Practices working within a very short distance of each other found that some were included and some not, and the financial amounts were very considerable. Payments were not related to any demonstration of improvement and regrettably some practices found that the additional remuneration was so substantial that there was little need for them to work to improve services and to achieve other quality payments such as for immunisation levels. These payments remained until the introduction of the 2004 Contract. Obviously they did not solve the underlying social problems which central government and local authorities would have to face up to and address and did nothing to improve care services by other providers except by drawing attention to the problems.

Interestingly with the improved wealth of the population even in deprived areas some people there have the trappings of luxury such as cars, mobile phones and satellite dishes but often it is the social opportunities and welfare facilities which are lacking. They may be better classified as socially marginalized and much work remains to be done to solve the problems in these areas. Social inequalities and deprivation remain one of the major issues to be tackled before a healthy nation is achieved

Acheson in a further report in 1998 suggested that "the pursuit of a free market economy by successive governments since 1979 has probably been the most significant factor in widening income inequalities which have a linear relationship with health inequalities." This opinion obviously needs further study but we are now moving into the realm of politics and perhaps leaving it as a quotation without comment is the best approach.

Care in the Community

The concept of Care in the Community, the philosophy of allowing the mentally ill, persons with learning difficulties, the frail elderly and those with physical handicaps, to live their lives as independently as possible in the community and outside of hospitals has been around for several decades now. The concept of the community has however differed between various organisations and providers. For many patients it has involved a change from a hospital institution into another residential or nursing home institution, without at times any benefit to the patient.

There were many very large hospitals around the country, often in old workhouses, where the frail elderly and the psychiatrically ill were spending their last years. From time to time major scandals erupted about the conditions and lack of care in these, with a major scandal arising in Ely hospital in Cardiff. There was obviously a need to improve conditions for these unfortunates, although it must be said that some who had spent much of their lives there had a relatively comfortable existence and were happy and integrated into the day-to-day running of the hospital, working in the laundry or on the farms. The discharge of patients from the North Wales Hospital in Denbigh from the late sixties onwards is discussed later.

Problems arose because of the differing concepts and the differing funding arrangements of the alternative providers, the NHS, social services, social security and the independent and private sectors. The Audit Commission in its report "Making a Reality of Community Care" in 1986 highlighted these conflicts between government departments and at a local level between providers of services. It also highlighted the "perverse incentive" arising from an open-ended social security budget for people in private homes care.

In 1986 the BMA published "All our tomorrows - growing old in Britain" and said "the true meaning of community care seems to have been forgotten in many quarters. Community care should mean the provision of welfare services tailored to the needs of people within the community. In practice, elderly people are often abandoned, with totally inadequate social services support, to fend for themselves or to be looked after by wives, daughters or daughters-in-law whose own well-being is jeopardised by the strain. Evidence suggests that far from people neglecting their elderly friends and relatives, society takes advantage of the goodwill of individual carers." In spite of many initiatives the situation remains much the same today. Although the contribution which carers make is acknowledged and a Carers Association has been formed it was not unusual in our practice to find a frail daughter of sixty-five uncomplainingly caring for a parent, or often two, in their nineties with very little support. Sometimes help had been offered in the past, refused because of a sense of pride, and not offered again.

Sir Roy Griffiths, deputy chairman both of Sainsbury's and of the NHS Policy Board, was asked by the government to review community care policy. His report "Community Care: Agenda for Action" published in 1988 was radical. He proposed that local authorities should be the single body responsible for organising "social care" for the elderly, people with mental health problems and people with disabilities. They would be funded by money transferred from the social security budget for care in homes and that this money should be specifically ear-marked, or in modern jargon "ring fenced". The government`s response was published in 1990 as a White Paper "Caring for People: Community Care in the next decade and beyond". A separate but virtually identical document - the Proposals for Wales - was issued by Peter Walker, the Secretary of State for Wales, and the NHS and Community Care Act followed.

Local authorities were given responsibility for designing and purchasing care packages for individuals and for ensuring that services were delivered, using maximum use of the independent sector. They were required to provide financial support for those who would previously have claimed income support. A requirement to establish inspection and registration units was also included. All in all a very major shift in responsibility at a time when social services departments were operating with inadequately trained staff. One of the Griffiths recommendations, that there should be a minister "clearly and publicly identified as responsibility for community care", was not accepted by the government.

The implementation scheduled for April 1991 to coincide with the introduction of the NHS reforms was delayed until 1993, cynics believing that this was because they would have led to a substantial increase in community charge bills at a time when opposition to the so-called Poll Tax was at its height. The BMA took an active interest in these developments which it welcomed as they addressed some of the concerns which had been raised over the past years. It established a new Committee on Community Care to look carefully at how the legislation addressed existing problem areas, seeking advice and comments by questionnaires to doctors, health authorities and community health councils, and it published a comprehensive "Priorities for Community Care - a BMA Report" in 1992.

The years since 1991 have seen the policies implemented, for better or worse, in local authorities across the country. Inadequate funding has resultedin much frustration amongst doctors in the health service and in workers in social services departments trying to implement the concept. Unfortunately other and new problems keep cropping up to frustrate good intentions, a major factor has been the demographic explosion in the elderly, while the increase in the abuse of drugs and alcohol have created massive additional problems. GPs and their primary health care teams are probably in the best position to assess how the policy has worked as they have had to bear the brunt of additional workload arising from absent services, by day and out-of-hours. Accident and emergency departments also shoulder a considerable burden arising from the inadequacies of others.

Social workers have come in for considerable criticisms from various quarters, both because of major scandals highlighted in the media arising from inadequate care arrangements and from other health care workers at local levels because of perceived inadequacies. Part of the problem was that they use different language and jargon which tends to create barriers. Certainly in the early years many of the social workers had no formal qualifications and appeared inadequately trained for the job or in the need for good communication. The BMA report suggested that there appeared to be marked cultural differences between health and local authorities. In management terms the former were more performance and target orientated while local authorities were more open to local pressures and focussed more on user involvement. Poor understanding of the way the "other side" works led to the development of unhelpful stereotypes. From a GP point of view our patients were referred to by social workers as clients, which irritated some GPs beyond reason.

The other major difference in terminology was the word "urgent". GPs have always worked on the principle that urgent means the same day, and often means leaving a waiting room of patients to deal with a situation. An urgent referral to a social worker frequently had to wait for a department meeting days later to decide to whom the case should be allocated, then further delay before the situation was assessed. In one case to my knowledge a request for a visit to a young person with terminal cancer had still not been responded to after three weeks and in spite of three further telephone calls. It was not a case where I was personally involved or someone would have jumped. Such examples were not uncommon. At the end of the process there was frequently no feedback to the GP about the proposed action. Differing ideas about confidentiality and reporting back to line management upset many GPs. Care in the community with more disabled people in their own homes or in residential care has caused a considerable increase in workload for doctors and the primary health care team which many feel has not been adequately recognised and resourced.

A major problem was that local authorities and health authorities were not co-terminous, leading to border problems at that level in reaching agreement. This was rectified in the 1974 boundary reorganisations which created larger co-terminous authorities in North Wales as elsewhere. Regrettably the later 1994 reorganisation with a reversion to six smaller local authorities co-terminous with Local Health Boards in North Wales has not been helpful in this respect, particularly so with general practices which have traditionally tended to serve communities which often straddle borders.

The major issue of funding of care and who has responsibility for it was and remains a major problem with conflicts between hospitals trusts and social services. Very considerable amounts are involved, often on-going for individuals for years. It was necessary to agree Eligibility Criteria which basically say that if a patient being discharged from hospital to a home required continuing nursing care then the health authority should be responsible for financing it, if not then social services should do so. Life is not that simple and many patients can be considered to require a degree of nursing but the majority of care can be considered social care, defined as the care which might be provided by a caring relative at home. Hospital financed continuing care is not means tested whereas social care is. Luckily GPs are not involved in these decisions which are made at administrative level. Relatives often are, especially those who are financing the care from their own resources, and they bring their concerns to the surgery.

One of the criteria of continuing NHS care was that the patient needed to be under the supervision and care of a consultant during the whole period. In fact this rarely happens in practice and care becomes the responsibility by default and without agreement of a GP under normal arrangements. Care of patients in residential and nursing homes has been a source of considerable annoyance which has not yet been resolved in spite of efforts over many years and is discussed in detail later.

The other major problem in community care has been that resources have not followed the patient and care workers have been thin on the ground, partly from finance but also because sufficient numbers have not been trained. Patients with mental illness, and particularly those with personality disorders who many psychiatrists now claim are not their responsibility because they cannot be treated, are vulnerable. Some are labelled as "bad not mad". They live isolated in the community and have a greater tendency to commit criminal offences, sometimes relatively minor but occasionally involving severe violence. When this happens it is often possible to demonstrate inadequate supervision and follow-up. Every time it is said that "lessons will be learned" but this does not seem to happen.

The Care in the Community policy certainly has helped many to live better lives but there remain anxieties as to whether the policy is correct to the extent it has been carried out.

Many carers are under continuous twenty-four hours a day, 365 days a year, strain and some are only able to cope by the provision of respite care. In earlier days this would be arranged on a regular basis every few weeks or months within long-stay or community hospitals. More recently it was decreed that hospitals were not for respite care and other arrangements had to be made. It was certainly not unusual for GPs to "manufacture" a medical reason for admission to overcome this decree. Others were admitted to social services residential homes but as these were closed down in many areas another avenue was shut-down. Admission to private homes could be arranged through social services, although sometimes this had to be funded by the patient or family.

Respite for a few hours on a day care basis is sometimes available at day centres or day-hospitals but these again are being closed down in some areas on cost grounds. Organisations such as Crossroads, where available, provide an invaluable service. Many carers struggle on to avoid admission and themselves suffer. It has not been easy to get across the concept that respite care may obviate the need for long-stay admission to hospitals or homes. The issues of Care in the Community are complex and difficult but have to be faced and resolved so that good care is provided.

The North Wales Hospital, Denbigh

The North Wales Hospital for Mental Illness to use its full title was one of the larger mental hospitals in the country and was an institution universally known and probably universally feared by the people of North and Mid-Wales. It was situated at Denbigh and was generally known by this name, and the stigma of "Denbigh" for many years was very great. It was opened in 1848 following a gift of land by Mr J. Ablett of Llanbadarn, with seventy beds, and within a few years it had 200 patients and was suffering from overcrowding. What's new in the health service?

Mental illness at that time was quite different from that which we see today, very loosely defined and largely incurable. People went into hospital and frequently never emerged again. Some went in as young people perhaps with depression after an illegitimate child, were unsupported by their families and never left the hospital. Others suffered from varieties of mental handicap and were placed in the hospital, living there for the rest of their lives with many happily doing useful work within the hospital and on the attached farm which provided for many of the needs of the hospital. The farm was sold in 1958 which resulted in less occupational and remedial therapy for patients.

Since many of the patients were not severely disturbed there was over many years a tradition of social events such as a drama club and sporting fixtures were held against teams from other institutions. A highlight was the annual Christmas Ball for patients, staff and local residents, started in 1842 and continuing until 1970. Top international Big Bands played there and tickets were sought after and hard to come by.

On the other hand some patients were very disturbed and extremely violent and the padded cells and restraints were in frequent use. Surgical leucotomies were introduced as a means of altering the personalities of patients and making them more manageable, and electro-convulsive therapy was often used for the depressed. The fifties saw the introduction of powerful new drugs like largactil and stelazine which had similar calming effects but much less invasively.

Considerable overcrowding persisted over the years and the LMC minutes in 1960 record that this was by 200 beds and that there was considerable difficulty in getting patients admitted in emergency. Following on from the Royal Commission on the Law Relating to Mental Illness and Mental Deficiency, the Mental Health Act of 1959 introduced fundamental changes, one of which allowed for the first time patients to be admitted to mental hospitals voluntarily.

In 1960 Mr Enoch Powell, the Minister of Health, visited the hospital and announced its eventual closure, confirmed the following year in the Hospital Plan for England and Wales which proposed the formation of District General Hospitals and the attachment of psychiatric units to these, and the discharge of patients back "into the Community". The first District General Hospital in North Wales at Bodelwyddan did not however materialise until 1980.

"The Mental" as it was known in Denbigh was in the forefront of this movement of patients into the community, considerably ahead of the field and with an enlightened approach achieved the objective successfully, but not without its human problems. Many patients were perfectly suitable for rehabilitation and were discharged into multiple occupancy homes and bed and breakfast accommodation, particularly in the Rhyl area. Unfortunately many were not welcome within their boarding houses during the daytime and spent hours wandering the streets and cafes. Others with more severe problems and with learning difficulties were resettled into small homes with a carer. Regrettably there was no requirement for registration of these premises and there was always a shortage of support workers, community psychiatric nurses and social workers, to help them with their problems. One of the consultant psychiatrists who was involved and who expressed concern about the situation in these unregistered homes was Dr. D.O. Lloyd, the father of Huw Lloyd from the Old Colwyn practice. Huw has maintained the family interest in mental illness and has for some years been active in promoting developments in community care of mental health both through the RCGP in London and in Wales.

The Hospital was always run by a Medical Superintendent who was the administrator as well as a clinician. Dr J.H.O. Roberts was appointed in 1940 and continued in post until he retired in 1963 to be followed by Dr T. Gwynne Williams and between them they oversaw major changes in medical management of illness and treatment regimes, together with the introduction of psychiatric nurse training and of new assistants such as psychiatric social workers and occupational therapists. An eponymous T. Gwyn Williams lecture was held annually at Ysbyty Glan Clwyd Postgraduate Centre for some years but has now come to an end as a result of changes in the structure of continuing education at the postgraduate centre.

One of the leading lights of this resettlement programme was Dr D.A. Jones, a consultant Psychiatrist appointed in 1964 and known to all including the general public as Dafydd Alun or simply D.A, a larger than life individual with a tremendous capacity for work in many places at the same time, even though it was often difficult to catch up with him, and then only for a few minutes before he was off elsewhere. An ardent supporter of the Welsh Language and everything Welsh, he stood for parliament on behalf of Plaid Cymru but was not elected. His ability to consult in a patients first language was much appreciated especially in the western areas where English was still a difficult language for many. He was well respected by all and many forgave his erratic timekeeping. He was always ready to assist with a medical or psychiatric report on those unfortunate to fall foul of the law or other authorities, or if early retirement on health grounds was being considered. A great lover of big fast cars, a number of which ended up in accidents, he also flew his own plane which he used amongst other things to maintain links with the community in Brittany. On one occasion a light aircraft landed in a field in our practice area and two men were seen to jump out and run to a waiting car. At the time there was a problem with illegal immigrants entering the country from Pakistan , but it turned out to be D.A. arriving late to see patients in Llandudno.

As mentioned Denbigh hospital, indeed any psychiatric hospital or outpatients, was for many a place to be avoided at all costs at that time and so D.A. developed an extensive private inpatient and outpatient practice, first at the West Shore Nursing Home in Llandudno and later at the North Wales Medical Centre as well as seeing outpatients all over North Wales and even way into the English Borders. The Medical Centre as discussed later provided an alternative (private) inpatient facility, particularly for the treatment of depression and alcoholism, for those wishing to avoid admission to Denbigh.

Later he developed a keen interest in the management and treatment of post-traumatic stress disorders, a new field which came into prominence after the Falklands war, and developed a specialist nursing home in Llandudno to deal with patients with these symptoms, the only institution of its kind in the U.K. Regrettably it has recently closed as funding from the Local health Board was no longer forthcoming.

With the increasing problem of hard drugs moving into North Wales in the nineties, especially in the Deeside area at that time, he developed with some success a management regime using diamorphine as a substitute, although it must be said that there were two opposing views on management in North Wales, methadone substitution therapy and drug withdrawal, and a consensus on the correct management has not yet been reached.

In all a hospital of over 1600 beds in 1970 was gradually reduced and eventually was a single ward by 1995. In 1970 Dr D.A. Jones gave a paper to the three-day annual conference of the National Association of Mental Health which met in Denbigh to debate the new concept of care in the community and its implementation. I attended on behalf of the LMC to listen to this and the implications appeared very worrying from a GP point of view.

During the earlier years of the process acute psychiatric admission and readmissions carried on as usual, but gradually the arrival of new drugs and changes in treatment patterns and in particular the management of acute illness within the community with Community Psychiatric Nurses and social workers resulted in fewer admissions. For doctors in practices however the available support was for years very inadequate and certainly not often available with any degree of urgency.

The need for specialist psychiatric services for the elderly was recognised and the significant Health Advisory Service report The Rising Tide in 1982 , the title recognising that the mental disorder of old age threatened to overwhelm the health and social services.

Admission in emergency particularly out of hours and at weekends became very difficult, particularly if the Police were involved because of anti-social behaviour and drunkenness, and for the elderly confused. One often had to make several calls to locate the duty psychiatrist, and we later discovered that they held lists of problem patients who were nor for re-admission. One outcome of this was the opening of the Ablett Unit which at the time was a major relief to on-call GPs faced with a, usually elderly, confused and difficult patient on a Saturday night. Often the on-call doctor would not know the patient nor the patient the doctor. The hospital would not accept the request for admission and suggested the Social Services who would then refuse to accept responsibility and refer back. On frequent occasions the patient had been drinking alcohol and any suspicion of this was sufficient excuse for social services to refuse to consider any compulsory admission under Section. The family would be insisting in the time honoured words "something must be done" and hours went on during which time, while still dealing with this problem, the doctor had others to attend to. After much pressure agreement was reached to open the Ablett Unit on the Denbigh site, where patients would be accepted and with the understanding that within three days a management decision would be made - admit to a hospital ward, to a Social Services Home or back to their own home.

In time inpatient units were developed within the three North Wales DGHs and eventually the whole hospital could finally be closed in 1995.

The subsequent history of the hospital site has been the subject of considerable controversy. Parts of it were listed. After some years and a number of false starts during which the North Wales Health Authority were paying out large sums annually for maintenance and security of the empty building, and supported and encouraged by Welsh Office, the Authority sold the property to a private developer at what is generally felt locally to be a ridiculously low price. Unfortunately it has proved very difficult to get agreement and planning permission on the development of the extensive site and the hospital building, the front of which is listed, has fallen into disrepair and been vandalised. Latest developments suggest perhaps a solution may at last be in the offing.

Psychiatry, and particularly access to care for mental illness, has become much more complex and difficult to access since the closure of the North Wales Hospital. Arrangements have been fragmented across the three Trusts, all of whom operate different structures. Indeed within each Trust arrangements over access and who makes the initial assessment vary between various teams and many of these seem to be operating understaffed and resourced. Retention of staff is reported as a problem, many being trained locally but then moving away across the border. Separate teams operate for adult mental illness, children, adolescents, the elderly , the elderly mentally infirm, and for drug and alcohol abuse but for individual patients considerable overlap occurs. Patients with severe personality disorders are labelled as untreatable and therefore no one accepts responsibility. The BMA through its consultant and GP committees have set down principles which should be adhered to in all referral management arrangements but consultation when introducing them is rarely adequate.

All this at a time when mental illness of all degrees of severity is increasing and is likely to affect most people at some time in their lives. There is evidence that the diseases of unhappiness are on the increase and that many patients are finding it difficult to cope. Much of general practice is now spent dealing with mental problems, very often associated with other conditions and .much effort is being expended at RCGP and at Assembly government level on developing strategies to support primary care and to support patients, with Dr Huw Lloyd from the LMC being actively involved at all levels.

Community Hospitals

Community hospitals have arisen from the older GP and cottage hospitals. The oldest in Wales and which is still functioning is my local community hospital, Denbigh Infirmary, or to give it the original name The Denbigh General Dispensary and Asylum for the Recovery of Health, opened in 1807.

The first "cottage hospital" in England was opened in 1858 at Cranleigh in Surrey by Dr Albert Napper in the same year as the Medical Registration Act. He defined a cottage hospital as "literally a cottage, with an optimum of six to eight beds, differing only from a patient's home in cleanliness, warmth, proper hygiene and absence of overcrowding" and being an alternative in rural areas to the large county hospitals which were often feared because of their high mortality rates. They developed rapidly in the early twentieth century, many of them having been built by subscription by their communities as War Memorials. Surgery and maternity were often the main activities. At the outset of the NHS the new consultants felt that there was a danger that GPs would undertake surgery which they did not have the facilities to perform and were not trained to do. In fact many of the GP surgeons were very good and knew their limitations so that their results were often as good as the nearest county hospitals before the NHS. In Colwyn Bay Hospital when I started there the GP surgeons and anaesthetists, Drs Herbert Lord, Kenneth Evans and Alwyn Millar were still about.

The Bonham Carter Report in 1969 on "The Functions of the District General Hospital" stated that "we do not think there is any good case for retaining small hospitals from which it is easy to reach the District General Hospital" and that services should be concentrated on large multidisciplinary DGHs. This view caused anxieties and problems in many areas and in particular in the Oxford Region which is predominantly rural and contained a large number of small hospitals which could not sensibly be closed down and the concept of a new type of Community hospital was developed and the first purpose-built one opened in 1973 at Wallingford in the Thames valley. The concept would include inpatient beds, rehabilitation on a day-patient basis and a health centre for the GP team with facilities for visiting consultants. Inpatient facilities would cater for acute medical cases which did not require the facilities of a DGH, postoperative and early discharge cases from the DGH, some post-assessment geriatric and psychiatric patients, holiday relief for chronic sick treated at home, and terminal care. They would not provide a full accident and emergency service and would not carry out surgery or admit children.

At that time cottage hospital beds as they were known were viewed in two ways by G.Ps, those who had them would fight tooth and nail to keep them while those who had never had them were very reluctant to consider taking on a another major workload especially as remuneration was very poor.

In North Wales the new District General hospital at Ysbyty Glan Clwyd, Bodelwyddan, was opened in 1981 on a greenfield site which attracted widespread local criticism because it appeared to be away from everywhere. In retrospect the open unbuilt surroundings have allowed for considerable extension and development, while the building of the A55, the main artery across North Wales, has made it very accessible. Prior to the new hospital acute services locally had been provided at hospitals at the West Denbighshire Hospital at Colwyn Bay, the Royal Alexandra at Rhyl, the old Sanatorium at Abergele, and the old workhouses at H.M.Stanley at St Asaph and at Lluesty Holywell.

At this time the Clwyd Health Authority had Dr David T. Jones as its Chief Administrative Medical Officer, a former GP with vision who later went on to become its Chief Executive on the retirement of Mr Donald Cope in 1987. The Authority in 1976 had adopted the policy written by David Jones and Wyndham Evans of having the two District General Hospitals supported by a network of active Community Hospitals providing care nearer to patients homes. As part of the package the closure of Llangwyfan Hospital was proposed together with the running down of the Mental Hospital in Denbigh.

There already existed in Clwyd at that time eleven community hospitals, more than in most areas of Wales. Colwyn Bay Hospital was proposed as a new community hospital of forty two beds on two floors, one floor for G.P. Beds and one for beds under the care of the geriatrician, Dr June Arnold. By this time those older GPs in Colwyn Bay who in the early years of the NHS and before had acted as GP/Surgeons and GP anaesthetists and had an association with the hospital had retired or died. Meetings of the local GPs from the catchment area showed marked variation in interest in the new concept. My partner Dr Patrick Edwards had had experience in the use of a community hospital in Denbigh while working as a trainee at Beech House and his experience was invaluable in persuading waverers and later in developing policies and protocols.

Some twenty-five GPs were likely to be potential users of the hospital and only 21 beds were on offer. To be worthwhile and to avoid disputes there had to be sufficient beds so that appropriate cases which GPs wished to admit could be accommodated. Unless sufficient beds are available allowing immediate or early admission of cases which do not require the facilities of a DGH and which can be looked after under the care of their own GP then the purpose of the local hospital is lost Management do not accept this and look upon a lower bed occupancy rate as wasteful Experience elsewhere indicated that about two beds per GP would be required. After long discussion it was decided that interest would be expressed but only if all the beds were made available to the

GPs. If not the geriatricians could have the lot - but with local GPs being very unlikely to provide cover for them as clinical assistants. Eventually all beds were designated as GP beds, the first new GP community hospital to be set up from scratch in Wales for many years.

Certainly the GPs were not in it for the money. Community Hospital beds have always been paid for from a Bed Fund calculated as £'s per bed per year. With forty-two beds at Colwyn Bay the total bed fund for providing care 24 hours a day, 7 days a week and 52 weeks a year was ridiculously small, divided between the twenty-one doctors. The hospital did however provide considerable increased job satisfaction to offset against the increased workload.

There was considerable local anxiety and disquiet amongst the public at what was seen as loss of facilities and the downgrading of their hospital. The Health Authority accepted that casualty, outpatient clinics, x-ray and laboratory facilities would be retained and this helped to ease the disquiet.

Various guidelines and protocols were set up during a series of meetings particularly on admission and discharge policies, and on length of stay. There was evidence that many other community hospitals had long stay patients and were in effect nursing homes with little active rehabilitation and with most of the beds blocked.

The discharge policies came under some pressure at the outset because one of the consultant physicians, Dr Geoffrey Lloyd, on vacating the hospital left behind an elderly patient who he had promised could stay as long as she needed care and whose family for two years resisted all efforts to discharge her, and allowing some other patients and their families to try to follow suit. A GP/Nurse review committee was set up to monitor individual cases and proved invaluable in supporting doctors who felt patients were ready for discharge but who were facing resistance from the patient or relatives. Obviously there were a few teething problems and anxiety particularly amongst the nursing staff some of whom had been used to theatre and acute surgery work but in all the transfer went smoothly. Much credit must be given to the matron Mrs Nethercott in facilitating the change. Many of the other community hospitals have since been upgraded and extended and Colwyn Bay Hospital itself was completely gutted and refitted in the late nineties.

Within Gwynedd Health Authority there was much less enthusiasm and for years no thought about actively developing them. The Authority did set up a review chaired by Mrs Margaret Merchant, chief nursing officer and Dr Jeremy Corson, an ex-GP turned community physician in 1993 but little change resulted.

There were considerable anxieties about which complaints procedures GPs were working under until it was established in 1990 that GPs working and paid in the Bed-fund were not covered by Crown Indemnity but that their Defence Bodies would cover them. If however they were employed as clinical assistants then they came under the Hospital Complaints regulations.

Some years later while I was a member on the Welsh Medical Committee advising Welsh Office it was decided to carry out an in-depth look at Community Hospitals across Wales and I was asked to chair a multi-specialty group to look at the present position and what their potential role might be. The group consisted of Dr. Sandy Cavenagh, a GP from Brecon who was a leading figure in the UK Community Hospitals Association and who was working in a Community Hospital which because of its geographical location was considerably more developed than most and still carried out fairly major surgery at that time, Dr Gareth Hughes the Consultant Geriatrician from Aberystwyth, Mr Aled Williams, the Consultant Obstetrician and Gynaecologist from Wrexham, Dr Alan Spence a specialist in Community Medicine and myself. The group worked very well together and held its meetings while visiting hospitals across Wales, discovering that while the hospitals were very different most had similar problems and were underdeveloped. Some were virtually full of long stay patients, some awaiting transfer through Social Services to a Local Authority Home. We encountered the ultimate folly in one area in a South Wales valley. Before a patient could be transferred to a Residential Home he or she had to be admitted to the Home for a two week period to assess suitability, and if deemed suitable had to return to the Hospital to await a vacancy in the Home which was sometimes up to a year, during which time the patient's condition had often deteriorated. In due course we reported to Welsh Medical Committee which received our report with considerable enthusiasm, apart from the paediatricians who brought in the big guns to condemn it because we had dared suggest that there was a place for the occasional admission of a child to a Community Hospital. Welsh Office then commissioned work by Helen Tucker who had previously published in 1987 a Project Paper for the Kings Fund on the Role and Function of Community Hospitals with Sandy Cavenagh and myself involved to look in more detail at the economics and costings.

In the past much maternity work was done in the local hospitals but with the majority of this work now taking place in specialist maternity units local doctors have become de-skilled and have withdrawn from the work. Some units such as Bryn Beryl, Pwllheli, and Dolgellau Hospital are still functioning as midwife-led units but how long this will continue remains to be seen. Emergency back-up at a distance of forty miles from a DGH is very difficult.

With the formation of the North Wales Health Authority in 1994 the community hospital policy continued but with its demise and the transfer of responsibility to the much smaller Local Health Groups and the development of the independent Hospital Trusts further problems have arisen in North Wales.

The whole future of Community Hospitals and their staffing is now back in the melting pot after a period full of promise.

Over the last few years changes in practice in the District General Hospitals and pressure on their beds has resulted in very early discharge of post-operative cases to Community Hospitals with a much different workload for both doctors and nursing staff. Originally patients came back to the care of their own GP but now patients are being discharged to community hospitals outside their hometown and with no connection with their GP. New guidelines for the nursing staff and the requirement for GPs to attend specially merely to sign authorisation for changes in therapy have increased demands and made the work less effective. This together with the changes in out-of-hours cover arrangements by GPs is making community hospital work less attractive and some GPs are pulling out with perhaps more to follow. The wholly inadequate remuneration issue has dragged on for years in spite of recurrent requests to address it and remains unresolved. Difficulty in getting commitments from the Health Authorities and later the Trusts added to the dissatisfaction felt about working in the community hospital.

The ability of doctors under the new contract to join out-of-hours organisations or to opt out of evening and weekend work altogether means that Trusts need to agree separate out-of-hours contracts with the Local Health Boards who now have responsibility for providing out of hours care. The longstanding low remuneration together with bureaucratic requirements and changes in the ability and willingness of nursing staff to make decisions have contributed to this. Already at Colwyn Bay the beds have been given back to specialists and the GPs have withdrawn. The total cost may prove to be considerably higher than what was paid to the GPs. Minor casualty facilities are likely to become nurse-led in all hospitals, supplemented by video links to the base hospital, while because of low staffing levels and staff security issues in the smaller units they may be withdrawn completely out of hours.

While community beds are being reduced there is no apparent plans to increase the bed numbers elsewhere, adding to the existing pressures on DGHs not to admit. All this at a time when DGHs discharge patients very early and where patients still need the now rarely mentioned periods of convalescence but in an environment where they are possibly less at risk from severe hospital acquired infections.

The Wanless Report published in Wales in 2003 suggested that a unit of less than thirty beds was not viable. Many community hospitals across Wales have less beds than this but the issue should not be judged only by the number of beds but by distance from the DGH and also by the other services which are or potentially can be provided on site. They should in fact be seen as community resource centres. As a result many local hospitals are under threat and local communities are very concerned, especially since a number of these were originally built by local public subscription as Memorial hospitals.

A new Community Hospital is currently under construction in Portmadoc which is intended to replace the Bron-y-garth Hospital in Penrhyndeudraeth and Ffestiniog Hospital - interestingly it was designed with less than the thirty beds suggested as a minimum for viability. The saga of this new hospital with major delays over site problems, the nature of the roof cladding and particularly finance makes interesting study. When it was first mooted the LMC and the local communities were opposed to a single site hospital and wished to retain the hospital at Blaenau Ffestiniog, seeing the Portmadoc hospital as a direct replacement for Bron-y-garth. and this view remains active amongst the local community. Time will tell which GPs will feel able to work in it and on what terms because of the distance and the time factor. The concept of patients being cared for locally by their own GP now appears to be disappearing rapidly.

The Hospice Movement

One of the important functions of the small community hospitals was the provision of terminal care for cancer and other diseases locally by their own GP supported by staff who were often already known to the patient. and sometimes with the support of a MacMillan nurse. For patients in larger communities who often did not have access to community beds the DGH and other hospitals like Llandudno were available but they did not provide wards with the quiet and relaxed atmosphere which patients often wished for. Many patients were admitted into private nursing homes.

The Hospice movement itself was started in 1967 by Dr Cicely Saunders, a former nurse and social worker who later trained as a doctor, when she created the St Christopher Hospice at Sydenham. It was the first hospice to combine clinical care, research and teaching, and jointly emphasised medical and psychosocial care. There had been hospices to care for the terminally ill before then, usually run by nuns providing nursing and tender loving care. Her concept was to develop a situation where a more active approach by doctors and nurses was taken with the development of better controlled pain and symptom relief in quiet and peaceful surroundings and with more emphasis on a positive attitude to the illness. She was rewarded for her revolutionary pioneering work by the award of the Order of Merit and was created a Dame.

Palliative care has traditionally been undertaken in general practice, sometimes much better than others. Wales was a prime mover in the improvement of palliative care, with Professor Nigel Stott and Dr Ilona Finlay in a general practice in Cardiff developing continuing education and then setting up the first Diploma in Palliative Care. She later moved into secondary care as a consultant and has since been created a Baroness.

Moves to establish hospices in North Wales started around1986. The St Kentigern Hospice was first put forward at a public meeting held in Bodelwyddan castle and chaired by Lady Langford in April 1986. Plans proceeded and in 1992 the opinion of local GPs, consultants and district and Macmillan nurses was sought by questionnaire. Nearly 60% of GPs and 14% of nurses felt existing arrangements were adequate, perhaps reflecting the availability of GP hospital beds, but none of the consultants did. However there was general support for a development in the Bodelwyddan area and the St Kentigern Hospice started to move forward. Funding was always difficult and was very largely by public subscription and fund-raising. In due course a day-centre with ten places was opened on the H.M.Stanley site in 1995 and after many setbacks and delays an inpatient unit was opened in 2000.

In the Wrexham area interest started following the appointment in 1977 of

Dr Graham Arthurs as consultant anaesthetist and the establishment by him of a Pain Clinic at the old War Memorial Hospital. In the early eighties Dr Arthurs` Terminal Care Fund was set up to finance the first two Macmillan Nurses In the area. The Nightingale House day Hospice was opened in the old Nightingale ward at the Maelor hospital, a ward I had often had to visit during my house physician days in 1955. In 1992 a Foundation was launched to raise funds for a purpose-built hospice and in due course this opened in 1995.

A similar movement was taking place in the Llandudno area in 1989 led by a group from Penrhyn Bay. Dr Oliver Galpin, the local Consultant Physician, was asked to become medical adviser in 1993 and he became chairman on his retirement from the NHS in 1994. The purpose built hospice on West Shore Llandudno was opened by the Prince of Wales in 1999, first the day hospital, now with ten places, and later four inpatient beds which has since been increased to ten.

Volunteers in North-west Wales went down a different path and instead of a hospice building they developed the Gwynedd Hospice at Home scheme. The first discussions took place in 1989 and Dr Jim Davies, the retired Principal of the Bangor Normal College, was again involved in another very successful appeal process which reached its target of £500,000 in two years. Specially trained palliative care nurses provided care and support to patients in their own homes, working alongside the District Nurses. Mr R.H.P. (Hywel) Oliver the much-respected consultant surgeon at Ysbyty Gwynedd became chairman after his retirement. A day hospice, Hafan Menai, was opened in the grounds of Ysbyty Gwynedd close to the Alaw oncology ward, another development in which Dr Jim Davies played an important fund-raising role. The scheme became part of the North-west Trust in 1996 with costs being shared between the Trust and the Charity and came under the supervision of a consultant in palliative care.

The need for high staff/patient ratios in hospices mean that running costs remain very high and the bulk of these are covered by local fundraising with relatively small amounts from NHS sources and it remains a mystery to many why the NHS does not support them to a greater extent. Costs are considerably less than palliative care carried out within a District General Hospital.

The local fund-raising position in North Wales is complicated by the needs of another Hospice, this time for children, based at Oswestry and known as Hope House which was set up in 1995 with eight beds. The extent of need for the care of children, both for respite care for severe physical and mental handicap and for terminal care has surprised everyone. A movement was started to open another one closer to central and north-west Wales led with great enthusiasm and skill by Mrs Sarah Kearsley-Wooller who had a handicapped child of her own. Ty Gobaith yng Nghymru, the Welsh translation for Hope House in Wales, was opened in 2004 with five beds on a fabulous site overlooking the Conwy river and has enthusiastic support from its patron Bryn Terfel.

All these hospices in their different ways have provided a valuable facility and support for patients and relatives which was not previously available in the area. The fund-raising support which they engender speaks volumes for the way they are appreciated. It is somewhat unfortunate that other local charities have perhaps suffered as a consequence.

Care of the elderly

A significant part of my professional life has had an involvement with the elderly, who have until recently been defined as the over 65s. The improved health and wealth of the nation, social and lifestyle changes together with the major demographic shift towards increasing numbers in the older age groups has required a redefinition. While concessions of various kinds are available to the over 65s, in health terms the major problems are now seen in the over 75s and in particular those aged over 85 and in their nineties. Last year saw a 33% growth in persons over ninety in North Wales. The term pensioners is no longer appropriate either as many are now choosing to retire and take a pension in their fifties, and then go on to start another career or interest.

Medical Care of the Elderly, previously called Geriatrics, has changed beyond recognition. During my medical school days geriatrics in Cardiff consisted of several wards of chronic long stay patients in the old workhouse at St David's Hospital. Discharge home was rare. Consultants then were usually specialists who had made a sideways move for a variety of reasons. The consultant at St Davids had no junior staff, his care being supported by final year medical students, myself included, honing their clinical skills part-time for a few weeks.

As discussed elsewhere, when I moved from Ruabon to Penrhyn Bay one of my first impressions was of the difference in the fitness and general activity levels in the retired residents there, reflecting clearly the influence of previous occupations and lifestyles. For the receptionists making appointments was often a negotiation based around their hair, coffee morning, or golf commitments. The other major difference was the number of them. The numbers remained around 40% of the practice being over 65 and 22% over 75, to my knowledge the highest in Wales by far. I recall on one occasion discussing the workload of the elderly with a GP from Porthcawl, the retirement centre for South Wales, who was bemoaning his 23% of over 65 year olds. The second big impression was the large number of nursing and residential homes in the new practice area, a topic which discussed in a later chapter.

Geriatrics started to become a specialty following the pioneering work in England of Dr Marjorie Warren and of Dr Exton-Smith. In the seventies a new generation of dedicated geriatricians were coming into post in North Wales, in particular Dr Glyn Penrhyn Jones at Bangor, Dr. June Arnold and later Dr. Bim. Bhowmick at Ysbyty Glan Clwyd, and Dr Beulah Simpson at Llandudno.

Bed blocking, that is the inability to discharge patients who are ready but for whom suitable alternative arrangements cannot be made immediately has been in the news recently as one of the causes of long waiting lists and patients waiting in ambulances outside hospitals. It is not new, both Dr June Arnold and myself wrote articles about it in the journal Geriatric Medicine in 1983. I believe it was she who originally coined the phrase "bed-blockers". Discharge to nursing and residential homes and the problems associated with them was reviewed by me in another paper in the same Journal and my research on this issue is discussed later.

At the same time a new specialty, psycho-geriatrics, was coming into being, albeit very patchily, to deal with the confused elderly and the elderly mentally infirm. Obviously there was considerable overlap, and considerable buck passing occurred at times. We as GPs would often spend considerable time especially at night and at weekends, under considerable pressure from families or neighbours and sometimes also the police, trying to persuade one or other departments to accept confused patients needing urgent care. Junior staff had to refer to their consultants and we finally understood that there were unofficial blacklists of patients in the psychiatric hospital and to get anyone on such a list admitted as an emergency was virtually impossible.

Dr DA Jones had in 1972 suggested to the Welsh Office the setting up of a unit to deal with the urgent admission of confused elderly patients without mixing them with the patients in Denbigh Hospital. In due course the Ablett unit was set up at H.M.Stanley hospital, St Asaph. The concept was that all emergency admissions of the confused elderly would take place to this unit and that after assessment and, if not fit to be discharged, they would be accepted within days into geriatric, psychiatric, or into residential or nursing homes under social services for further care. Ten years later in 1982 he was anxious about the difficulties in placing these patients in registered homes due to the financial problems arising and also the supervision of them afterwards.

The care of elderly patients in the community was a very active topic at that time with Clwyd Health Authority setting up active Health Care Planning Teams. I proposed to Dr Bridie Wilson, the responsible Community Physician, that there was a place for an organisation of volunteers to be set up with responsibility to act as unofficial watchdogs over the care of individual frail elderly, physically and mentally infirm patients in the community and in residential homes as there was evidence that individuals were falling through the supervisory net and being overlooked and neglected. This proposal was discussed informally at the Welsh Office by Dr David Jones, the CAMO, but nothing subsequently transpired.

An issue which has not received sufficient attention is the increased mortality following transfer of the frail elderly between hospitals and care homes. It was raised in 1998 in the Select Committee on Administration, chaired at that time by Mr Rhodri Morgan, by the Health Minister Mr Frank Dobson who asked the NHS executive for more information and statistics on deaths soon after transfer. The outcome is unknown. With all initiatives there seems to be a problem in that while policy is decided centrally at national or district level local implementation is left to middle management who often do their own thing, either from inertia or from lack of resources and funding.

My interest continued by being involved in 1985 on behalf of Welsh GMSC in the Welsh Office document A Good Old Age which looked at care in a wider perspective than just health and in the symposia which followed its publication. The BMA Board of Science and Education published a report All our Tomorrows-Growing Old in Britain in 1986 and made numerous recommendations many of which related to social conditions and which have taken years to implement. One of its interesting aspects was a comparison of the level of old-age pensions in the UK as a proportion of average gross earnings compared with other countries such as the Netherlands, France, and Belgium where they were twice as high.

My involvement in the care of the elderly had developed further when in 1977 I began to undertake two morning sessions a week in the Day Hospital in Llandudno Hospital with Dr Beulah Simpson the new geriatrician who was developing an excellent service for the elderly in the area.

What exactly are Day Hospitals and what do they do? They must be clearly differentiated in their aims and functions from Day Centres run by Social Services departments. The concept of a Day Hospital was an excellent and forward looking one aimed towards earlier discharge from the wards with treatment and supervision both medical and nursing continuing as an outpatient on two or three days a week. They provide medical, investigative, nursing and physiotherapy services as a one-stop shop for elderly patients within a convenient distance from their homes, together with a degree of social care provision and carer respite for these patients but these only. Physiotherapy and occupational therapy could continue while the availability of kitchen and similar facilities in the unit allowed assessment for independent living to be made. They provide opportunities for further observation, examination and investigations for the elderly prior to or instead of admission to a hospital bed and also provide a half-way stage between hospital and home allowing earlier discharge while still maintaining the treatment regime and continued monitoring of progress.

Other patients who were being cared for at home came once or sometimes twice a week to continue treatment and also very importantly to allow their carers a few short hours break. Until that time very little thought or recognition had been given to the needs of the carers, many of whom were themselves very elderly and infirm.

Patients would arrive from about 10.00a.m and leave at about 3.30 p.m. by ambulance transport which was considered better than being brought in by relatives which sometimes caused disruption. If a patient's home was near the end of the ambulance run he or she was probably all right. On the other hand if at the start of a run he or she might be picked up at 8.00am and have a long and tortuous journey picking up others en route and often arriving at the day hospital tired and exhausted. One of the pioneer consultants of day hospitals herself went on the ambulance "milk run" and decided that changes were necessary. The ambulance journeys were identified as the commonest cause of failure to continue to attend the day hospital.

At the same time as day hospitals were being developed Social Service departments were running day centres which provided food, warmth and the stimulation of company for clients but in most cases no active treatment. They did provide a vital period of much needed respite for carers if only for a few hours. There was a very definite social stigma attitude shown by some patients and their families about day centres, the day hospital was socially acceptable, a day centre less so in their eyes.

As my interest in Day Hospitals developed I was fortunate in 1978 to be awarded an Upjohn Travelling Scholarship allowing me to travel and visit some ten day hospitals across England and Wales run by consultants known to have a keen interest in the field. Different populations had given rise to considerable variation in the way the service was provided and I hope I was able to bring ideas back. In some areas I visited day hospitals and social service day centres were run in tandem but this in itself was not always successful. Day hospitals only function well if there is an adequate complement of support from physiotherapists, speech therapists and occupational therapists to aid the rehabilitation process. My clinical assistant contract was terminated summarily after three years because of the wish to appoint an additional registrar in the department. It is my opinion that there is benefit in having an input into care of the elderly by doctors who have actually worked outside hospital walls and in the community.

More recently day hospital care has been developed in the mental illness field and we as a practice provided the general medical back-up support for the Bodnant unit at Llandudno Hospital for both day and in-patients over a number of years.

Another excellent and innovative development in the seventies is now in danger of imminent demise. Within the NHS there come times when financial strictures start to bite and management looks around for something to cut. The mechanism is that parts of the structure of a service are gradually whittled away over a period by non-appointment of casual vacancies until the service is no longer produced effectively, then it is argued that the facility should be withdrawn or closed down. Day hospital facilities have been downgraded at peripheral units. The last day hospital in Gwynedd at Dolgellau was due to close within a week but the GP who worked in it had not yet been told. In fact it was apparently never closed, services just stopped being provided there and the facility lies empty. In the climate of very early discharge from hospitals before rehabilitation has even started the need for a half-way stage is even greater.

Nursing and residential homes

Over the last thirty or forty years long-term care of the elderly and infirm has gradually moved from long stay geriatric wards in hospitals and into residential or nursing homes. The early eighties saw a considerable interest in the concept of Care in the Community and one aspect was the problem of accommodating the elderly infirm within the community setting.

The latest thinking is that many more can be cared for in their homes with mobile carers. In addition the provision for the less infirm has moved from residential homes run by local authorities and into privately run homes. Some areas and counties moved much more rapidly than in others. This move of course resulted in care of the patients being transferred from hospital doctors and staff and on to GPs and community services. Since the administrative and funding mechanisms are different for both this change has taken place largely without any coordination or assurance that appropriate facilities and services were available.

The care of residents in these Nursing and Residential homes has long caused problems for GPs, for some more than others because of the massive concentration of these homes in some areas. The Llandudno and Colwyn Bay areas have always been retirement areas, the elderly moving there away from their families in Manchester and other areas, some finding it difficult to integrate and many losing their partner soon after moving. Failing health then meant they needed residential care. The area had many large private properties suitable for conversion and a large number of Homes were opened even before the boom elsewhere in the 1980's. The migration of the elderly from England had not reached the north-western counties to such an extent at this time, prior to the building of the A55, and the number of homes there was much less of an issue.

In various fora and meetings I kept bringing up in discussion the problems as seen by GPs but receiving a lukewarm response with many doctors not experiencing or acknowledging a problem. Yes, they had a nursing home or two in their area but they were not really a problem.

There obviously was a problem in our area and in 1985 I entered into a research exercise with Dr John Kassab from the Statistics Department of UCNW, Bangor, looking at the number of Homes and the number of beds in them and by two questionnaires studying the issues arising from them.

At that time within the three mile radius area surrounding our Penrhyn Bay practice there were over one thousand beds in the private sector in twelve nursing homes and forty-three private residential homes but only a hundred and thirty-nine in four local authority homes. Since the practice visited patients in many of these homes we were able to check the responses to the questionnaires against our personal knowledge.

On inquiry it appeared amazingly that 26% of all private nursing homes and 33% of all private residential homes in the whole of Wales were to be found within this three mile radius Many more homes were to be found along the coast in Rhyl and Prestatyn.

A report of our research was published in Journal of the RCGP. No previous papers on this subject had been published anywhere but subsequently the issues raised were looked into and researched by others and we received considerable feedback. I spoke at a number of conferences including one run in South Wales by Welsh Office and at an RCGP research symposium at Chester and was also asked to contribute an article on Health Care in Homes for the Elderly in the 1986 RCGP Members Reference Book.

The rapidly increasing problem of the elderly was becoming an important issue in the 1980`s with the number of elderly in the 75-85 age group estimated to increase by 80% by 1986 compared with 1980. The Care in the Community initiative was developed by Welsh Office based on their statement "Most people who need long-term care can and should be looked after in the community, this is what most of them want for themselves and what those responsible for their care believe to be the best". To be precise, care in the community meant not in a hospital bed.

Drs Bhowmick and Arnold at H M Stanley in the Geriatric Medicine Journal in 1984 advocated homes "as the solution to the blocked bed syndrome which had been a thorny subject ever since the establishment of geriatric departments". And bed blocking is still a frequent topic of discussion.

The first NHS Nursing Home was opened in Sheffield in 1985 although little was heard of its success or failure afterwards. Significantly it was already in operation but without any agreement having been reached about any payment to GPs for providing medical care.

In 1981 Mr David Jones, the progressive Area Nursing Officer of Gwynedd Health Authority, set up a working party "to examine the feasibility of setting up within the NHS nursing Homes similar to those provided in the private sector". The working party whose membership was purely nursing and with no medical input or consideration of the medical requirements recommended that a NHS Nursing Home be set up in Gwynedd funded by Welsh Office for five years. As far as I am aware nothing further was heard of the proposal.

The problems associated with the care of the elderly was not just an UK issue. The BMJ in 1984 ran a series on Care in the Netherlands and in Denmark and concluded that their services were superior to ours.

Issues surrounding the financing of patients in homes have been very prominent politically over the years with different arrangements in Local Authority residential accommodation, private and voluntary residential homes and nursing homes. Suffice it to say that they were means tested and many residents were required to pay the full fees whereas had they been kept long-term in hospital their care would have been free. Some would be paying hundreds of pounds a week while the majority in the same home were being state funded in some way or other.

To fully understand the issues arising from Homes it is important to appreciate the differences between the two types of Homes. Nursing Homes are registered by the local Health Authority while Residential Homes are registered with the Local Authorities and do not require any nursing staff to be employed. The distinction appears not to have been fully understood in many quarters and a GMSC document written by John Lynch for an independent review of residential care. carried out on behalf of the government identified that the review did not mention nursing homes in its terms of reference.

In practice residents moved into a residential home, their health deteriorated to the extent that they required nursing care but since the Home was now their personal home there was understandably a reluctance to insist they moved elsewhere. Home owners for financial reasons were reluctant to let them go, relatives did not want them moved because the cost would be higher, and GPs often did not want to rock the boat.

The line between residential care and nursing care became so tenuous that in 1984 the concept of Dual Registration was introduced in the Registration of Homes Act and was taken up by some homes, allowing some beds to be designated as nursing and some as residential and avoiding patients having to move when their condition deteriorated.

Obviously residents in homes, by definition almost, required above average medical attention and this nearly always meant a visit to the homes. Some were paying large fees for their accommodation and expected other benefits to follow. Home owners were very reluctant to use their staff to bring patients to surgery even when well enough to do so. A personal communication from Dr PS Kelly in 1996 showed that in his Wrexham practice covering twenty homes residents made up 0.69% of the practice list but generated 20% of the total daytime calls. Relatives would descend on a fine summer weekend, not having been seen for months, think Auntie looked rather pale and weaker since they last saw her and insist on a visit by the doctor and a report before they left for home again that afternoon.

Standards of care in homes was very variable. Some were first class but in others care was often provided by changing and frequently untrained and outdated staff working shifts, not always willing to accept clinical responsibility, and who would ask for out of hours and emergency calls to cover themselves. Registering authorities were required to make two inspections a year, one announced and one unannounced. `We certainly never saw any reports on these inspections and court action by the authorities was never easy as magistrates were loathe to take action except in the most severe infringements. A star-rating system was proposed by a councillor in a social services meeting in 1983 and officials were asked to investigate this proposal. Nothing further transpired.

The large number of Homes available did present another problem, for doctors that of having one or two patients in a number of different Homes, and for the proprietors having a number of different practices and doctors visiting, often with differing views on the management of insomnia and sedation and on the control of incontinence.

The use or abuse of sedatives including the newer psychotropic drugs as a means of patient management, the so-called "liquid cosh", was not infrequent. Doctors visiting and prescribing were dependent on the not always honest reports of the nurse in charge when deciding on prescribing, and there was suspicion that drugs were not always used for the patients for whom they were prescribed. Talk of the use of the liquid cosh in Homes is still taking place now.

The 1980's saw a boom in Homes as more and more patients were discharged from long-term care in geriatric and psychiatric hospitals, and also because the length of stay of acute patients, both medical and surgical, became shorter and shorter and in the absence of a relative to support them required a period of recovery before returning home. Unfortunately the support services available in hospital such as physiotherapy and speech therapy were not available in the community and especially in the private homes thus delaying recovery. Anxiety about standards resulted in the suggestion by Professor Tom Arie of Nottingham in 1984 that the Health Advisory Service should monitor nursing homes but again nothing happened.

There was considerable anxiety amongst GPs about the standards of care which some residents were receiving and the North Wales Medical Committee in 1999 set up a Nursing Homes Subgroup meeting with the officers of the Health Authority responsible for Registration and Standards to discuss the quality of care in nursing homes with particular reference to staff training and medical cover. The work came to an end when the Health Authority was fragmented into six Local Health Boards and the N.W. Wales Medical Committee ceased to exist.

Another cause for concern for doctors was that whereas district or community nurses could go into residential homes as required and on request they were not allowed to go into Nursing Homes. Very often one felt that the district nurse had special skills not available in the Home from which the patient could benefit but from which they were barred.

As registration procedures and supervision became tighter new guidelines and requirements were introduced, in themselves increasing workload on GPs. And all this for the same capitation fee as for an elderly patient of the same age spending his life on the golf course. All residents in a private home are entitled to NHS treatment and to be accepted on to a GPs list and such a patient may not be charged a fee even if the service provided is in addition to those normally provided. Efforts were made over a number of years and at various levels to have the care of patients in homes recognised as above average demand and remunerated appropriately. Demands were often for the convenience of the Home management. This led some GPs to request a retainer fee from the owners of the Homes but this was not without its legal risks of a suspicion of impropriety or illegality. In 1986 GMSC sought legal guidance and thought it necessary to issued a Memorandum of Guidance on the provision of GP services to registered nursing homes and on any financial arrangements with the homes. Certainly in our area to my knowledge no GPs were receiving retainer fees.

As additional demands on the doctor increased efforts to obtain additional remuneration within the payment schedule continued unsuccessfully over the years. Within the last ten years Bro Taf LMC in South Wales were successful in persuading their Health Authority to agree an additional fee for patients in nursing homes but in spite of continual efforts North Wales Health Authority refused to follow suit.

Until 1990 the financing of care of patients in nursing homes, if not funded by themselves, was the responsibility of the Department of Social Security whereas the provision of the care either at home or in registered homes was the responsibility of the local Social Services. The NHS and Community Care Act transferred financial responsibility and funding to Local Authorities which meant that they were now able to develop individual care plans, either within Homes or alternatively provide greater services to patients in their own homes. It led at last to the development of a joint Health Authority / Local Authority inspection and registration arrangement for all homes which hopefully may achieve a better system of residential care

However the Act and the more rigorous regulations appertaining to improved standards in Homes has given rise to other problems. With the great increase in the number of nursing homes and bed numbers in recent years some of the smaller privately run homes were running into difficulties arising from bed vacancies, particularly if they fell out of favour with the placing social services. Previously the patient or relatives would be guided by their GP as to a home which would suit them, and finance if required would then be sought from Social Security. One or two empty beds in a small home of say ten beds could be catastrophic whereas vacancies in larger homes tend to even out over a period. This on top of much more stringent requirements in the way of staffing levels and training requirements, fire precautions, and the requirement for single-occupancy rooms meant that many smaller Homes have closed. The knock-on effect is that it is not always easy to quickly place a patient ready for discharge into a suitable Home close to their locality and can result in hospital bed-blocking. The wheel has turned full circle since the time in the 1970`s when Dr June Arnold and myself were writing articles in the Geriatric Journals about "bed-blockers", which came almost to be a derogatory term. Obviously with the over 75s population going up by about 15% in a year and the over nineties by a staggering 30% the problems will not go away.

The sort of problems which can arise from staff working part-time in homes and not always being fully briefed on patients is illustrated by an occurrence which happened in our practice some years ago. An elderly resident who was terminally ill and expected to die shortly had been seen by a partner during the day but died in the early hours. The night staff rang the partner on duty to say she had died, he confirmed with the staff member that this was not unexpected and that she had been seen by his partner the previous day and so gave permission for her to be moved to a Chapel of Rest. (Homes always liked patients to be moved during darkness hours and without disturbing other residents). Unfortunately he was not told that she had had an operation within the last thirty days and therefore the permission of the coroner was required before she could be moved. In due course an inquest was held. The coroner was not at all pleased that she had been moved, insisted that the partners attended the inquest and said so in no uncertain terms. Had he, or rather the coroner's officer, been rung there would have been no problem. The press had a field day.

Similar instances of poor communication and of differing levels of seriousness occurred not infrequently. Of course not all such problems arise in the community, the hospital service has similar problems over recording and communication. Many of the problems are associated with understaffing, working under pressure and inadequate training or updating.

More recently the severity of incapacity of the patients being transferred out of hospital has increased and it is not at all usual to have patients requiring intragastric Peg feeding and similar complex nursing requirements arriving at the Home, not infrequently without any previous consultation with the practice. We did some years ago have a patient in one Home who remained in a coma for at least three years, but at least she was quiet and no trouble. Nursing standards have had to be improved.

Health Authorities have a continuing responsibility for patients requiring continuing NHS in-patient care with on-going specialist clinical supervision but have since the 1977 NHS Act been able when appropriate to arrange for this provision in an independent sector nursing home. They are required to provide for the full cost of this and to continue to be responsible for on-going specialist clinical supervision. In such circumstances the GP should have no clinical responsibility for the patient unless a contract and specific arrangements for supporting the specialist have been made. This requirement did not seem to occur. It was often impossible for the GP to be certain under what funding arrangements patients were in the homes and to be clear of their responsibilities. Yet another source of frustration to them.

The new 2004 Contract is now providing the opportunity for negotiated payments recognising the additional time and expertise required for the care of these residents, but the journey has been long and hard since our report in 1985.

The Promotion of Health

The 1946 Act setting up the National Health Service in 1948 was based on the Beveridge reports written for the National Government during the later stages of the war and setting out a vision for the post-war period. It was introduced by Mr Aneurin Bevan, the Minister for Health in the Labour government with the stated objective of providing a comprehensive health service for all, delivered free at the time of use. It was also envisaged that the cost of the service would decrease as the health of the nation improved.

Whether these lofty aims have been achieved remains debatable. Certainly the cost has escalated beyond wildest dreams and while many of the traditional diseases like tuberculosis have been largely eradicated many would argue that the fitness levels of the population today with an epidemic of obesity and alcohol abuse compares poorly with that of war-time Britain. Without doubt the gap between the health levels of the upper classes and the poor appears to have widened over recent years. The Black Report and the Acheson Report emphasised the links between poverty and social conditions and health and that improvements may arise more from tackling the problems of social deprivation rather than concentrating on health services. I became personally aware of this when moving in 1967 from the Ruabon practice in a relatively poor area to the more affluent retirement area of Penrhyn Bay, Llandudno.

The National Health Service has frequently been referred to, and with some justification, as the National Illness Service because most of the efforts have been directed at the treatment of sickness rather than directed towards the prevention of disease. Nevertheless considerable amounts of effort have been put into health education and the promotion of health over the years, by individuals, by organisations and by government and it is appropriate that these be reviewed.

In the earlier years up to the 1974 reorganisation the Medical Officer of Health of the county, the district or the town, was a pivotal figure and had considerable standing in the community. As well as the environmental issues of water and sewage he had responsibility for providing clinics for infant welfare and maternity, and he employed the district nurses, the midwives and the health visitors who had major contributions to be made in the field of preventative medicine and health promotion. He had an oversight of the local cottage hospitals and was supported only by a number of often part-time clinic doctors.

Following the 1974 reorganisation bringing health services under one authority for the first time they were renamed community physicians. As the number of infant welfare, family planning, and cervical cytology clinics were drastically reduced in number as the work was taken over by general practitioners and as they had become largely advisory to the Health Authorities their numbers and influence declined for a while. When increasing emphasis started to be placed centrally on developing preventative strategies their role became more influential again.

GPs have always played a very significant if low-key and understated part in advising and educating in the ways of healthy living during the course of routine consultations, often helped by their knowledge of the patient's family history. Many surveys have indicated that patients respond better to this personal opportunistic intervention than to programmes devised by others. It has also been a very cost effective means of communication. The increasing contacts of patients with the practice nurse both for on-going treatment of chronic illness such as hypertension and diabetes and for preventative measures such as immunisations and cervical smears gave her ideal opportunities to discuss ways to improve health.

District nurses have had a limited role in this area which was primarily the function of health visitors. It is an open secret that my personal opinion of the working of health visitors in general, and there are some exceptions, is not favourable. There are a number of reasons why I believe they have been far less effective than they might have been, certainly in relatively affluent areas. One is that they, or their managers, resisted for years attempts to get them practice based rather than working a patch covering a number of practices and based at a clinic. They therefore did not have regular contact with other members of the team allowing them to pick up problems or potential problems opportunistically. Where they have been practice-based and running their own clinics in the surgery it has not been unusual for them to be withdrawn without consultation or notice and not replaced for months at a time. There has been difficulty for the LMC over the years in getting from management exactly what their job description covered. The perception of their role certainly varies amongst health visitors themselves. Some see their role solely with babies and the pre-school child whereas others see a wider role amongst the socially deprived and the elderly.

School nurses originally were the "nits" nurses but now have an important educational and pastoral role for a very vulnerable group of children facing considerable conflicts and anxieties and are probably an underdeveloped and under-utilised resource.

As early as 1981 WGMSC set up a working party under the chairmanship of Dr Hubert Jones and prepared a Report on Health Education At around the same time in 1983 the RCGP in Wales produced its document " Stitches in time" and the Welsh Office launched its campaign to reduce the incidence of heart disease, Heartbeat Wales.

Various reports from Welsh Office including A Good Old age (1985) and the report Nursing in the Community (the Edwards Report 1988) have highlighted areas for the improvement of health while the 1987 White Paper was entitled Promoting Better Health.

Welsh Office have from time to time developed major strategies for improving the health of the nation, which it acknowledged compared unfavourably with that of many other European countries. In1993 the Welsh Health Planning Forum which had been established in 1988 with only one GP amongst its 24 members, one not known amongst the medical establishment, published a series of Protocols for Investment in Health Gain with the slogan "the NHS in Wales aims to add years to life and life to years" and its aim as "working with others the NHS aims to take the people of Wales into the 21st century with a level of health on course to compare with the best in Europe". These protocols covered wide areas from Cardiovascular Disease, Cancers and Respiratory Disease through to Maternal and Early Child Health, Physical Disability and Discomfort, Mental Health Problems and on to Healthy Living and they set a large number of Health Gain targets in percentage terms and a series of general targets for the health service. To my knowledge no coordinated statistics has been produced to demonstrate that this lofty aim is being achieved, and some especially in the field of alcohol and misuse of drugs in young people have failed miserably. Binge drinking has now become a fashion. Reduction in the number of teenage pregnancies is another area where expensive programmes appear not to be having any impact and the reasons for this are complex and perhaps more related to social factors rather than to health. Obesity in children and in adults is approaching an epidemic with the subsequent alarming increase in diseases such as diabetes. From a time before the NHS when families had too little food we have moved to a time when there they consume too much. In other areas there have been some considerable improvements such as smoking, except in younger people, and in breast cancer through Breast Test Wales. Recent legislation resulting in the banning of smoking in public places will continue this trend.

Health Promotion is however not the sole prerogative of the medical and nursing professions. Much more needs to be done within the schools setting and in local communities. Over the years various voluntary or private organisations have been set up and have contributed considerably to the health education and promotion scene, with many of them such as weight watchers having a social and competitive component adding to their effectiveness. The demographic explosion in the elderly population means that a major effort will need to be made to ensure that they enter old age in a healthy state and that they take steps to maintain their activity and fitness to allow them to live independently.

In 2001 as part of Putting Patients First NHS Wales introduced Health Improvement Programmes (H.I.P.s) to institute broader strategic planning for the health improvement agenda. Each Health Authority was required to take the lead in improving health and health services in co-operation with local partners, the local health groups, local authorities, NHS Trusts, community health councils, the voluntary and independent sector, and the public. Principles of social inclusion and equality of opportunity, recognition of the needs of all social groups particularly the young, older people, ethnic minorities and disabled people were to be fundamental to the programmes.

In other words "the HIP is about a collaborative and inclusive planning process involving all stakeholders". It is interesting to note that once again there was no direct representation of doctors and other health workers at the coalface, and as far as I am aware there has been no sharing of a completed HIP with the LMC, the Royal College or other groups.

Social marketing is a concept being introduced into health promotion on a population level, using commercial strategies to influence consumers. It was defined by Andreasen in Marketing Social Change in San Francisco CA 1995 "as the application of proven concepts and techniques drawn from the commercial sector to promote changes in diverse socially important behaviours such as drug use, smoking, and sexual behaviour". It uses a wide range of mass-media communication strategies. It is effective but doctors need to continue to reinforce the messages during direct and indirect contacts with patients.

To return to the contribution of GPs and the primary health care team. The 1990 contract amended the terms of service to make clear that health promotion and illness prevention fell within the definition of general medical services, and in fact laid down the areas expected to be undertaken and the ways in which this should be done. As discussed elsewhere, to qualify for a new Postgraduate Allowance a GP's continuing education had to be undertaken by attending courses in three defined areas, one of which was health promotion. The contract encouraged GPs to hold "health promotion clinics" with a minimum of five patients at their surgeries, an obligation carried out in the spirit rather than in the requirement in many practices.

The 1990 contract also required GPs to offer a visit annually to all patients over 75, although this could be delegated to a nurse from the practice. The intention was to ensure that the elderly were at least seen and reviewed annually and appropriate advice and action taken. This requirement may have been sensible in some deprived areas but was certainly a distraction from more effective work in most of North Wales.

GPs and the practice team have probably over the years been the most effective and acceptable medium of health promotion through opportunistic advice given during routine consultations with doctors and with practice nurses. They were not at all happy with the bureaucratic way in which it was suggested they work and as always were resourceful in undertaking requirements in ways that best suited their individual practices. Posters and leaflets are probably more effective in a surgery setting as there is someone available to give further information and encouragement. The difficulty now is that there are probably too many of them to impact properly.

Opportunistic health advice related to their present state and carried out by all members of the practice team will remain probably the most effective avenue of health promotion.

Wales has always had the high incidence of ill-health and morbidity already described but has been active in trying to rectify this and has a justifiable reputation in the UK and internationally for taking a public health partnership approach through Health Challenge Wales, which called upon the government, professional organisations and other bodies to create the conditions necessary for healthy living, and Designed for Life, which outlined the vision for health and social services in 2015. The recently appointed Chief Medical Officer, Dr Tony Jewell, is an ex-GP with ten years at the coalface in East London and has set this as a priority for everyone. In so doing he is continuing the excellent work done by his predecessors, Dr Gareth Crompton, Dr Deirdre Hine and most recently by Dr Ruth Hall.

The changing face of infections

By the time I started medical school the scourge of tuberculosis had been brought largely under control but with isolated pockets still to be found, particularly in poorer areas and in the ethnic population. The sanatoria had been very considerably reduced in size and their treatment regimes had become more tolerable to patients. This followed the introduction of newer effective drugs, originally streptomycin which caused deafness as a side-effect and later Isoniazid and PAS in huge one-inch diameter cachets which had to be swallowed intact. Thankfully other drugs followed. Control was enhanced by the successful development of the routine testing and immunisation programme. The testing and subsequent vaccination was made easier by the development of the Heaf gun by Professor Heaf who was one of my teachers at Cardiff. Small pox had been virtually eliminated following routine vaccination and in 1996 the World Health Organisation officially declared it eradicated from the world and ordered all stocks of vaccine to be destroyed.

Diphtheria was another killer disease which had virtually disappeared by the fifties as a result of childhood vaccination and is a condition I have never seen although it was necessary always to bear it in mind in the early years. Tetanus is now rarely seen following routine vaccination with boosters at the time of injury. Before that we had to give anti-tetanus serum produced from horses` blood at the time of injury, and which sometimes gave rise to reactions.

Diagnoses of possible whooping cough, measles and polio still struck fear into many parents at that time. Whooping cough was still around but not such a problem as it had been. In an immunised child it was much less debilitating but still very distressing to watch and nurse. Measles was common and at times a very worrying disease with severe complications and at times death, particularly in debilitated children. All became less troublesome as children generally became healthier.

Less serious infections such as bronchitis and tonsillitis were being dealt with by the new antibiotics which were starting to become available. Penicillin was only starting to come into general use in the late forties and the fifties, and the old M&B sulphonamide drugs were still in use.

Poliomyelitis was still a major cause of death and of serious disability and while working at Wrexham Maelor Hospital in 1955 there were a number of patients to be cared for in the so-called "iron lungs", the huge early respirators not unlike coffins. With the introduction of the Salk and then the Sabin vaccine in the fifties, the former by injection but the later Sabin vaccine given orally, an intensive vaccination programme carried out by GPs and in infant welfare clinics proved very effective. Ensuring that all children were immunised required considerable effort, involving both GPs and health visitors often working independently, and recording systems were less sophisticated then. As with later injections such as the MMR vaccine, they were at times subject to media scares and controversy.

With the increase over the next decades in foreign holidays and travel to exotic parts of the world tropical diseases such as malaria and other parasites started to appear in practices where they had never been previously considered. Now missing malaria is likely to be considered negligent.

Sexually transmitted diseases have made a comeback, gonorrhoea and syphilis had largely disappeared but are making a come-back with the addition of thrush following increased use of antibiotics and of clamydia which was previously not recognised. The fact that these are often asymptomatic make transmission to others more likely. 1980 saw the arrival of a potentially catastrophic new infection into North Wales, the HIV/AIDS virus with two possible modes of transmission, by sexual contact and by the sharing of equipment by drug misusers. While the misuse of drugs of addiction had not been a previously been a major problem in North Wales some communities including Llandudno were seeing a significant increase. Much of this was coming in from England. and the issues are discussed in more detail in another section.

Most recently on the scene, and one which causes the most worry to patients going into hospital is the development of MRSA., the staphylococcal infection which has become resistant to antibiotics and where death rates from this infection are officially reported as having increased thirty-fold in the last decade. Similar problems are arising with the Clostridium difficile organism, the spread of both being associated with inadequate cleansing and hygiene procedures in hospitals. Efforts to eradicate the organisms are proving difficult.

The Pharmaceutical Industry

The Pharmaceutical industry over the years has had an immense influence for good and for bad on medical care. Most members of the public and probably most medical managers would if asked feel that the pharmaceutical companies were potential "baddies " in their contacts with general practitioners and the techniques used to advertise and promote their wares. They would not be aware of the many ways in which the industry and individual companies have encouraged and promoted good practice in practices and the record perhaps needs to be put straight. While obviously their aim, as in any industry, is to promote the use of their products the ways by which this has been done has often been constructive and laudable.

The public would be aware through media coverage only of promotional trips abroad particularly in the Seventies at the expense of drug firms or of free lunches and dinners for GPs and sometimes their wives, although it must be said that most business men and managers would have recognised this as being normal practice.

Undoubtedly there were occasions when hospitality was excessive and where the sales pitch was hard but this certainly in North Wales was not the norm. Perhaps the representatives recognised their audience. Doctors normally can afford to pay for their own meals or trips, and their off duty time is limited, and so most attend for other reasons. Promotional meals were often the only times when local GPs met socially and developed relationships, and at the same time became aware of developments in treatments and therapies and able to discuss these amongst themselves. Many reps admit to finding the going much tougher promoting a product to a group than to a single doctor in the surgery.

The postgraduate centres at the DGHs have over the years benefited immensely from support from the pharmaceutical industry and indeed would not have succeeded without their contribution.

Many of the medical reps in North Wales have been around for many years, although not always with the same company, and have become well known and respected and their information on their products appreciated. Reps like Charles Williams, Ian McAlpine, Kelvin Thomas, Bill Williams, Sue Griffiths, Sue Jones, Alan Jones, Joan Knight, and Anwen Jones become friends without in any way unduly influencing the use of their products. One famous character from the past was Jimmy Gibb who would breeze in with his long overcoat with poachers` pockets from which he would produce a variety of goodies. Very often the actual product did not feature large in the discussion, but what was said was listened to and they also become involved in many other ways. Their companies through them are frequently on hand to provide sponsorship for meetings run by GPs but also for organisations such as the RCGP and at times even for Health Authorities.

Following on various criticisms in the past they operate to a strict code of protocols at sponsored meetings which does include separating their input, usually limited to a stand outside the lecture hall and which people can visit if they wish, from the actual clinical part of the meeting. Providing refreshments on site is very helpful for doctors coming straight from work and who if they had to go home first might decide not to attend. Organisers of GP meetings, unlike many other organisations, do not have a fund from which costs can be met. The A.B.P.I., the Association of British Pharmaceutical Industries, has for many years been very anxious that the drug industry acted ethically in its advertising and in its dealings with doctors and detailed guidelines have been developed and regularly updated as appropriate. The fact that its Medical Directors, Dr Frank Wells and afterwards Dr Richard Tiner, were both former GPs who had practical experience of the issues and potential problems as well as both having been members of the GMSC with an understanding of the medico-political implications made for good relationships and communication with general practice.

While some reps. have been around for years many others come and go, often only seen once. They are usually the bright young things who come in with a set pattern of words spun out at great speed and if one interrupts them they sometimes have to start again at the beginning. They have no understanding of how doctors and practices work and usually they do not last long.

Medical reps also act as informal transmitters of local news between practices, hatches, matches, dispatches, movements and retirements as well as who is available for locums and as potential replacement partners.

Access to the doctor meant first getting past the so-called "dragon at the gate" caricatured in the media, the receptionist who was often bought off with pens, sticky pads, diaries and notepads, all things which the doctors neglected to supply them with. In the early days of appointment systems in practices one of the companies produced all the necessary appointment sheets and cards together with guidance on their use. As always it is much easier to introduce changes if someone else does the thinking and organisation for you.

The input of pharmaceutical companies into GP education and practice management has been very much wider than this. In the sixties and seventies there was little easily digested up-to-date material on medical subjects available to busy GPs, the sort of thing one could read over breakfast. Two weekly newspaper format publications appeared, Pulse and General Practitioner, followed later by Doctor. They are still produced and required reading by many doctors. In addition to printing medical and medico-political news and views they also provided a forum for advertising for locums and for practice vacancies As they developed they started to produce supplements on specialised subjects bringing up-to-date information in a collated form and written for a GP audience.

A very successful early educational initiative was the production of audio-cassettes, at a time when these were comparatively new, containing three or four short items on specific diseases or medical issues and which could be listened to at home or while driving in the car. Sometimes the cassette would concentrate on one topic in depth. Patients have often wondered why the doctor continued to sit in his car outside their house, he was waiting for the topic to finish.

The advance of medicine is so fast that most textbooks are out of date before being published and the learned journals such as the BMJ and The Lancet did not often produce material in this easily read form. Some reps would produce reprints of articles from the Journals on the topic under discussion although one had to be aware that the articles had been carefully selected to support their product. Representatives often brought newly published medical books with no mention of any drug firm near them for the practice library, a very useful service for us in North Wales where there were no medical bookshops to browse in.

At one time I used to write a regular column in GP (or it may have been Pulse or both) about issues in Wales. A photographer arrived to take a series of photographs of me in various locations within the practice area and these would appear alongside the articles. They were all of course taken on the same day, leading in due course to comments by colleagues that it was time I bought a new suit.

Another very important publication for some years was Update, each issue having a series of well written and easily read informative in-depth articles on current thinking and treatment. Over and above the newspapers new journals started to appear such as Modern Geriatrics which dealt with topics geared to GPs and were paid for by advertising.

Travelling Scholarships in this country and abroad were given by companies such as Upjohn and as described I was fortunate to be awarded one of these to study the newly developing concept of Geriatric Day Hospitals in the UK.

Another company, Syntex, for years sponsored awards for each Vocational Trainee Scheme in Wales for the best work produced by a Trainee in the Scheme during the year and contributed to the early stages of introduction to project work and practice audits. I am glad to say that trainees from our practice were frequently successful. In North Clwyd we always managed to link the presentations with a good social bonding evening.

Reps on their visits used to leave samples, both of the new drug they were promoting and also other drugs which the company produced. While effective as an advertising ploy these samples were invaluable in the surgery or in the visits bag to start treatment immediately when no pharmacy was open in evenings and weekends. One does have to wonder exactly what state the drugs carried by doctors were in when they had been in the visits bag in the car boot for some months, in the heat of the summer and then in the cold of the winter. Such considerations did not seem as relevant then as they might be today.

At times a rep might leave an item of equipment, new on the market, and some would also take responsibility for servicing and calibrating blood pressure machines and similar instruments, again a service not otherwise easily available in North Wales.

One of the oldest promotional aids produced by a drug firm was the Appointments Diaries for visits by Burroughs Wellcome. I have in my possession one dating back to 1912, although I hasten to add not used by me personally, the format virtually identical but the clinical information obviously very different. The diaries carried considerable valuable reference information pages and while the content has changed over the years they are still made available today. Looking back on my old ones reminds me of the extent of home visiting done in the Sixties and particularly of the frequent repeat visits to the same patients to check on progress, a habit which seems to have largely disappeared now with the increased use of telephone contacts and an increasing expectation that the therapy will work.

One publication which had a major impact was the monthly issue of MIMS which was sent free to all GPs and which listed all available drugs, whether available on the NHS or not, their format and strengths, all listed under categories and including their price. This was for many years the most frequently used prescribing bible in practices, frequently referred to by reception staff and copies were much sought after by district nurses.

When it became a requirement for drug companies to issue Data Sheets for each drug listing all relevant information and side-effects these were conveniently made available in a Compendium. The official BNF, the British National Formulary, which had been in existence for decades was far less comprehensive and outdated. The other official publication, the Drug Tariff, at that time in its old loose leaf form with amendments which never seemed to get filed correctly, was far too difficult to use and less informative. By the nineties however the new format BNF, updated six-monthly, was produced with clinical treatment information as well under each drug grouping and rapidly became the reference of choice.

As the concept that patients needed to know more about their illnesses and treatments gained ground information leaflets for patients were often produced by the pharmaceutical companies long before hospital departments started to appreciate the need for these.

In all these ways the Industry contributed greatly to easily accessible postgraduate education for busy GPs and deserves considerably more praise than it receives.

Prescribing and dispensing

Prescribing for doctors` registered patients, the cost and the frequency and the availability of drugs, has been a major issue since the start of the NHS and has received more and more prominence and pressure as drugs have become more complex and expensive. GPs have been constantly badgered to reduce their treatment costs even though much of the prescribed treatment may be initiated by others from within the hospital service.

Wales for reasons which have been debated at length over many years has always had a much higher per capita prescribing cost than England, for many years by half as much again. Many other indices such as unemployment, long term illness and low incomes have also been traditionally much higher in Wales than in the UK. There is no doubt the two issues are interrelated as has been demonstrated by work and reports on deprived areas although it has been difficult to quantify the relationship, one suspects at times because of the political implications.

In 1973, a typical year, the Welsh national cost average was 690p per patient on doctors lists whereas in England it was 512p. The highest cost was in Merthyr Tydfil at 855p while the highest in England was Bournemouth, with its high elderly population. WGMSC set up a working group to identify the issues and possible savings, but the overall situation remains the same today as it was then.

Investigations have shown that the cost of individual items is close to the UK average but that it is the number and frequency of items which is high in Wales.

For many years the two areas of Wales with the highest prescription costs were always Caernarfonshire and Merthyr Tydfil, alternating from quarter to quarter. They were invariably at the top of the list for the whole of England and Wales, both areas were similar in having heavy industry in coal and slate and the consequent high morbidity rates. When in 1974 Caernarfonshire was merged into Gwynedd and Merthyr Tydfil disappeared as an administrative entity Gwynedd moved to the top of the UK list, and stayed there. Since I was working in Caernarfonshire and then Gwynedd the topic was always to the fore in discussions in the Health Authority.

As a result a study was carried out in 1970 comparing prescribing in Caernarfonshire with Cardiganshire, attempting to correct for all relevant factors such as age, gender, number of temporary visitors. At the end of the study the only conclusion which emerged was that doctors in Caernarfonshire prescribed more Amoxil (a new antibiotic at the time) and more Lasix (the new and powerful diuretic) than their counterparts. Perhaps one reason for this was the influence of the local drug-firm representatives. On the other hand it might also indicate a more up-to-date and effective provision of care by local GPs.

Many of the newer more expensive and also long-term use drugs are originally initiated by hospital consultants who can have a considerable influence on GP prescribing. There was always the feeling that drug firms supplied new drugs to hospitals initially as loss leaders knowing that these drugs would later become transferred to the general practice budget. Hospitals varied widely as to whether they supplied drugs to outpatients and this was a source of considerable discussion over many years. There have never been any published statistics of the combined hospital and practice prescribing budgets in areas and this might have thrown up interesting results.

Traditionally before the NHS all family doctors dispensed drugs from the practice dispensary, usually employing a dispenser who had no formal qualifications. Its content was very limited and very often the requirement was to remember which colour medicines the patient had had before and which were their favourites. The "bottle", which in early days was carefully wrapped in white paper and sealed with wax, was very important and satisfied the expectations if not the medical needs of patients. One elderly lady was found on her death to have a complete chest full of unwrapped bottles going back several years. Obviously she did not feel she needed the medicine but it was part of the ritual of her need for regular visits and reassurance by her doctor.

With the advent of the Health Service and of independent pharmacies on the High Street doctors in all except some rural areas lost the right to dispense. The whole subject of the right to dispense, of what is considered as "rurality", and of the right of doctors to use unqualified assistants to dispense while pharmacies always have to have a qualified pharmacist on the premises when a dispensed prescription is given out has given rise to continual conflict ever since between the representatives of the two professions nationally and locally. Indeed it could be the subject of a treatise by itself. The Clothier Report in 1978 went into the problems of doctor dispensing at some length and laid down guidance but disputes still arise. It is a complex area which I never ventured too deeply into even during my time as WGMSC chairman, leaving it to those actively involved in dispensing in their practices.

Doctor/pharmacy issues have been prominent for many years and figured largely in LMC conferences and in the various freebee newspapers with considerable criticism of the efforts of GMSC in this field, led very vociferously by Dr David Roberts who was a thorn in their flesh for some years. He founded the Dispensing Doctors Association as a pressure group and after a number of attempts eventually managed to get elected to the GMSC. Later the DDA was have felt to worked too closely with GMSC and the pharmacists and in

1998 he was involved in the setting up of another group, the Country Doctors Association.

Obviously dispensing at the surgery provides a service appreciated by patients who can pick up their medicines on site rather than make a visit to a pharmacy which may be some considerable distance away and may not be open at the same time as the surgery. The practice benefits from the additional income which arises and this may be instrumental in allowing an additional partner to be employed. In isolated single handed or two doctor practices the ability to have an additional doctor would make a very significant difference to the on call commitment.

Doctors were only allowed to prescribe in areas defined as having "rurality" and only for patients living more than a mile from the nearest chemist and from the main surgery. This definition of rurality itself gave rise to considerable arguments over the years, especially when large building developments took place in previously rural areas, and usually had to be resolved by tribunals followed by appeals. The one-mile rule also gave rise to an interesting argument in Clwyd where a village was divided by a river crossed by a bridge raising the question whether the definition of one-mile from patients home to the chemist was as the crow flies or by road.

Another interesting situation arose in Cerrig-y-drudion where the local practice had always dispensed for its patients. A pharmacist opened a business in the village which meant that many patients had to be taken off the doctors` dispensing list and on to their prescribing list with considerable loss of financial stability to the practice and with considerable concern to patients. The pharmacy proved not to be viable and within a short time closed, requiring the practice to reorganise and start dispensing to all its patients again.

Prescriptions were originally written by hand, allegedly often illegibly, taken to the pharmacy and dispensed. Prescriptions then had to be sorted by hand into separate piles for each of the doctors, in some pharmacies this might be twenty or thirty, and sent on to the Health Authority, who would forward them to the Prescription Pricing Authority (P.P.A) in Cardiff. Here each item was priced manually by a group of young women who achieved fantastic rates of prescriptions per hour. Something like 130,000 per day were processed in the department in 1988. Dr Hugh Cairns, a Cardiff GP and chairman of the PPA and who was a fellow member of WGMSC, arranged for us to visit the PPA on one occasion and we could not believe the speed and also the accuracy achieved by them. Legibility of writing was never a strong point with doctors. With the introduction of computer generated prescriptions and computerisation of their pricing, the process changed but not always for the best. A computer blip one year caused considerable delay in the payments to both doctors and chemists, as well as delays of some months in obtaining up-to-date prescribing figures and costs at a time when drives to reduce these was in progress, one of many attempts to reduce these over the years.

Much time has been spent over many years, and much resentment caused amongst doctors and patients, in attempts to reduce the cost of the drug budget. The LMC together with the FHSA in Gwynedd formulated a guidelines document to try to reduce inappropriate prescribing and this was subsequently adopted on an all-North Wales area basis. Prescribing advisers were appointed by the FHSA. Since the drugs available, the indications for them, the advice coming out from the lo cal hospitals and the unit cost of individual preparations were continually changing it was always difficult to identify the success of the various initiatives. The one certainty was that the total cost of medication continually and inexorably rose.

In earlier years the only information which could be made available to doctors by the administration was a three monthly report giving the total number of items prescribed and the average cost per item, both compared with the county average. At this level there were too many variables to make comparison of any use. Figures were produced on an individual doctor rather than a practice basis but since prescriptions and particularly repeat prescriptions were frequently written on others partner's prescription pads this diminished their usefulness.

The Welsh Office employed Regional Medical Officers (RMOs) to visit doctors to discuss their figures and any other matters of concern such as the level of prescriptions for drugs of addiction. The RMO service played a useful role and was operated very sensibly in Wales, initially by Dr John Parry and later Dr Graham Moses, both respected ex-GPs. North Wales was the responsibility for a number of years of Dr Nigel Thomas, who was a partner in the Colwyn Bay practice with whom I worked a rota until he left to join Welsh Office and to attend to his family business.

PACT data (Prescribing Activity and Cost Trends) was introduced for individual doctors in 1989 to allow them to monitor their costs but again since in many practices the doctors shared the care of patients and the writing of repeat prescriptions the data was only of use to the practice as a whole rather than to individuals. Delay of some months in receiving the data also meant it was of limited practical value as ideas and practice might have changed in the interim.

As the ability to treat more medical conditions increased, with more care being transferred from hospital clinics to general practice, and with many patients with several diseases, related or quite separate, on long-term medication the number of drugs prescribed each month increased. Doctors were requested not to write more than five items on a single form to improve legibility.

Repeat prescribing without seeing the patient each time became a necessity as well as practically sensible for those on regular medication. The workload was still considerable for doctors and their staff but the introduction of computerisation made monitoring and subsequent audit of prescribing easier. Unfortunately it was sometimes too easy to authorise more repeats without adequate review.

On taking over a new practice in the early days I found it was the usual practice to leave repeat prescriptions on a windowsill in the hall for patients or their relatives to root through and take the right one. Not an acceptable practice both from safety and for patient confidentiality, but perhaps previously necessary in practices where no receptionist was present at all times during the day.

Various and repeated attempts have been made over the years to deal with the burden of the repeat prescribing problem. The idea of prescription forms with two carbons to allow three months supply without review to be issued seemed very sensible as a means of reducing workload and at the same time avoiding giving three months of tablets at one time. It was very nearly accepted nationally on several occasions but finally ran into trouble with pharmacists representatives. It still resurrects as an idea from time to time.

In 1988 researchers at Exeter developed a Smart-card repeat prescription facility which seemed promising. At about the same time a trial of a similar card involving a pharmacy in Pontypridd and the pricing authority in Cardiff and which held much prescribing information and could be used as a swipe-card seemed very promising but like many innovations foundered on cost implications. The cost was calculated as about £5 per patient which if introduced across Wales would have been very high but the potential savings must have been considerably higher. Another idea ahead of its time and one which is sure to re-emerge.

In 1984 the Government introduced the Limited List of Drugs, not a list of those available for prescribing but rather those which were black-listed. The profession foresaw the problems and favoured a White List of prescribable preparations but as usual were not listened to. The problem with any blacklist is that if something is not on it then it is permissible. As a consequence additions and amendments had to be continually added. Items such as Fishermen's Friend lozenges, possibly by doctors trying to make a point, appeared on some prescriptions and had to be specifically excluded, and this could only be done by parliamentary legislation.

Some drugs which were also considered to be foods were classified as Borderline Substances and could only be prescribed for certain conditions and if the prescription form was endorsed ACBS (According to the Committee for Borderline Substances). Periodic checks were made to ensure GPs were not abusing the system.

At about this time there was a great increase in so-called generic non-proprietary drugs, drugs on which the patents had expired allowing other manufacturers to produce and sell them at a considerable cheaper price. These drugs could be manufactured anywhere, often with no quality supervision, and many were imported. Some were frankly of very poor manufacture and often disintegrated. There was considerable political pressure on doctors to prescribe "generically" and this has continued.

For patients the names were different, often more complex and not so easily remembered, the colour and appearance might be different and might vary each month depending on where the pharmacy had purchased them or if the prescription was dispensed at a different pharmacy. Confidence in them was low because they were considered a cheap option and patients felt they did not work as well as their original tablets. At times they would ring up to say they had received the incorrect tablets, and without seeing them it was impossible to say whether they had had a different generic or whether as sometimes happens a genuine error had been made at the pharmacy and they had actually received an incorrect drug. Later when most prescriptions were produced by computer the programme routinely printed a generic form unless over-ridden. To add to the confusion the generic names have had to be changed recently to confirm to the European nomenclature.

A scam practice which came to be known as Parallel Importing developed. Drugs were bought wholesale in Britain for export at a lower price, were shipped abroad and then re-imported to the UK and resold here. Doctors representatives expressed considerable anxiety about the adequacy and quality of the storage arrangements while the drugs were travelling around the continent.

In time the problems were acknowledged. Under the Consumer Protection Act of 1987 manufacturers were responsible for any harm or injury arising from defects in their products and this applied equally to prescription drugs. To fight a claim, possibly years later, the source of the product and the manufacturer had to be identifiable. Dispensing doctors, and to a lesser extent non-dispensing doctors using vaccines and other injections amongst other products, were therefore obliged to keep detailed records including batch numbers of all drugs which they handled. If any medicine was made up or even diluted by the doctor then they could be considered to be a manufacturer and therefore be liable in law.

1989 saw the introduction of "original pack" pre-packaged tablets which avoided the need for tablet handling and counting and made the dispensing process for monthly repeats much easier. At least it would have done if all manufacturers used the same definition of a month. Some produced 28 day packs and some 30 day packs, causing considerable difficulty if a patient was receiving drugs in both package sizes. After several difficult years twenty-eight days was agreed as the standard, theoretically avoiding patients completing packs on a weekend.

It had always been the advice that no more than a months supply should be issued at a time and most doctors stuck to this, at least until patients were well stabilised on a drug. Often the cost of the drug was less than the patient had to pay as a prescription charge but the doctor could not write a private prescription for them The one month rule did cause increasing problems in recent years as more and more patients spent extended periods abroad in the winter months. The official advice originally was that these patients were then outside the NHS supervision and that they should only be issued with a month's supply and should buy any further supplies abroad, ignoring the fact that identical products were often not available locally. Some of these patients in any case commuted backwards and forwards between home and abroad, and the easiest way was to use commonsense and ignore the advice. Later this was modified to allow medication regularly used to be prescribed. With increasing travel to exotic destinations patients started to request prescriptions to take with them prophylactically in case they were taken ill. These were not allowable under the NHS but GPs were also not allowed under their terms of service to write private prescriptions for patients registered with them. A further difficult problem was with merchant seamen perhaps spending many months or more away and where the responsibility had to be passed to the shipping company.

As the cost of their prescribed drug budget became more and more a pressure area by the Health Authority, and as comparisons were drawn with neighbouring practices doctors looked for ways to justify their high individual costs. One of the major variable factors was the number of elderly patients with high medication requirements cared for by the practice and the number in nursing homes serviced. This was of particular interest to our practice with its exceptionally high over 65 and over 75 year old population. After considerable discussion a system of ASTROPUs (covering age, sex, temporary residents) was agreed nationally and went someway to make comparisons fairer.

The amount of repeat prescriptions requested daily required special arrangements to be introduced into practices. Pressure on telephone lines, and in an attempt to reduce possible mistakes in transcription, meant some practices would only accept requests in writing. Others developed a recorded telephone request line. Many practices required at least 24 hours notice, later increased to 48 hours, for repeat requests.

To reduce the need for patients to pick up their forms from the surgery before taking them to the chemist and then having to wait or return later to collect the drugs many pharmacies started to collect prescriptions daily, or in our case twice daily, in bulk from the surgery in order to have them ready dispensed for collection by patients or their representatives. It did require identification of whether or not the scripts were to be sent and to which pharmacy, and this did at times lead to considerable aggressive behaviour when the system had broken down for some reason and the prescription was at the wrong place.

It has always been the position that patients did not have to register with a named chemist but could take their prescription to any pharmacy. This had some advantages for them in that they could at times perhaps use one closer to their home or to their place of work. It did mean however that no single pharmacy had a complete record of their past medication and the ability to check or query potential errors or interactions. Most patients do use the same pharmacy most of the time and in recent years pharmacists have seen an extended role for themselves and have been keeping their own computerised record of medication dispensed, allowing them to spot potential errors. There is no doubt that developing a good relationship with the local pharmacy pays dividends for the practice. From time to time one has been spared an embarrassing situation by a quick telephone call from our friendly pharmacists. Regrettably continuity of care in the pharmacy as in the surgery is threatened by part-time working and the employment of managers and locums by the large pharmaceutical companies. Very few pharmacies are now privately owned, most having been bought out by the large companies although often still trading under the old name, and the ability to obtain urgent medication out of hours is now rare in most places. Pharmacies in supermarkets with extended opening hours have been a help in this respect. In the past doctors often carried an emergency supply of simple drugs like antibiotics, frequently supplied as samples by drug reps. But awareness and anxiety about the storage conditions in the doctor's bag and car have changed this.

Charges to patients for prescriptions has been a political issue from the early years of the NHS and were first proposed by a labour government in the budget in 1951 at the time of financial austerity and when defence costs were escalating because of the Korean war. Clement Attlee the Prime Minister in1949 justified prescription charges "as a deterrence against extravagance rather than as an economy".

Together with charges for dental and optical treatment they were seen as an attack on the "free at the time of delivery" concept of the NHS and Aneurin Bevan threatened to resign. Initially they were set at one shilling (5p) a prescription and later per item. The new Tory government confirmed that they would be permanent and that further charges would be introduced. Although abolition of the charges was part of the Labour Party manifestos from 1951 onwards this never happened and the charge per item has continued to escalate. Various ploys have been introduced to alleviate hardship over the years, both by exempting certain categories of patients such as the elderly, the disabled and those on low incomes and also by exemption of certain specified medical conditions. These disease related exemptions have been criticised regularly over the years as being completely illogical. Patients suffering from heart disease or from cancer and on multiple drugs were not exempted but patients requiring long-term medication for thyroid disease, often one tablet a day, were exempt. It has been impossible in spite of repeated efforts by the GP leaders and by patient groups to force a change in the nominated diseases. It is officially recognised that because of the various exemptions about 87% of all prescriptions are not chargeable. With some patients regularly on say five items they may have to fork out considerable sums each month. Chemists say that some patients ask which are the important items and ask for these only. Those who are required to pay have the option of buying an annual exemption certificate which is good value for some provided they can afford the lump-sum payment. Exemptions have not been reviewed since 1968, at a time when some illnesses such as HIV/Aids had not surfaced. The House of Commons Select Committee in2006 has published its Report suggesting a review of the whole system of charges, something the BMA have been pressing for in the interest of fairness to patients for some years.

Whether the bureaucratic arrangements for signing and for checking exemption claims on each prescription form with so few chargeable are worthwhile is perhaps debatable. Nevertheless it has been estimated that prescription fraud in various ways costs the service some £70 million a year Certainly it has for many years been a bone of contention with doctors in rural dispensing practices who are required to "act as tax-collectors for the government" and collect the fees from patients and submit them to the FPC or FHSA. Ethical problems do arise when a patient says he or she does not have the money to pay, or only enough to pay for some of the items.

The Welsh Assembly following the devolvement of health matters to it has adopted a different approach to England and has been reducing the cost per item by £1 each year with a view to abolition in 2007. Abolition has been controversial, could the money have been better spent elsewhere in the NHS.

The misuse of controlled drugs

One of the problems which has increasingly become a problem in the community, in some much more than in others, is the misuse of drugs by addicts and habitués, the latter sometimes including little old ladies who loved their sleeping tablets. There was some abuse of the amphetamine group as far back as the 1960s, the "purple hearts" being popular. Barbiturate sleeping tablets were frequently overused and addictive. Thalidomide was introduced and widely used as a very effective and safe alternative, until it was implicated in multiple congenital deformities in babies. Mandrax and Modadon followed safe as sedatives, then the "non-addictive" benzodiazepines including valium and its derivatives. Abuse of the benzodiazepines drugs was highlighted at the 1984 LMC Annual Conference, along with glue sniffing, and voluntary restrictions on their prescribing and use were adopted by the profession to try to curb these. At that time drug-barons and the import of drugs from abroad had not developed to the extent it has today and much of the misuse was misusing prescribed medication. Various excuses and ploys were used to obtain them and keeping an easily identified record was not easy in pre-computerised days.

The legal prescribing and the illegal abuse of controlled drugs, the drugs of addiction, has been to the fore over many years and subject to a number of Acts and Regulations. It is an area where attitudes have varied markedly in different times and in different countries and communities. In Victorian times the use of opium or laudanum was widespread and was even given to sedate babies and infants.

Abuse by the traditional drugs of addiction, opium, morphine and heroin was rarely seen in most practices. If it was it was sometimes the doctor who was the abuser. The use has escalated in recent years with cannabis, cocaine and its derivatives becoming encountered frequently. Doctors used to carry traditional bags and had "Doctor on call" stickers in their car windows and were rarely bothered, now there is a considerable risk in some areas of doctors and nurses being mugged for their case, thought to contain drugs and of their cars being vandalised. They no longer carry an identifiable bag. This, together with the very much tighter regulations about storing and accounting for controlled drugs since the Shipman inquiry including keeping the drugs and the register in different places, has made many doctors stop carrying these drugs. It was always a requirement to keep them in a locked container in the car, the locked glove compartment was for some reason not considered adequate by the authorities although in practice it was considerably safer than any other locked container likely to be in the car.

I recall while in Prestatyn losing my medical bag, at least I thought I had lost it. I rang the last house where I had been to see a patient in his bedroom and where I had used the case. The family checked and said it was not there so I concluded it must have been taken from my car in the road outside and reported the loss to the police. They naturally wanted to record how many ampoules and tablets of the range of drugs of all sorts it contained, impossible to answer correctly and guesses had to be made. Luckily some three hours later the family "found the case" at the side of the patient's bed. It would have been very difficult if the police had found it with different numbers of tablets from those I had given them.

Recent years have seen an explosion in the use of these drugs in North Wales, both for so-called recreational and occasional use and for more regular addiction. Closeness to Merseyside with its problems has not helped.

The misuse by mouth or by injection of drugs can be considered to be a life-style issue rather than a health care one and has to be fitted into the local social cultures. Dr David Williams always argued that a distinction in management had to be made between the social problems of drug misusers which were for the community at large to deal with and the medical problems of drug addicts which were the province of the health services.

Control of heroin misuse has been controversial for years with some arguing for non-prescription and others for controlled maintenance therapy with alternatives such as methadone. Different areas of North Wales have adopted conflicting policies over the years. Entrenched attitudes to drug misuse still exist, some communities across North Wales adopting a more liberal and progressive approach than others. Addicts being very devious and resourceful and also very mobile makes it very difficult to control their supply adequately.

Our local pharmacist at Penrhyn Bay, Mr Gron Bennett-Williams began to become involved in 1982 when drug misusers started to turn up at young peoples group activities. He set up a drop in centre at Eryl Wen in Llandudno for individuals who needed and requested help and with a number of lay and some trained volunteers an abstinence programme with support and counselling was put in place.

Substitution or maintenance therapy has been organised in some areas by allowing addicts to receive their daily fix in a liquid form which they were required to drink under the supervision of the pharmacist. Some were found to be holding the liquid in their mouths until they had left the pharmacy and subsequently spitting it out into a container and passing it on. Obviously not all pharmacies wished to have a series of addicts queuing up at their premises alongside their regular clientele and there was no opportunity for more than basic advice and counselling.

A problem developed over the danger to the general public and to refuse-men during collections from discarded needles and for addicts themselves from sharing needles. Headlines from America were highlighting the risks of HIV/ AIDS and its proliferation. The dangers of sharing needles and equipment were emphasised. The first needle exchange scheme (clean equipment in exchange for returned used material) was started from a pharmacy in Sheffield in 1986. Until then the Royal Pharmaceutical Society had imposed restrictions on the sale of syringes and needles to the public.

A Gwynedd Drugs and Alcohol Committee was set up in the Health Authority but the majority of members were initially opposed in principle to any exchange scheme. A pilot scheme was proposed in 1987 but it took two years for agreement to be achieved. The appointment of Dr Hugh Jones as consultant in Infectious Diseases probably tipped the balance.

Mr Bennett-Williams was appointed as a member of the new Gwynedd FHSA when it was formed in 1989 and with the support of its chairman, Dr Arthur Kenrick, an embryonic non-funded pilot was instigated involving nine pharmacies where there was proven evidence of need. Misusers could receive free sterile syringes and needles and have their used ones replaced on their return.

The following year Welsh Office provided funding to health authorities for needle-exchange schemes. Neither of the two North Wales Authorities operated an exchange through their Community Drugs Services and community pharmacies remained the only route. The pharmacies who were voluntarily involved deserve to have their major contributions acknowledged. Their role was not seen merely as an exchange of clean for dirty equipment, it included providing advice and guiding misusers to other services. This excellent service starting from small beginnings has probably prevented a major spread of HIV/AIDS in North Wales into the sexually active but non-drug misusers community.

Waiting lists and rationing

Rationing, by whatever name one calls it, will be a large factor in medical care thinking over the next few years. Resources are bound to be insufficient for the wants, if not the needs, of the public and new developments in surgery and in medication will result in hard decisions having to be made. GPs over the years have practised a form of rationing by ensuring that the clinical needs rather than the wants of patients have been catered for in referral to secondary services. Patient power in the form of protests against the availability of drugs is already becoming significant but the profession need to be aware of the potential hazards to both patients and themselves of using treatments before they are fully appraised and registered.

Doctors in at the start of the NHS reported great relief that they no longer had to consider a patient's and their families circumstances before advising and arranging treatment. The extent of the previously unmet need became apparent after 1948 with the huge demand for dental treatment and dentures, spectacles, wigs, and corsets, all of which had previously not been affordable. While there were examples of waste and excess demand the need was very apparent in many communities. The political trumpeting of care for all, free at the time, meant that any attempt at moderating unnecessary demand and of rationing was not easy.

It was said recently with considerable truth that " before the NHS the patient had to worry about the cost of treatment, after its introduction neither patient nor doctor had to worry about it, now it is the doctors who have to consider the cost".

Rationing, by whatever name it has been called, is not new and health authorities have for years adopted various strategies to try to live within their allocated budgets These have included hospital and ward closures on a permanent or temporary basis, failure to replace staff leaving, restrictions in access to and delays in providing investigations and treatments, and transferring work and costs to someone else's budget. Changes occur without consultation or even notification and they have contributed greatly to agendas within committees at all levels and resulted in confrontation rather than cooperation between primary and secondary care.

Waiting lists may be considered a form of control of demand or rationing and particularly in surgical specialities and waiting list targets within the NHS have dominated much of the thinking and indeed of the additional investment for some years now. How much of the extra investment has gone into clinical work on patients on waiting lists rather than on the administration associated with it and whether the correct patients have been targeted is very questionable.

Waiting times for specialities such as dermatology which can be over a year do not often figure in discussions

Thinking back to my early days waiting times were not a major problem. Admittedly there were less patients needing hospital investigation and care, or at least fewer being referred because the facility was not there, but there were also far fewer consultants. Waits were only a few weeks and if one felt a patient needed to be seen urgently a quick call to the consultant's secretary would usually produce a slot at the next clinic, although I do recall that at some time in the sixties the LMC highlighted there was a problem with long delays with orthopaedic referrals in the Wrexham area. At that time there were many less sophisticated diagnostic investigations, with the resulting delays and waiting times arising from these and from the need to see the consultant again to review these. Many patients were dealt with on a one-stop basis, and at that time many operations were carried out on a look inside and see basis. Undoubtedly some patients had unnecessary operations in this scenario but on the other hand the risk of a cancer spreading during a period of waiting and prolonged investigation was less than it is now.

Waiting lists in themselves have considerable implications, financial, budgetary and in workload terms, for the GP who has to continue to treat symptoms and support the patient and the family during the wait including reassessment to review any deterioration and possibly one or more phone calls to try to expedite the appointment or admission. This period also has considerable financial implications for the NHS as drugs are usually required to deal with continuing symptoms, while patients may be off work and on benefits.

Initially all political emphasis was on the total number of patients on waiting lists, more recently emphasis quite rightly has been on the time individual patients have to wait. Wales has not been done as well as England in this respect, and failure to reduce them quickly enough has been the cause of a number of political casualties. This in spite of various ploys to massage the figures, by delaying putting patients on a waiting list developing some sort of a pre-waiting list, by regularly writing to patients asking whether they still want treatment and removing their names (often erroneously) if no response is received, and asking for a re-referral by the GP if a patient cancelled an admission amongst others. There was also the long wait from referral by the GP until actually seeing the consultant for the first time and for investigations to be carried out, all before a patient attains a place on any waiting list. For years GP representatives have argued that the correct waiting time to be counted should be from the time of first referral by them rather than from going on to a consultant's list for operation or treatment, and this has at last been accepted.

It was because of the delays in getting patients seen that GPs have actively pressed, sometimes long and hard, in the early years for access to diagnostic facilities such as X-rays and blood tests and later for more complex investigations such as barium tests and echocardiograms. It was always the same story, the departments could not cope with GP demands, ignoring the fact that these tests would be done anyway if ordered by a consultant or indeed often by a very junior doctor. Sometimes tests done meant that a referral was not required or if it was then the specialist would have a fully investigated patient before him and could proceed immediately to discuss treatment options with the patient. Similar problems arose with getting access to services such as physiotherapy and occupational therapy, both often benefiting from early active treatment without waiting for an out-patient appointment. Battles for direct access have taken an undue amount of time on all committees over many years and if won in one hospital had to be fought again in another.

Problems have arisen for GPs practising on the Welsh borders and having to refer to English hospitals which have different waiting times for patients on the same waiting list depending on whether they lived in Wales or in England, the difference sometimes many months, and attributed by management to different contractual funding arrangements. Subtle pressure is applied from time to time on GPs on Deeside to refer to Wrexham rather than to Chester hospitals because they are cheaper

Suggestions for charges for certain services such as for hospital stays and for visiting the GP have surfaced regularly over the years. While the latter has been seen by a minority of GPs as a means of restricting access charges would fall more heavily on those most needing care and doctors would not be happy to collect charges on behalf of government. They have been comprehensively rejected by GP leadership and by GPs as a body.

More recently political suggestions that certain operations considered unnecessary and including tonsillectomies and varicose vein operations might no longer be carried out to divert funds elsewhere. While undoubtedly some operations may be done without sufficient reason, patients who suffer from these conditions would disagree, certainly few submit themselves to operation without due thought and anxiety. An even more ridiculous suggestion is that GPs could undertake operations on hernias and varicose veins in the surgery. I was not practicing in the age of operating on the kitchen table but I recall that we did inject varicose veins in the surgery, until it was considered too dangerous.

Patients at times opt to pay for a private consultant appointment but with the intention of having any subsequent treatment on the waiting list. By so doing they could enter the waiting list often months sooner. Various attempts have been made over the years to stop this, especially when private practice was under attack by the government of the day, setting out that patients should go on to the list when they would have done so if they had been seen at an NHS clinic rather than privately. Other patients opt to pay for all the treatment themselves or through paying into private insurance schemes and the saving to the NHS through this must be substantial. Many, particularly the elderly not covered by medical insurance opt to pay considerable amounts from their life-savings to be free of pain or to maintain the ability to live independently for the time they have left.

Various national strategies to deal with long waiting times in some specialities have been adopted. In the late eighties Welsh Office decided to set up specialist treatment centres to fast-track care for orthopaedics particularly hip-replacements, for cataract surgery and for hernia repairs. Certainly in our area there did not appear to be the need for the last. The treatment centres for the whole of Wales were at Bridgend for orthopaedics and hernias and at Bangor for cataracts. What was not taken into account was that patients never travelled from North to South Wales, or vice versa, for care because of the distances and inconvenience involved, traditionally opting to go into England rather than South Wales if treatment was not available locally. While they dealt to some extent with a local waiting list the overall concept was flawed and failed. Some patients have opted to go abroad for treatment funded through the NHS but this has had little impact in Wales, no doubt it is far easier for patients living in the South East of England to cross the Channel.

More recently much resources have been pumped into additional weekend and special operating sessions done on an extra-contractual basis by consultants and by locums from outside the area but this very expensive arrangement has not yet reduced waiting times to an acceptable level and new ideas are required. Much work is being contracted out to private and commercial organisations, at considerably extra cost, and this process is now being questioned by politicians and by the public

Resource management centres are the latest idea to manage demand. GPs referrals are not necessarily going to the named consultant but being allocated, sometimes by non-medical staff, to whoever they consider appropriate and who is available, not always a doctor. Referral letters are sometimes being sent back to the GP labelled inappropriate. It has always been one of the strengths of the referral system that the GP is able to select the consultant considered most appropriate for a particular patient, not always on clinical grounds but sometimes on assessed compatability between patient and consultant. Very often the idea of a referral to hospital has to be "sold" to an anxious patient and a discussion on who they will see and an endorsement is part of the process. I recall an attempt to introduce the concept of referral to the gynaecology department in Ysbyty Gwynedd was raised some twenty-five years ago and successfully resisted by both consultants and the LMC.

Attitudes by successive governments and by Trust administration over many years has also had a considerable effect on the morale of hospital consultants and of their attitudes to their work and which will take much to restore. It has recently been suggested by consultants that Trust should be spelt as "trussed". The new consultant contract may provide a way forward providing early teething problems and attitudes are resolved. Attempts to tie down consultants to specified working hours are countered by reminders of the many unpaid hours worked under previous contracts. GPs have been luckier in that because of their independent contractor contracts they have been able to deal better with issues than their hospital colleagues in spite of various attempts to rein them in.

Whatever is done waiting lists are unlikely ever to disappear.

Priority Setting, that is Rationing, has been under discussion for many years. A major conference on the topic under the banner of the BMA, the Kings Fund and the Patients Association and involving politicians was held in 1993.

Rationing in one form has been labelled the "post-code lottery". Increasingly, access to treatment is varying from authority to authority, not just in waiting times but in whether the treatment will be funded at all. In many cases emotive conditions such as cancer or IVF treatments are at issue

One of the organisations which has become well known to the public in recent years because of demands by individuals and groups to receive new drug treatments claimed to be effective but not yet fully assessed is NICE although its remit and way of working is less well understood. The National Institute for Health and Clinical Excellence was set up in 1999 and charged with getting the best out of NHS resources. It appraises both the clinical and the cost effectiveness of health technologies referred to it by the Department of Health and its recommendations are issued as mandatory guidelines on the use of technologies and the treatment of diseases to the NHS. Scientific assessment and the collation of evidence is carried out by independent academic groups and the NICE committees consisting of clinicians, health scientists, managers and patients representatives then make an appraisal based on this evidence which is often incomplete and inconclusive. While NICE has repeatedly stated that it does not have a threshold above which cost becomes unacceptable obviously the higher the uncertainty with regard to effectiveness the more cost assumes relevance.

The greatest pressure both nationally and locally involves the availability of the many newer and not fully tested drugs available for various cancers and where the cost per patient runs into five or six figures for what in many cases is a temporary prolongation of life. Within a budget the argument is whether the money might be better spent in providing facilities for earlier diagnosis and conventional treatment. The media and also individual members of parliament have not helped with harrowing stories of individual cases and dying patients being denied drugs leading to moral blackmail to provide treatment locally and so encouraging others to follow suit.

The moral and ethical issues for the NHS and for the public will continue to escalate as complex and expensive (in human resources as well as financial) technologies and treatments continue to be developed.

The Fundholding experiment

General Practice budget-holding, later renamed Fundholding, was the great idea of the Conservative government in the 1989 white paper Working for Patients which introduced the concept of the Internal Market and of "money following the patient" to control hospitals and their administration and to raise standards in those deemed to be performing badly. Instead of having a block grant some of their money was to be given (nominally) to fund-holding practices who would then commission services at negotiated rates and withdraw funds if performance was not satisfactory. Practices would as an alternative be able to commission the same services from other providers, including themselves or other practices with special expertise. The BMA from both sides, consultants and GPs through thi conferences and ARM, opposed the concept but it went ahead in some practices.

I chaired the GMSC group which produced a commentary for the main committee setting out the problems as envisaged and why the concept was flawed and unlikely to be successful. Budgets would impose cash limits on GPs who would be responsible for keeping to them even though no restriction could be imposed on the demand and they were still required to give their patients "all necessary and appropriate medical services". While initially voluntary it could later have been made compulsory. It was thought that a patient's confidence in the doctor could be affected if they knew they were working within a budget and especially if advised that a medication or investigation was not necessary. Hospitals could not accurately cost their procedures and disputes over costs were likely to damage relationships between general practitioners and hospitals. No pilot studies had been carried out and a King`s Fund publication by two American authors, supporters of the idea of budget-holding, contained damning condemnation of the proposals. Unsuprisingly proposals went ahead, initially in England with considerable sweeteners being provided for practices agreeing to take part.

There was never any real enthusiasm for Fundholding in Wales amongst practices and I suspect also at Welsh Office level. It usually required considerable persuasion by the FHSA to get practices to consider joining and much discussion amongst partners about whether to join or not as it meant considerable changes in practice administration and staffing and in the computer requirements and software. Many went into it because it was a new experience to try out rather than with any true enthusiasm for the concept, but recognising that it could perhaps lead to improvements in care for their patients, but also on the basis that first-timers in any scheme are usually given substantial incentives to encourage others to join later.

In Penrhyn Bay we were actually in a better position to provide alternative choices than many other practices as we already referred patients to Bangor, to Llandudno and to Glan Clwyd Hospitals. Fundholding involved considerable extra administrative work and our practice had to employ a new practice manage, Mrs Beth Roberts, who spent half of her time with routine practice work funded by us and the other half on fund-holding work and funded through the scheme.

Theoretically the fund-holding concept involved money following the patient with Trusts only receiving payment for commissioned work done on behalf of the GP rather than receiving a block sum direct from the Health Authority. Since the Trusts and hospitals had traditionally received money in fairly large blocks without too much detail being specified as to the detail of the commissioning it was not easy for fund-holding to make major changes in their ways of working. Initially only certain services were available for commissioning by GPs. Each practice received a notional annual budget for commissioning but because the scheme was experimental and in the early stages there was considerable and tight oversight of budgets and how they were spent, both by the FHSA and by Welsh Office.

Clwyd FHSA were much more pushing of the concept than the FHSA in Gwynedd The first practice in North Wales to become involved in the first wave was the Russell Road practice in Rhyl led by Dr Gwyn Pierce Williams. In the second wave the following year they were joined by Beech House Denbigh and by the St Asaph practice, and then by Pendre, Holywell. Even though I had been prominent in the GMSC resistance to the concept, once it was up and running pragmatism set in and we applied to join in the fourth wave in1994

The western end of North Wales was much less adventurous and more cautious and no practices took up the concept for several years, possibly reflecting the degree of enthusiasm and pressure and persuasion applied by the respective FHSAs, but also because in that area there was only the one hospital, Ysbyty Gwynedd to provide services and in practice very little real patient choice without considerable travel.

Commissioning gave GPs an opportunity to put pressure on local Trusts, to introduce changes which had been suggested to them unsuccessfully in the past, but carried out in a spirit of goodwill and co-operation and with the realisation that all practices had to be treated equally so that improvements resulting from Fundholding benefited patients of all practices. A successful consortium of the practices in North Clwyd developed under the chairmanship initially of Dr Gwyn Williams and later Dr Gruff Jones with Dr Nick Taylor of St Asaph as secretary together with Mr Peter Clarke and later Mr Brian Pickles seconded from the Health Authority. Obviously the practice managers played a vital part in the fundholding process and were an integral part of the consortium and of the negotiations They were initially Judith Parry from the Rhyl practice, later joined by Jane Edwards from Beech House and Beth Roberts from our practice Evening meetings were held at the Farmers Arms in Rhuallt and proved enjoyable socially as well as effective.

One of the stated intentions of fundholding was the ability to develop alternative and innovative facilities. In our case we developed with Mr Puvuna Chandra, a weekly Ophthalmology clinic at our Penrhyn Bay premises. He brought his own Sister from the hospital to assist him but we provided the reception facilities. We were able to purchase the necessary equipment which remained at the practice and was available for practice use if required. The equipment was in fact better than he had available at some of the hospital clinics. We had hoped to take advantage of his presence to update our knowledge and skills of ophthalmology but somehow there was never the convenient time. Obviously appointments were not confined to our practice and patients from other practices could be seen there. Its usefulness was such that it continued for some time after Fundholding ended when the new Labour government was elected in 1990

A fresh initiative on similar lines was proposed for England in 2004, known as Practice Led Commissioning and which would allow GP practices to receive an indicative budget from their Primary Care Trusts (equivalent to LHBs in Wales) and to directly commission care and services tailored to the specific needs of their patients. Since budgets were to be indicative the PCT would pick up any overspend but practices would be expected to balance the books over a three year period. It is obviously to early to assess the effect of this development. Wales decided not to go down this route, devolution of health matter to the Assembly does allow considerable differences to develop.

The South Wales Scene

South Wales has played a major part in the development of general practice medicine over the fifty years during which I have been involved, in both the medico-political and the educational fields and there have been many personalities from there who have contributed immensely. Obviously I have not been as intimately connected with what has gone on there as I have on North Wales but as mentioned elsewhere Wales is really a medical village where most of us have known each other personally although those from the North and those from the South have not been fully aware of contributions within the local areas. Many of the national commitments have been described in other parts of this narrative but it may be appropriate to collect them together and add a few more.

Two practices seem to stand out as having made major contributions in the educational field, the Llanedeyrn (Cardiff) practice on a new housing estate which developed into the professorial and academic centre under Robert Havard Davis, and later Nigel Stott and Simon Smail, and the Riverside House practice in Bridgend which has made a great contribution to vocational training in Wales. David Coulter and Derek Llewelyn edited the first textbook for general practice, The Practice of Family Medicine, based on contributions from twenty-two practitioners in Wales, and were also involved in the setting up of vocational training in Wales. The pilot scheme was run there and one of the partners, Derek Llewelyn was appointed the first Postgraduate Adviser for Wales in 1972, followed in 1990 by another partner Terry Reilly.

Dr John Owen of Portcawl, a North Walian who had moved south contributed considerably in research and in his interest in the development of nursing within general practices. He also chaired the sub-committee in general practice for several years in the early eighties.

Further west research was being carried out by Dr. W. O. Williams, at first as an individual and later as Director of the Swansea Research Unit based in the University and funded by the RCGP. Later Dr Alun Jones from Gorseinon acted as his deputy but the RCGP withdrew funding on W.O.s retirement'.

A proposal to develop a second Welsh medical school based at Swansea was made in the seventies and championed by Margaret Thatcher who was Secretary of State for Education at the time. As part of the developing process an active Postgraduate Department was extended with Bruce Lervy and Neil Upton being actively involved in the development of audit while a second District General Hospital adjacent to the University campus was proposed in addition to Morriston Hospital only a few miles away. The proposal ran into trouble when at a public meeting it was disclosed that the development of the medical school would result in loss of services and the probable closure of a number of smaller hospitals including Neath and Llanelli and local councillors withdrew their support. In the end Swansea lost out to Southampton. The Postgraduate department has gone on from strength to strength.

The BMA has probably been more active at Divisional level in South Wales as compared with the North. One name springs immediately to mind, that of Dr David Parry from Portcawl who spent many years on WGMSC and BMA Welsh Council and also represented Wales on the General Medical Council He was awarded the BMA Gold Medal for his contributions.

The Port Talbot area has been to the fore, originally with Dr Hubert Jones and more recently by Dr Bryn John, while Gwent has been well served by Dr Greg Graham and by Dr Tony Calland and before that by Dr Bill Murray Jones, the first chairman of WGMSC, by Dr John Crossley who went on to the Welsh Office, and by Dr Dipak Ray who while on WGMSC was always going to send me a paper on the current problem but never did. Dr Hefin Jones has been active in providing leadership in the Merthyr Tydfil area and the valleys as chairman of the LMC and later of Welsh Medical Committee. Dr Hugh Cairns from Cardiff represented the profession well for years on the Welsh Pricing Bureau, and Dr Denzil Davies from Barry was active on WGMSC and provided considerable support to me on the Sub-Committee of the Postgraduate Education Committee dealing with vocational training. Dr Gilbert Clark has been acknowledged for his work on the Medical Practices Committee in London. Dr Julian Tudor Hart of Glyncorrwg is mentioned elsewhere for his original thinking and research which demonstrated the value of effective team working in a very deprived mining community.

West Wales has also played its important part. Dr John Hughes from Aberystwyth was an active BMA member who at times courted controversy over his views on abortion and the pill and who successfully battled the University authorities over the issue of confidentiality for students. An early stalwart was Dr Hugh Herbert of Aberaeron, whose footsteps are being followed by his daughter Helen, who I first met as the representative of trainees on the Subcommittee in general practice in 1983 and who was recently chairman of RCGP Welsh Council, while Dr Gwyn Jones a firebrand from Cardigan contributed much to Welsh GMSC in the early days. Dr Simeon Ovis from Llandrindod was the sole representative from Powys on WGMSC for many years. An interesting WGMSC member and character was Dr Chris Tiarks from the Vale of Glamorgan who stood unsuccessfully for parliament as an Independent and then went off to Scotland to become the GP for a few hundred people on the Western Islands of Eigg, Muck and Rhum. In spite of this relative isolation he still managed to appear regularly at BMA meetings and become a member of BMA UK Council.

If readers think this was a very male dominated field, unfortunately it was.

It has been difficult over the years to attract women doctors on to the various committee structures at all levels. Mention must be made of the considerable contributions of Drs Agnes M Hood and Susan Pierrepoint to WGMSC and other committees. Dr Kay Richards from Cardiff has been a frequent contact during her Welsh Office days and now remains active in a Cardiff practice and in the RCGP.

And there were many others, to whom I apologise unreservedly for failing to mention them and their contributions, as well as their fellowship and support over the years.

Designing around the patient

Much has been made by governments from both parties and by others about making a service more suited to patient needs, if not their wishes, and obviously this would appear a laudable aim. The process probably started in earnest with the requirements of GPs introduced in the 1990 contract and with the publication of the Patients Charter in 1991 with the intention of explaining how the NHS works to allow them to make best use of it. Additionally the Charter enabled patients to put pressure on the NHS so that it became more responsive to their wishes. At around the same time legislation and guidelines concerning access to medical records and to health records and about confidentiality of patient information and consent to treatment continued the process. The raising of expectations in circumstances when they could not be always be achieved led to a substantial increase in complaints to FHSAs and to hospital trusts.

Designed for Life-Creating world class Health and Social care for Wales in the 21st Century and published by Welsh Assembly Government in 2005 sets out a long-term strategy which states that "High quality design is durable, safe, and effective - it delivers to people what they want".

Concern has been expressed that the pursuit of patient choice at all times may not necessarily be in the best interests of the NHS. Before one goes too far and too quickly down this road one has to look at the potential downsides as the law of unintended consequences may once again figure large. Better and more effective services can often only be developed by amalgamation and centralising of services resulting in increased patient travel and inconvenience. One of the problems of recent re-organisations and guidelines has been the attempt to create a "one size fits all" solution.

Much is also made of consulting the public and seeking their views but in practice public meetings, questionnaires and focus groups tend to have a poor response and one which is not always a true representation of needs and wishes. Focus groups in particular are attended largely by middle class professionals in good health rather than patients with chronic disease or social problems. The alternative agenda sees doctor and patient as joint stakeholders in a partnership based on mutual respect and shared objectives.

GPs, unlike the hospitals who have only comparatively recently experienced competition and money following the patient, have always been in the market place, going back to the time when competition between practices was fierce and more patients meant more income, and they have always tried to provide a service which suits their individual area and circumstances. Surgery opening times varied between areas, in industrial practices surgeries were often very early to suit patients coming off or going on to their shifts while retirement area practices started later in the mornings and ran early afternoon surgeries so that elderly patients could go home safely during daylight.

Things have moved on very considerably since I started in practice when appointments were unknown, although we did start with a partial system soon afterwards. Not so long before that doctors were known to go into a crowded waiting room, look who was there and tell up to half of them to go home and come back another day. One early system which we adopted in Ruabon and similar to that found in supermarket counters was a numbered token which patients collected at the surgery and if there appeared to be a long wait they could go and do some shopping. Regrettably many tokens were lost or not returned resulting in gaps in the numbering and making it difficult for patients to know exactly how many others were before them. In the early days few patients had telephones in their home and they had to visit the surgery to make an appointment, now many have phones but report difficulty in getting through. Running a system was made much easier when one of the pharmaceutical companies provided loose leaf books with appointment slots already included - as always introducing a system which works requires someone to set up protocols and easy mechanisms for them.

A flexible system allowed doctors to change surgery times to allow for individual circumstances, holidays, days off and school events which had to be attended. It became increasingly necessary because of the need to fit in postgraduate work and team training, and for various committee commitments.

It allowed patients to select days and times suitable to themselves. Over time, as individual consultations became longer while working days became shorter resulting in fewer slots, making an appointment at a convenient time became more difficult. even though reduction in home visiting had allowed more consultations to be made available.

Regulars would book appointments a week or two in advance resulting in slots for new or acute conditions becoming more difficult to obtain. As frequently happens outside guidance, or interference, was not helpful. and the law of unexpected consequences again came into play. A government requirement that patients should be able to see a doctor within 48 hours resulted in some practices doing away with the majority of advance appointments and requiring patients to attend or ring for a slot on the day. Queues are forming outside the door at opening time and the phones are red-hot, leaving many patients dissatisfied when all slots have been filled. Only major changes in the way days are organised and how patients are seen will help to improve the situation. Whether this will satisfy more patients is debatable. As with the rest of the NHS developments lead to increased demand which becomes difficult to manage.

Complaints of difficulties in accessing the GP are common but all surveys still show satisfaction by the majority of respondents with the care received when seen. Patients are certainly welcoming the additional services being provided on-site including blood tests and other investigations rather than having to travel to clinics, as well as the local access to other professionals. Many surgeries are fulfilling the original concept of health centres.

Nurse triage, a new term which has recently entered the vocabulary, involves the first contact, either face to face or on the telephone, being with a qualified and specially trained nurse who will decide whether and when treatment is required, the degree of urgency and who is the best person to provide it. This happens in A&E departments, in out of hours services, and increasingly in practices where perhaps it is an improvement on the arrangements where in some practices a receptionist would take it upon herself to make this decision Patients are becoming aware of the advantage, as well as of the potential for error, in the developing of nurse triage, both within the practice and by the national NHS Direct organisation set up in 1999 to offer 24hours a day advice on health matters. NHS Direct is currently under criticism in many parts of the country because it is an expensive system which often fails to provide as good a service as it should. Some patients are very happy with its nurse triage as a means to a quicker and better service, others complain of difficulty in getting through and get quite irate when a "mere nurse" makes a decision which does nor correspond with their wishes. As in most fields dissatisfaction is widely voiced whereas satisfaction is rarely voiced publicly and it will always be difficult to get a practical and affordable balance between patient wants and patient needs.

Within general practice efforts have been made through the RCGP to encourage practice participation groups to provide a forum to discuss and air problems and to discuss developments within the practice. The difficulty has been that they tended to attract those with a grouse rather than with a positive attitude and sometimes careful selection was necessary. One of the few groups in our area was that developed by Dr Huw Lloyd at the Cadwgan surgery in Old Colwyn. He has maintained an interest in this concept and has been involved in its development within the College centrally. Other surgeries, particularly in rural areas have developed Friends of the Practice as a liaison forum and these have sometimes raised considerable sums of money to provide expensive equipment. Practice newsletters are now being developed to keep patients informed about changes.

Patient choice - one of the pillars of the current reforms - and the development of Choose and Book which is at present only being introduced in England may be relevant in some areas where there is the possibility of genuine choice of hospital or other providers. In the periphery patients are much more likely to wish to obtain quicker and better treatment in their local hospital rather than to have to travel far with all the subsequent inconvenience for themselves and their families.

The imposition by central government of the same guidelines and targets on every GP surgery irrespective of the very wide variation in communities and their needs destroys flexibility and local autonomy. There is a major difference between the urban practice reported recently to be taking on four hundred new patients a month, many from eastern Europe, and a small rural practice with a static practice list. If as we know one-size fits all creates problems within general practice then it is highly likely that problems will be similarly created in other parts of the health service.

Dr Michael Wilson, the GMSC chairman, when addressing a Special Conference in 1986 asked "Was it too much to hope that ministers had learnt that the British system of primary care had evolved to meet the needs of patients and required development to meet the rising demands rather than divisive and radical alternatives to satisfy political dogma"

Designing around the patient has also being markedly influenced by the raft of legislation coming into being over the last few years in particular the wide-ranging Human Rights Act of 1998 with in particular its Articles on the right to life, the right to liberty and security, the right to respect for private and family life, and the prohibition of discrimination in various forms. All these aspects now need to be taken into consideration daily in the practice of medicine, both in the overall provision and organisation of services within the NHS, and in the way services are provided to patients on an individual basis. On many occasions decisions may have to be made at short notice with the threat of legal challenge ever present and in many cases what is correct in law may be uncertain, may be multi-factorial and depend on circumstances at the time.

Certainly all the above will result in additional time being spent in considering the various issues and may further require time to consult widely before decisions are made, cause anxieties to doctors, and may result in considerable additional costs.

End piece

Writing these recollections has made me realise more fully how much has changed over the last fifty years and has brought back to mind issues which had receded into memory and which may be of historical interest to those now actively engaged in the provision of health care. It has also made me more aware of prejudices which I have developed over the years and which show through at times within this narrative.

Ten years ago, on the eve of his 1997 election victory Tony Blair famously said there was twenty-four hours to save the NHS. Has it been saved, indeed was it ever in mortal danger? Opinion is divided as to whether it is in better shape now than then. Undoubtedly some parts are better, some are worse. The total investment has increased enormously. However Wales and the UK remain at the bottom end of league tables which compare health across Western Europe. Perhaps it will be useful to end this view from retirement ten years on by looking at some of the major current issues for the public and for doctors

The Review of Health and Social Care in Wales (the Wanless Report) in 2003 set out the current problems and its overall vision and objectives to which Wales should aim and the methods by which these might be achieved, perhaps the most important being the need for health and social care organisations to sing from the same hymn sheet and to collaborate more closely. Achieving better results and at the same time getting better value for money will involve considerable change in working methods and relationships. It is very difficult to get different parts of the health service to work cooperatively, let alone to do so with other agencies but it must be attempted. Very often it seems that in the past financial and budgetary frontiers have been at the bottom of failure to work together.

General practice has been evolving into Primary Medical Care over the last decades and now needs to evolve into Primary Care. The European definition of general practitioners is that they provide "comprehensive and continuing care to every individual seeking medical care" and are "normally the point of first medical contact within the healthcare system, providing open and unlimited access to its users, dealing with all health problems. This may or may not be true in practice in Europe and is probably more a wish statement than a statement of fact. It may no longer be as true as it was in the UK but there seems to be an increasing need for a single person, or at least a single base, to be the patients` navigator through the increasingly complex health-care system.

General practice as we have known it with the GP acting as gatekeeper to services and holding the only complete record of a patients medical history and care is under threat by the plethora of different providers of health care developing separate pathways and often without communication between them, aggravated by changes in the availability of doctors themselves. General practice may be seen as increasingly a Monday to Friday nine-to-five service. Alternative providers include A&E and minor injuries departments, hospital out-reach nurses, increasingly the ambulance service and paramedics, occupational health services, social workers and psychiatric social workers, pharmacists screening clinics, NHS Direct, TESCO and other stores, BUPA, alternative medicine practitioners, the internet and TV programmes. All are providing care and information at different levels, not always appropriate to the understanding of patients and their carers needs but quite adequate in the circumstances. They are not being provided by the patient with a full picture either because it is considered unnecessary or because it is too confidential. The national system of computerised and patient held records which is currently under discussion is unlikely to contain a complete record and obviously access will need to be restricted in parts to maintain confidentiality. Many of these alternative providers currently have a more significant role in urban conurbations and commuter areas but all may be relevant at some times, even in North Wales.

Pressure on time during consultations and the disruption to others arising from a doctor leaving surgery to deal with an emergency call is increasingly resulting in cases which are likely to need emergency investigation being sent immediately to hospital by ambulance. Before we had appointment systems patients did not mind the doctor going out and would either wait patiently or go home and come back to the next surgery. Now they tend to grumble and wait.

The argument for delegation of care to nurses and other assistants employed by the practice is that they can undertake much of the routine work leaving the GP time to deal with more complex cases and problems which arise. In some ways this is a flawed concept in that complex cases often start out with simple symptoms and if these are not adequately assessed and their significance realised care can be delayed, sometimes tragically. Extending prescribing rights to nurses may escalate the problem. There is the further argument that good personal care is built on a continuing relationship and trust developed over a period, perhaps dealing with minor illness or with other members of the family, and with the knowledge that whatever is discussed will be completely confidential. If this has not been established rapport during more complex illness and in times of crisis may not be present, the patient may not feel at ease to discuss all his symptoms and particularly to voice his or her anxieties. One sees this at present when patients go to hospital clinics and return feeling unhappy that they have not been able to present themselves adequately to a stranger, or to ask questions. In these circumstances they should always be made to feel free to return for further discussion and advice.

The RCGP Welsh Council in 1988 commented "General practitioners should be ushers guiding patients to the most appropriate care, not gatekeepers rationing their entry" and this should remain a fundamental principle on which care is based while not precluding a continuing emphasis on providing good health care effectively in the most economical way.

Since the new contract allowed doctors to opt out of working after 6.30pm and at weekends with the responsibility of commissioning services at these times being that of the Local Health Boards, a fact which is frequently not understood, there is developing within the working public anxieties about the difficulties of access to their own doctor, or even to the practice partners. GPs will need to look at this situation if they are not to lose their position as the accepted gateway to medical care. There may be a need to consider the need for an evening or Saturday morning session strictly limited to those who genuinely are unable to attend during normal hours because of work commitments, and on the understanding that this does not include any visits or other commitments.

The increasing expectations of patients and of governments and administration with the increasing threat of complaints both locally and to the GMC may result in a working-to-rule type of consultation. The plethora of guidelines and protocols to which one must defer may result in a medical painting by numbers. I was amazed to find recently that there is a monthly publication, several hundred pages in all, detailing the guidelines for managing medical conditions. The worry is that if a doctor does not follow the guidelines fully then potentially he or she may be subject to a claim for negligence in the event of some mishap.

A further issue for GPs arises from the new contractual position between the practice and the LHB. The new ability of LHBs to terminate contracts following practice breakdowns as a result of unresolved disputes between partners has already been demonstrated locally as perhaps has been the inexperience of the LHB in dealing with such problems. In England following alleged poor service in one area the Primary Care Trust invited tenders and appointed an U.S-based health organisation to provide services, surely a first within the NHS and an area which will be watched with interest. This will have to be counteracted by continuing to strive for quality, by the adoption of good practice ideas and by earning a good reputation both with the administration and with the public.

Performance indicators and targets have dominated much of the thinking in the last few years. However most indicators of healthcare performance do not give answers but instead should encourage further enquiry and investigation. By themselves they give an incomplete and inaccurate picture of the whole. There is some evidence that setting targets does improve efficiency and care in general but that this may be only in the areas targeted. The need to record details across various fields, prompted by various "pop-ups" on the screen, does have an effect on focussing on the condition which the patient wishes to discuss with the doctor. The use of targets as indicators presumes that the priorities targeted reflect the whole picture, and that what is omitted does not matter. Many of the qualities most appreciated by patients can not be easily quantified. There is no doubt that targets do result in playing games with data being manipulated by administrators whose job and career prospects depend on them and by clinicians who want the administration off their backs. Services which are not targeted may be postponed or cancelled to concentrate on target areas. Visits to Districts by CHIMP, the Commission for Health Improvement, identified examples of such gaming. Whether the naming and shaming of under performing trusts is effective will only become clear in the longer term.

Change is on-going and inevitable and the profession has to respond and react to it. Harold Wilson once said "He who rejects change is the architect of decay, the only human institution which rejects progress is the cemetery". Many management manuals and courses have been developed in the last few years on the management of change. Many managers appear to have read or understood only parts of the reasoning. It may be confrontational or consensual. As also happens in cases of alleged sexual assault consensual can often be misconstrued and consent believed to be present when it is not. Change usually meets resistance from at least some quarters and this is usually more vociferous if change is imposed too rapidly and where the reasoning for it is not explained or where the explanation is not credible. In many cases changes are seen as being driven by financial reasons and a need to balance budgets. As in sport there are three elements to consider, the opposition which one can not influence directly, the referee who is difficult to change but who one tries to influence and succeeds occasionally, and one's own team which has to respond and react to changing circumstances'. Much of medical management of change is focussed on the last, in both the clinical and the medico-political fields. Many of us have found this a fascinating area in which to become involved. Many other doctors have no interest in the details unless and until it affects them personally and get on with the work of the practice leaving the committee work to enthusiasts. At times they may have felt that we were on "jollies" but the reality was long hours and hard work and preparation, together with catching-up work back at the practice. Spin-off benefits for the practice arise from better knowledge of the regulations and from experience gleaned from other parts of the country.

General practice has experienced a changing role over the last decades but the underlying principles have remained the same. In the mid-eighties the RCGP described this as "patients traditionally have consulted their general practitioner when they are ill, or think they are ill, for advice, diagnosis and treatment. There is also a clinical service for people who consult the doctor when they are well, for example when seeking advice on contraception, for maternity care and for immunizations. Anticipatory care is relatively recent and depends on members of the practice team searching out groups of patients in the practice who are vulnerable e.g. screening for diseases such as hypertension and cervical cancer". These general principles should not change although the ways in which this is achieved will change substantially with bigger units and an evolving multidisciplinary approach. There is likely to be a considerable blurring of the edges between primary and secondary care with closer working and with much of the work now done in hospitals which will have fewer beds being undertaken in the community and with day-case working considerably expanded. Specialist units as well as general practices are likely to be amalgamated on single sites aiming for better care but often resulting in greater patient inconvenience.

There remain serious doubts as to whether under the new and shorter training programmes, both undergraduate and postgraduate, tomorrows doctors will reach the standards we would all expect and this is particularly felt within the consultant body and especially by the surgeons where the total number of hours experience required before certification as fully accredited has been drastically reduced.

Since its inception power broking in the NHS has always been a balancing act between central policy making and local delivery. Recently it has shifted too far towards the centre. Power struggles develop between hospitals and hospitals, between doctors and nurses, between consultants and managers, and between doctors and in particular consultants themselves. There is a strong feeling that the whole health service is under managed but over administered On the other hand if all administrative arrangements and decisions are left to bureaucrats alone, rather than involving doctors with experience in the field, then they are likely to come up with decisions which have unintended consequences which are of no benefit to anyone.

The Assembly in Cardiff which has devolved powers for health will hopefully continue to develop policies which more closely reflect the needs of Wales. Whether its decision to phase out the charges for prescriptions is a good use of scarce resources is open to question. It may be appropriate to include a quote from Dr Brian Gibbons, the current Health Minister for Wales. "Professional people join the service to work with patients not to have meetings and to be worrying about their jobs. There is a lot of evidence that nothing annoys clinical staff more than bureaucracy". It would be wonderful if his legacy on leaving his portfolio was that this aim and vision had been achieved

Overall funding of the NHS is likely to remain funded by taxation, available to all on the basis of need. Radical alternatives have been considered over the decades and rejected. The funding problems are not confined to the United Kingdom and other countries have had to consider whether they can continue to provide services from the cradle to the grave Attempts such as those in New Zealand and Sweden, and in Oregon in the USA have shown even more weaknesses

In considering all the apparent deficiencies within the NHS it is appropriate to recall the observation by Enoch Powell, a former Tory Minister of Health that ; "one of the most striking features of the National Health Service is the continual, deafening chorus of complaint which arises day and night from every part of it, a chorus only interrupted when someone suggests that a different system altogether might be preferable, which would involve the money coming from some less (literally) palpable source. The universal exchequer financing of the service endows everyone providing as well as using it with a vested interest in denigrating it, so that it presents what must be a unique spectacle of an undertaking that is run down by everyone engaged in it".

There are increasing demands for the NHS to be taken out of politicians and run by some corporate structure. Whether it is too late to reverse the move into the "managed market" based on an industrial model rather than a clinical one which has been developing over the last decades and particularly the last decade remains to be seen. It is probably more likely to come from pressure by the public rather than from other sources. One of the problems for the leaders of the professions is to recognise which are the important issues on which to battle and go to the barricades. Medical professionals, as well as other health professionals, have probably been guilty of failing to react vigorously enough to the changes. Many now know nothing different.

In spite of all the problems the practice of family medicine still retains much of its basic ethos and the attractions including the continuity of care of individual patients which brought most of us into it at the start of our careers. Its basic scenario remains unchanged and challenging, based on a succession of undifferentiated presentations which may or may not turn out to be significant. Marshall Marinker wrote that "the role of the GP is to tolerate uncertainty, explore probability and marginalize danger. In contrast the role of the secondary care specialist is to reduce uncertainty, explore possibility and marginalize error". One of it's strengths is that it does manage uncertainty when symptoms are inconclusive and get it right most of the time.

It gives me a feeling of pride and of satisfaction that I have been involved to the extent I have in the evolution of general practice and the management of change over the last fifty years and it is my hope that sharing these recollections will help others to understand what has been taking place in medicine during that time. It is perhaps significant that GP contractors are now described and recorded by LHBs as "performers on the list". Perhaps this symbolises the hoops through which they are now required to jump.

I think the era in which I practised had considerable attractions.

Acronyms and abbreviations

ACBS	According to the Committee on Borderline Substances
BMA	British Medical Association
CCSC	Central Consultants and Specialists Committee
CMO	Chief Medical Officer
EC	Executive Council
FPC	Family Practitioners Committee
FHSA	Family Health Services Authority
GMSC	General Medical Services Committee
GPAC	General Practice Audit Committee Wales
GPC	General Practitioners Committee
HA	Health Authority
HCSA	Hospital Consultants and Specialists Association
JCPTGP	Joint Committee for Postgraduate Training in General Practice
LA	Local Authority
LHB	Local Health Boards - in Wales
LMC	Local Medical Committee
MAAG	Medical Audit Advisory Group
MDS	Medical Defence Society
MOH	Medical Officer of Health
MPC	Medical Practices Committee
MPU	Medical Practitioners Union
PACT	Prescribing Analysis Cost and Trend Data
PCT	Primary Care Trust - in England
RCGP	Royal College of General Practitioners
TQM	Total quality management
WAG	Welsh Assembly Government
WGMSC	Welsh GMSC
WMC	Welsh Medical Committee

Significant dates

1948   NHS and Executive Councils started
1950   Collings report in The Lancet
1952   Formation of College of General Practitioners
1961   The Platt Report
1962   Pilkington Royal Commission.   Pay Review Body set up
1963   Annis Gillie report The Field of work of the Family Doctor
1965   MRCGP by compulsory examination introduced
1966   New GP contract introduced. Dr Jim Cameron
1967   Royal Commission - the Todd report. Merit awards proposed & rejected
1967   Fellowship of the College instituted
1967   Porritt Report - A Review of the Medical Services in Great Britain
        Hospital plan for England and Wales
1969   The Functions of the District General hospital - Bonham Carter Report
1970   An Enquiry into Prescribing Costs in Caernarfonshire
1970   Reorganisation of NHS
1971   Long term Policies in General practice produced by the Welsh Assoc of
Gps
1971   The Organisation of Group Practice - R. Harvard Davis report
1971   Inverse Care Law postulated by Julian Tudor Hart
1972   Appointment of Regional Adviser in Wales
1975   Medical Audit by Peer Review WGMSC chairman David Williams
1975   Report of the Working party on Prescribing Costs in Wales by WGMSC
        Chairman W. Murray-Jones
1997   NHS Plan - a plan for investment and reform
1997   The Development of Community Hospitals
1978   Health Education in Wales WGMSC working party - chairman Hubert
Jones
1979   New Charter working group - Report GMSC
1979   Discussion document on Devolution in Wales - the first and unsuccessful
        attempt
1979   Royal Commission on the NHS- the Merrison report
1979   Casualty, accident and ambulance services in Wales - Report of WGMSC
        chairman G Martin Jones
1980   Workload, manpower and net remuneration of General Practitioners in
        South Wales - Report of WGMSC working party chairman Bryan Davies
1981   Structure and management in the NHS in Wales
1980   Bilingual Death Certificates introduced
1981   15 Feb last date for exemption from VT regulations requirements
1981   First Welsh Clinical Review Conference at Llandrindod

1981   Economies and Priorities in the Health service -WGMSC report - chairman
        H.I. Humphreys
1980   Report on Inequalities in Health - the Black Report
1980   National Insurance certification - green paper published
1981   Working Party on Health Education WGMSC report chaired by
        Hubert Jones
1981   Acheson Report Inner London
1981   Care in the Community - consultation document
1981   Report on Community hospitals WGMSC document
1982   NHS Reorganisation - AHAs disbanded, FPCs formed with full autonomy
        Community services brought in
1982   Arthur Anderson Report of a study of family practitioner services
        administration and the use of computers
1983   General Practice - a British success GMSC document
1983   Separate Medical practices Committee for Wales mooted and rejected
1984   Commercial Deputising Services - Minister proposed banning them
1984   Limited list introduced - the Black list ACBS Dec 1984
1984   Parallel importing of drugs
1985   Product Liability the EC Directive adopted after 9 yrs discussion
1985   A Good Old Age Welsh Office document
1985   What Sort of Doctor RCGP quality statement
1985   Symposium on the Care of the Elderly Welsh Office
1985   Project 2000 launched - new training programme for nurses
1986   General Practice in Medical schools in UK- the Mackenzie Report
1987   Promoting Better Health - the white paper on primary health care
1987   Underprivileged areas identified
1988   Nursing in the Community - the Noreen Edwards Report for Wales
1988   Neighbourhood Nursing - the Cumberledge Report for England
1988   Guidelines on Audit in GP - joint report of GMSC and RCGP
1986   European Council Directive on Specific training in General practice
1986   Havard Davies annual lecture set up
1988   Community Care - report by Roy Griffiths
1989   Community Hospitals Report for WMC
1989   Formation of N.Wales Faculty RCGP
1998   Product Liability issues
1989   South Wales Valleys initiative commences
1989   Working for Patients - government proposals for a new GP Contract
1989   Fellowship of the RCGP by assessment introduced
1990   FHSAs formed and North Wales Health Authority appointed
1990   Terry Reilly succeeded Derek Llewelyn as Regional Adviser
1990   Kenneth Clarke's new Contract imposed

1990	Internal market and Fundholding introduced
1990	General Practice Audit Committee Wales formed
1991	Colwyn Bay Community Hospital opened
1991	Patients Charter published
1992	CME Tutors appointed
1992	Academic department for N Wales proposed
	Arthur Anderson report
1993	Patients Charter or 91
1993	Caring for the Future -The Pathfinder NHS Directorate document
1994	Reorganisation - new FHSA reorganisation /dha s/ into LHB`s
	NWLMC CHAIR
1994	Re-organisation of out of hours co-operatives introduced in Wales
1995	Primary Care - the future - NHS Executive document
1997	Welsh language policy formally adopted by Glan Clwyd Trust
	Deputising services document attempt to change terms of service
1997	Core Services document - GMSC defined what was included in the contract
1997	Mental Health - a Strategy for Wales
1999	Putting Patients First, then Better Health, Better Wales
1999	Concept of Health Improvement programmes (HIPs) introduced
1999	Fundholding discontinued
1999	Welsh Assembly assumed devolved responsibility for health
1999	NHS Direct set up
2000	NHS Plan - targets for performance & delivery, accountability and monitoring
2000	Local Health Boards functional
2000	The Future of Primary Care- a plan for the NHS and its partners
2000	Improving Health in Wales
2002	Appraisal introduced for GPs
2004	New Contract introduced for GPs

Significant Legislation

1815	The Apothecaries Act
1858	The Medical Act - which established the GMC register
1886	Medical Act -required qualification in medicine, surgery and midwifery
1948	NHS Act - introduction of NHS
1967	Abortion Act
1968	Health Services and Public Health Act
1974	Local Government Reorganisation
1974	NHS reorganisation AHAs formed . Exec councils replaced by FPCs
1976	NHS (Vocational Training)Act 1976
1977	The National Health Service Act 1977
1978	Medical Act
1979	The NHS (Vocational Training) Regulations effective from Feb 1980
1980	NHS Reorganisation in Wales
1984	Community Care Act
1984	Data Protection Act
1984	Police and Criminal Evidence Act - PACE
1984	Registered Nursing Homes Act
1987	Consumer Protection Act
1988	Access to Medical Reports Act
1990	NHS and Community Act Hospitals divided into purchasers and providers
1990	Access to Health Records Act
1994	The Vocational Training for General Medical Practice (European Requirements) Regulations 1994
1998	Data Protection Act
1999	Health Act - PCTs and LHB`s announced
2000	Freedom of Information Act in force from Jan 1st 2005